American Medical Asso

Physicians dedicated to the health of Amer

MW00846524

cpt® changes

An Insider's View

AMA
press

2005

Michael Beebe, Director, CPT Editorial and Information Services
Catherine Duffy, Director, CPT Education and Information Services
Desiree Evans, Project Coordinator
Todd Feinstein, IT Consultant
Ron Friedmann, Coding Consultant
DeHandro Hayden, Coding Consultant
Elizabeth Lumakovska, Coding Consultant
Marie Mindeman, Director, CPT Editorial Research and Development
Karen O'Hara, Senior Coding Consultant
Mary O'Heron, Senior Coding Consultant
Desiree Rozell, Senior Coding Consultant
Lianne Stancik, Coding Consultant

CPT® 2005 Changes: An Insider's View

www.ama-assn.org

For information regarding the reprinting or licensing of CPT 2005 Changes: An Insider's View, please contact:

CPT Intellectual Property Services
American Medical Association
515 N. State St.
Chicago, IL 60610
312 464-5022

Additional copies of this book may be ordered by calling: 800 621-8335 or from the secure AMA Press Web site at www.amapress.com. Refer to product number OP512905.

This book is intended for information purposes only. It is not intended to constitute legal advice. If legal advice is desired or needed, a licensed attorney should be consulted.

ISBN: 1-57947-585-X
AC24:04-P-004:11/04

Table of Contents

Foreword

The American Medical Association is pleased to offer *CPT® Changes 2005: An Insider's View*. Since this publication was first published in 2000 it has served as the definitive text on additions, revisions, and deletions to the CPT code set. In developing this book it was our intention to provide CPT users with a glimpse of the logic, rationale, and proposed function of CPT changes that resulted from the decisions of the CPT Editorial Panel and the yearly update process. AMA staff members have the unique perspective of being both participants in the CPT editorial process, and users of the CPT code set. *CPT Changes* is intended to bridge understanding between clinical decisions made at the CPT Editorial Panel regarding appropriate service/procedure descriptions, with functional interpretations of coding guidelines and code combinations necessary for users of the CPT code set. A new edition of the book is published annually.

To assist CPT users in applying new and revised CPT codes, this book uses clinical examples that describe the typical patient who might receive the procedure and detailed descriptions of the procedure. Both of these are required as a part of the CPT code change proposal process and are used by the CPT Editorial Panel in crafting language, guidelines, and parenthetical notes associated with the new or revised codes. In addition, clinical examples and descriptions of the procedures are used in the AMA/Specialty Society RVS Update process for conducting surveys on physician work and in developing work relative value recommendations to the Centers for Medicare and Medicaid Services (CMS) as part of the Medicare Physician Fee Schedule (MPFS).

We are confident that the information contained in *CPT Changes* each year will prove to be a valuable resource to CPT users not only as they apply changes for the year of publication, but also as a resource to frequently refer to as they continue their education in CPT coding. The American Medical Association makes every effort to be a voice of clarity and consistency in an otherwise confusing system of health care claims and payment and *CPT Changes 2005: An Insider's View* demonstrates our continued commitment to assist users of the CPT code set.

Acknowledgments

Thank you to these members of the AMA Press:

Anthony J. Frankos, Vice President, Business Products

Mike Desposito, Publisher

Jean Roberts, Director, Production and Manufacturing

Dan Reyes, Director, CPT Product Development

Erin Kalitowski, Marketing Manager

Pat Lee, Technical Developmental Editor

Rosalyn Carlton, Senior Production Coordinator

Ronnie Summers, Senior Print Coordinator

Boon Ai Tan, Senior Production Coordinator

Thank you also to Patrick Gallagher, Director of Physician Payment Policy and Systems, and Todd Klemp, Senior Policy Associate, both of the AMA, for their assistance.

Using This Book

This book is designed to serve as a reference guide to understanding the changes contained in *Current Procedural Terminology (CPT) 2005* and is not intended to replace the CPT book. We make every effort to ensure accuracy; however, if differences exist, you should always defer to the information contained in the CPT book for 2005.

The Symbols

This book uses the same coding conventions that appear in the CPT nomenclature.

● Indicates that new procedure numbers were added to the CPT nomenclature

▲ Indicates that a code revision has resulted in a substantially altered procedure descriptor

+ Indicates CPT add-on codes

⊘ Indicates codes that are exempt from the use of modifier 51, but are not designated as CPT add-on procedures/services

►◄ Indicate revised guidelines, cross-references, and/or explanatory text

Whenever possible, we tried to include complete segments of text from the CPT book; however, in some cases, the text has been abbreviated.

⊙ Indicates code which typically includes conscious sedation

The conscious sedation "bulls-eye" symbol has been added to the list of CPT code symbols for *CPT 2005*. This symbol is intended to indicate those procedures in which the provision of conscious sedation services is considered to be inherent and would therefore not be separately reported by the same physician performing the primary service. The symbol appears before each procedure in which conscious sedation has been identified as a typical component. It is expected that if conscious sedation is provided to the patient as part of one of these services, that it would be provided by the same physician who is providing the service. A complete list of all procedures identified by the "bull's eye" symbol can be found in Appendix G.

The Rationale

After each change or series of changes is a rationale. The rationale is intended to provide a brief explanation as to why the change(s) occurred, but may not answer every question that may arise as a result of the change(s).

Reading the Clinical Examples

The clinical examples/procedural descriptions included in this text are presented to give practical situations for which the new and/or revised codes in the *CPT 2005* book would be appropriately reported. It is important to note that these examples do not suggest limiting the use of a code, but only represent the typical patient and service/procedure. They do not describe the universe of patients for whom the service/procedure would be appropriate. In addition, third-party payer reporting policies may differ.

The Tabular Review of the Changes

The table beginning on page 257 allows you to see all of the code changes at a glance. By reviewing the table you can easily determine the level to which your particular field of interest has been affected by the changes in the *CPT 2005* book.

CPT Book Text/Guidelines

Guideline and revised CPT book text appears indented. Any revised text, guidelines, and/or headings are indicated with the ▶ ◀ symbols.

Evaluation and Management

Excluding minor editorial modifications, revisions to the Evaluation and Management section for CPT 2005 consist solely of clarification of the neonatal age, for consistency between the diagnostic and procedural code sets.

Evaluation and Management

Critical Care Services

Critical Care is the direct delivery . . .

Providing medical care to a critically ill . . .

Inpatient critical care services provided to infants ▶29◀ days through 24 months of age are reported with pediatric critical care codes 99293 and 99294. The pediatric critical care codes are reported as long as the infant/young child qualifies for critical care services during the hospital stay through 24 months of age. Inpatient critical care services provided to neonates (▶28◀ days of age or less) are reported with the neonatal critical care codes 99295 and 99296. The neonatal critical care codes are reported as long as the neonate qualifies for critical care services during the hospital stay through the ▶28◀th postnatal day. The reporting of the pediatric and neonatal critical care services is not based on time or the type of unit (eg, pediatric or neonatal critical care unit) and it is not dependent upon the type of provider delivering the care. To report critical care services provided in the outpatient setting (eg, emergency department or office), for neonates and pediatric patients up through 24 months of age, see the hourly Critical Care codes 99291, 99292. If the same physician provides critical care services for a neonatal or pediatric patient in both the outpatient and inpatient settings on the same day, report only the appropriate Neonatal or Pediatric Critical Care code (99293-99296) for all critical care services provided on that day. For additional instructions on reporting these services, see the Neonatal and Pediatric Critical Care section and codes 99293-99296.

✍ Rationale

An editorial revision to eliminate inconsistencies between Current Procedural Terminology (CPT) and International Classification of Diseases, Ninth Revision Clinical Modification (ICD-9-CM) coding related to the neonatal period has been made to the neonatal and pediatric critical care service codes 99293, 99294, 99295 and 99296. The most commonly utilized definition of the neonatal period is beginning at birth and lasting through the 28th day following birth. Formerly, CPT utilized 30 days of age or less, causing confusion for both physicians and insurance carriers. For example, a critically ill patient who is 29 days of age was previously reported using a neonatal CPT code and a non-neonatal ICD-9-CM code(s). The revisions to the pediatric and neonatal critical care codes resolve this discrepancy. The Critical Care Services and Inpatient Neonatal and Pediatric Critical Care Services guidelines were also revised to reflect this change.

Inpatient Neonatal and Pediatric Critical Care Services

The following codes (99293-99296) are used . . .

The initial day neonatal critical care code (99295) . . .

Codes 99295, 99296 are used to report services provided by a physician directing the inpatient care of a critically ill neonate through the first ▶28◀ days of life. They represent care starting with the date of admission (99295) and subsequent day(s) (99296) and may be reported only once per day, per patient. Once the neonate is no longer considered to be critically ill, the Intensive Low Birth Weight Services codes for those with present body weight of less than 2500 grams (99298, 99299) or the codes for Subsequent Hospital Care (99231-99233) for those with present body weight over 2500 grams should be utilized.

Codes 99293, 99294 are used to report services provided by a physician directing the inpatient care of a critically ill infant or young child from ▶29◀ days of postnatal age through 24 months of age. They represent care starting with the date of admission (99293) and subsequent day(s) (99294) and may be reported by a single physician only once per day, per patient in a given setting. The critically ill or critically injured child older than 24 months of age would be reported with hourly critical care service codes (99291, 99292). Once an infant is no longer considered to be critically ill but continues to require intensive care, the Intensive Low Birth Weight Services codes (99298, 99299) should be used to report services for infants with present body weight of less than 2500 grams. When the present body weight of those infants exceeds 2500 grams, the Subsequent Hospital Care (99231-99233) codes should be utilized. To report critical care services provided in the outpatient setting (eg, emergency department or office), for neonates and pediatric patients up through 24 months of age, see the hourly Critical Care codes 99291, 99292. If the same physician provides critical care services for a neonatal or pediatric patient in both the outpatient and inpatient settings on the same day, report only the appropriate Neonatal or Pediatric Critical Care code (99293-99296) for all critical care services provided on that day.

Care rendered under 99293–99296 includes . . .

The pediatric and neonatal critical care codes include those procedures listed above for the hourly critical care codes (99291, 99292). In addition, the following procedures are also included in the bundled (global) pediatric and neonatal critical care service codes (99293-99296): umbilical venous (36510) and umbilical arterial (36660) catheters, central (36555) or peripheral vessel catheterization (36000), other arterial catheters (36140, 36620), oral or nasogastric tube placement (43752), endotracheal intubation (31500), lumbar puncture (62270), suprapubic bladder aspiration (51000), bladder catheterization (▶51701, 51702◀), initiation and management of mechanical ventilation (94656, 94657) or continuous positive airway pressure (CPAP) (94660), surfactant administration, intravascular fluid administration (90780, 90781), transfusion of blood components (36430, 36440), vascular punctures (36420, 36600), invasive or non-invasive electronic monitoring of vital signs, bedside pulmonary function testing (94375), and/or monitoring or interpretation of blood gases or oxygen saturation (94760-94762). Any services performed which are not listed above should be reported separately.

Rationale

An editorial revision to eliminate inconsistencies between CPT and ICD-9-CM coding related to the neonatal period has been made to the neonatal and pediatric critical care service codes 99293, 99294, 99295 and 99296. The most commonly utilized definition of the neonatal period is beginning at birth and lasting through the 28th day following birth. Formerly, the CPT code set utilized 30 days of age or less, causing confusion for both physicians and insurance carriers. For example, a critically ill patient who is 29 days of age was previously reported using a neonatal

CPT code and a non-neonatal ICD-9-CM code(s). The revisions to the pediatric and neonatal critical care codes resolve this discrepancy. The Critical Care Services and Inpatient Neonatal and Pediatric Critical Care Services guidelines were also revised to reflect this change.

Inpatient Pediatric Critical Care

▲99293   **Initial inpatient pediatric critical care,** per day, for the evaluation and management of a critically ill infant or young child, 29 days through 24 months of age

▲99294   **Subsequent inpatient pediatric critical care,** per day, for the evaluation and management of a critically ill infant or young child, 29 days through 24 months of age

 Rationale

An editorial revision to eliminate inconsistencies between CPT and ICD-9-CM coding related to the neonatal period has been made to the neonatal and pediatric critical care service codes 99293, 99294, 99295 and 99296. The most commonly utilized definition of the neonatal period is beginning at birth and lasting through the 28th day following birth. Formerly, the CPT code set utilized 30 days of age or less, causing confusion for both physicians and insurance carriers. For example, a critically ill patient who is 29 days of age was previously reported using a neonatal CPT code and a non-neonatal ICD-9-CM code(s). The revisions to the pediatric and neonatal critical care codes resolve this discrepancy.

Clinical Example (99293)

A six-month-old female, former 28-week gestational age premature infant, now with chronic lung disease (CLD) (bronchopulmonary dysplasia) following her neonatal course is admitted to the Pediatric Intensive Care Unit (PICU) from home with respiratory distress and impending respiratory failure. She had been stable on a low flow of nasal oxygen until 2 days prior to admission when she developed a fever, cough, and increased oxygen requirement. She gradually developed tachypnea, wheezing and retractions despite increased bronchodilator therapy at home (in addition to her daily diuretics, supplemental oxygen and maintenance bronchodilator therapy for her CLD).

In the emergency room (ER) she was found to have an oxygen saturation of 83% on 1 L of nasal cannula O_2. An arterial blood gas (ABG) measurement revealed acute and chronic hypercarbia and hypoxia. A chest x-ray revealed bilateral diffuse pneumonia, as well as hyperinflation. She was transferred to the PICU for evaluation and management by the pediatric intensivist. Despite aggressive therapy to treat her pulmonary disease, she progressed to respiratory failure requiring intubation and mechanical ventilation. Central venous and arterial access was obtained by the pediatric intensivist after numerous attempts at peripheral arterial and venous catheterization were unsuccessful due to scarring from line placement during her Neonatal Intensive Care Unit (NICU) stay. Arterial blood pressure and central venous pressure monitoring revealed hypotension and intravascular volume depletion. Blood, urine, and respiratory cultures were obtained and broad-spectrum antibiotic coverage was instituted for presumed sepsis. The patient's hypotension responded to treatment with fluid boluses and low doses of pressors. Her respiratory failure worsened and she developed acute respiratory distress syndrome (ARDS), circulatory failure and fluid and electrolyte disturbances that required high frequency oscillatory ventilation and increased inotropic support for 7 days. She was eventually converted back to conventional ventilation and weaned to extubation. The pediatric intensivist spent many hours throughout the child's admission coordinating the activities of other subspecialists, nursing staff, respiratory therapists, nutritionists and social workers involved, as well as providing daily communications to the family and the patient's primary care physician.

Description of Procedure (99293)
A complete examination of the head, eyes, nose, mouth, chest, lungs, heart, abdomen, genitals, rectum, joints, spine, extremities, and a neurologic appraisal of movement, reflexes, cranial nerves, and degree of arousal and activity is performed. All attached monitors and tubes are checked for secure placement and proper function.

Clinical Example (99294)
A 1½-year-old male, who was in his usual state of health, now presented with acute respiratory distress to the emergency department. The patient's ongoing medications included home nebulized bronchodilator therapy and low-dose steroids for significant reactive airway disease. After evaluation and failure to clear with bronchodilator therapy in the emergency room (ER) he was admitted to the PICU with increasing respiratory distress and impending respiratory failure. Over the next few hours he demonstrated increasing oxygen requirements, tachypnea, cough, and a mild rash. He was placed on bronchodilator therapy, constant cardiopulmonary, blood pressure, and oxygen saturation monitoring, intravenous (IV) infusions, antibiotics, chest radiographs, blood gases, and intravenous steroids. He was placed on a nonrebreather mask and multiple laboratory examinations for bacterial and viral studies were performed. His response to therapy was variable over the first 12 hours and he then gradually deteriorated. The patient's deteriorating clinical state was discussed extensively with the family including the need to intubate the patient for ventilatory support. He required endotracheal intubation and mechanical ventilation for respiratory failure. His chest x-ray at that time showed a diffuse, interstitial pattern consistent with progressive diffuse alveolar disease. The patient was placed on IV continuous sedation to assist with ventilator/patient asynchrony. The patient's family and primary care physician were contacted daily for daily updates and therapeutic planning. The patient continued to show a deteriorating state of oxygenation and ventilation over the first 48 hours, and increasing lung congestion consistent with noncardiogenic pulmonary edema. Initially, this was treated with diuretic therapy and increasing the mechanical ventilatory support with positive expiratory pressure. The patient had associated glucose and electrolyte abnormalities, which were treated with additional diuretic therapy and changes in intravenous

Ⓢ=Modifier 51 Exempt   ⊙=Conscious Sedation   ✚=Add-on Code

solutions. Nutritional support was provided in the form of hyperalimentation. Over the next 72 hours, he continued to require increased oxygen concentration increasing ventilatory support resulting in high airway pressures, necessitating placement on high frequency oscillatory ventilation. Due to the child's unstable condition he required 1:1 nursing care. An arterial line and central venous pressure monitoring line were placed to closely monitor the patient's hemodynamics and his intravascular fluid status. During the course of high frequency oscillation, progressive anemia from blood obtained for laboratory tests and from hemodilution was treated with packed red blood cell transfusions. Over the course of the first week of high frequency oscillation the patient developed improvement of his chest radiograph and decreased oxygen requirements. By the end of the second week his respiratory status had improved and he was transferred to conventional mechanical ventilation with moderate settings on pressure regulated volume control. The family was given daily updates and discussion about his progress. His primary physician received daily calls with clinical changes discussed. At this time the patient was taken off paralysis and sedation was weaned down to minimum ventilator and oxygen levels. By the end of the third week the patient had been successfully weaned down to continuous positive airway pressure (CPAP) and subsequently extubated to a nasal cannula. His clinical condition was no longer considered critical, but he continued to require close observation and evaluation.

Description of Procedure (99294)
A complete examination of the head, eyes, nose, mouth, chest, lungs, heart, abdomen, genitals, rectum, joints, spine, extremities, and a neurologic appraisal of movement, reflexes, cranial nerves, and degree of arousal and activity was performed. All attached monitors and tubes are checked for secure placement and proper function.

Inpatient Neonatal Critical Care

▲99295 **Initial inpatient neonatal critical care,** per day, for the evaluation and management of a critically ill neonate, 28 days of age or less

This code is reserved for the date of admission for neonates who are critically ill. Critically ill neonates require cardiac and/or respiratory support (including ventilator or nasal CPAP when indicated), continuous or frequent vital signs monitoring, laboratory and blood gas interpretations, follow-up physician reevaluations, and constant observation by the health care team under direct physician supervision. Immediate preoperative evaluation and stabilization of neonates with life threatening surgical or cardiac conditions are included under this code. Neonates with life threatening surgical or cardiac conditions are included under this code.

Care for neonates who require an intensive care setting but who are not critically ill is reported using the initial hospital care codes (99221-99223).

▲99296 **Subsequent inpatient neonatal critical care,** per day, for the evaluation and management of a critically ill neonate, 28 days of age or less

A critically ill neonate will require cardiac and/or respiratory support (including ventilator or nasal CPAP when indicated), continuous or frequent vital sign monitoring, laboratory and blood gas interpretations, follow-up physician reevaluations throughout a 24-hour period, and constant observation by the health care team under direct physician supervision.

(Subsequent care for neonates who require an intensive setting but who are not critically ill is reported using either the intensive low birth weight services codes (99298, 99299) or the subsequent hospital care codes (99231-99233))

✍ Rationale

An editorial revision to eliminate inconsistencies between CPT and ICD-9-CM coding related to the neonatal period has been made to the neonatal and pediatric critical care service codes 99293, 99294, 99295 and 99296. The most commonly utilized definition of the neonatal period is beginning at birth and lasting through the 28th day following birth. Formerly, the CPT code set utilized 30 days of age or less, causing confusion for both physicians and insurance carriers. For example, a critically ill patient who is 29 days of age was previously reported using a neonatal CPT code and a non-neonatal ICD-9-CM code(s). The revisions to the pediatric and neonatal critical care codes resolve this discrepancy.

🩺 Clinical Example (99296)

A 3-day-old infant is under the care and direct supervision of the attending physician. The infant remains intubated and on intermittent mandatory ventilation. The infant has both umbilical artery and view catheters in place and is on continuous cardiac, respiratory and blood pressure monitoring. Blood pressure is being supported with dopamine. Hyperalimentation has been started. After evaluation, indomethacin has been started for a patent ductus arteriosus. Evaluation for intraventricular hemorrhage with ultrasound has been completed. A packed red blood cell transfusion is given. The infant is examined repeatedly and laboratory, x-rays and arterial blood gases are repeatedly evaluated. The parents are informed and counseled as to the infant's condition and prognosis. Medical records are maintained, including orders and progress notes. Fluids and ventilator changes are made frequently as required.

Preventive Medicine Services

Immunizations and ancillary studies involving laboratory, radiology, other procedures, or screening tests identified with a specific CPT code are reported separately. For immunizations, see ▶90465◀-90474 and 90476-90749.

✍ Rationale

The range of codes listed in the introductory notes for Preventive Medicine Services referencing immunizations has been revised to encompass new codes (90465, 90466, 90467, 90468) for immunization administration accompanied by counseling.

Anesthesia

Revisions of the Anesthesia section this year are minimal, with the addition of a single code, and the revision of the Anesthesia guidelines in tandem with the addition of Appendix G.

Anesthesia

Guidelines

Services involving administration of anesthesia are ...

The reporting of anesthesia services is ...

To report sedation with or without analgesia (conscious sedation) provided by a physician also performing the service for which conscious sedation is being provided, see codes 99141, 99142. ▶When any physician, other than the physician performing the procedure, provides anesthesia services as specified in *CPT* guidelines (conscious sedation or otherwise), the Anesthesia codes should be reported.◀

Intrathoracic

00560 Anesthesia for procedures on heart, pericardial sac, and great vessels of chest; without pump oxygenator

●00561 with pump oxygenator, under one year of age

▶(Do not report 00561 in conjunction with 99100, 99116, and 99135)◀

Rationale

Code 00561 is intended to describe the demanding and high risk administration of anesthesia associated with surgical repair of congenital heart lesions in children less than one year old. Establishment of this new code was necessary as code 00560, developed over three decades ago, was introduced to describe anesthesia for coronary artery bypass and valve replacement. The procedure described by the new code differs significantly in the complexity and stability of the patient, the age, the amount and intensity of anesthesia work in all phases of anesthetic care, and the risk of anesthesia.

Previously, correction of congenital heart disease defects was only able to be performed after the child was able to grow for several years to allow enough maturity to endure surgery. Advances in technology and improvement in surgical techniques have altered the landscape of the surgical approach for these corrective procedures. Since the state of health of the children who have these conditions has dramatically changed in the past two decades, the type and timing of the surgery has also been changed. Complete repair can now be performed at the earliest possible time, frequently shortly after birth. Due to the proliferation of surgical procedures and codes involving the heart and pump oxygenator, the corresponding anesthesia codes have been revised to better reflect these procedures. Code 00562 was established to report anesthesia services for coronary artery bypass or valve replacement. With advances in medical practice, code 00562 has evolved to report anesthesia for the newborn for repair of hypoplastic left heart, the elective repair of an atrial septal defect in a healthy five-year-old, and coronary artery bypass in a fifty-year-old.

Clinical Example (00561)

The infant was noted to have trisomy 21 and a heart murmur at birth. Subsequent studies determined the presence of an atrioventricular (AV) canal defect. The patient was followed closely after starting digoxin and furosemide by mouth. At his six-month check-up, the infant was noted to have tachypnea and failure to gain weight. The oxygen saturation was noted to have decreased from previous measurements, and radiologic examination of the chest noted signs consistent with cardiac failure. The repair of the congenital heart defect under cardiopulmonary bypass was scheduled.

Description of Procedure (00561)

Anesthetics were calculated based on weight and administered intramuscularly, after sterile preparation, into the deltoid muscle. Once the infant was noted to be under the influence of the anesthetic, he was transferred to the operating room. Monitors were placed for five-lead electrocardiogram, pulse oximetry, and blood pressure. A saphenous vein was cannulated with a 20-gauge catheter, and intravenous narcotic anesthesia and muscle relaxant were infused. Manual ventilation with 100% oxygen was begun. After appropriate demonstration of paralysis with a nerve blockade monitor, the trachea was intubated with the appropriate age-calculated and sized endotracheal tube (separately reported). Auscultation of breath sounds and capnography confirmed the correct tube placement. The endotracheal tube was secured with waterproof tape so as not to be disturbed by placement of the transesophageal echo probe. A radial artery was cannulated with a catheter and a left subclavian central line was placed under sterile conditions (both reported separately). Both lines were connected to the pressure transducers after calibrating to zero as recommended. Blood samples were drawn for blood gas analysis and activated clotting time (ACT). A 1 mL test dose of aprotinin was administered and after noting no adverse reaction, the continuous infusion was started. The remaining cardioactive infusion drugs were connected to the central line but not started. Intravenous medications to prevent infection and inflammation were administered. Anesthesia charting was performed. Ventilation was adjusted as indicated by the blood gas results. Surgery commenced and ventilation was momentarily stopped during sternotomy. Intermittent blood gas analysis and ACT were measured throughout the surgery. Narcotics and muscle relaxants were intermittently administered as necessary and blood pressure was titrated. After the surgeons adequately dissected the great vessels, anticoagulant was administered intravenously and ACT was measured to be over 400 seconds. Cardio-pulmonary bypass commenced soon after cannulation of the aorta and right atrium, and ventilation was discontinued. During bypass, the anesthesiologist, in conjunction with the perfusionist, administered anesthetic agents and relaxants as appropriate. Surgical repair of the atrio-ventricular canal ensued with graft closure of the septal defects and suture repair of the valvular insufficiency. The anesthesiologist and the surgeon worked together to assure venting of air from the heart prior to release of the aortic cross-clamp. Near the anticipated end of bypass and after adequate re-warming, ventilation was restarted and inotropic cardiac support was begun with infusions of dopamine and dobutamine. Afterload reduction was produced by an infusion of milrinone.

Heating the infant was partially accomplished with a forced warm air mattress controlled by the anesthesiologist. After discontinuing bypass, the pulmonary artery was cannulated by the surgeon and the pressure line was passed to the anesthesiologist for connection to a transducer. As is typically seen with atrioventricular (AV) canal repair in children less than one year of age, the pulmonary artery pressure was discovered to be high and inhaled nitric oxide gas was added to the inspiratory anesthetic circuit. Flows were adjusted to obtain the correct concentration as measured in the inspiratory limb. Once cardiac and pulmonary parameters were stabilized, the heparin anticoagulation was reversed with intravenous medication and the activated clotting time (ACT) was measured as normal. Blood gases were intermittently checked. Due to the patient's weight and the effects of cardiopulmonary bypass on the coagulation system, coagulopathies are commonly seen after discontinuation from bypass. After the conclusion of surgery, a portable monitor and ventilation circuit were connected to the patient for transport of the infant to the intensive care unit. The nitric oxide circuit was tested to ensure adequate delivery of the vasodilator during transport. The infusion pumps delivering cardiovascular medications were checked for proper function prior to transport. On arrival to the intensive care unit, hemodynamic and respiratory monitors were transferred to the unit's system. Ventilation was transferred to a bedside ventilator and parameters adjusted to satisfaction. The continued administration of nitric oxide was confirmed. Vital signs were monitored.

Surgery

Most notable of the revisions to the Surgery section are six new transplant series of codes and guidelines to report lung, heart/lung, intestine, liver, pancreas, and kidney transplantations. The conversion of Category III codes to Category I codes for CPT 2005 resulted in the addition of 10 Category I codes. These include new codes for endovascular repair of abdominal aortic aneurysm, endometrial cryoablation, carotid stenting, arthroscopic and open approach knee repairs, and endoscopic repair of the esophageal sphincter.

Guideline additions include breast excision procedures, the clarification of reporting spinal procedures related to exploration of spinal fusion and revision of previously placed instrumentation in the Musculoskeletal subsections of Spinal Arthrodesis, and Spinal Instrumentation. Also notable are new codes for skin debridement for necrotizing infections, gastric restrictive procedures, and further revisions and additions to the bronchoscopy codes.

Surgery

Skin, Subcutaneous and Accessory Structures

EXCISION—DEBRIDEMENT

▶(For abdominal wall or genitalia debridement for necrotizing soft tissue infection, see 11004-11006)◀

● **11004** Debridement of skin, subcutaneous tissue, muscle and fascia for necrotizing soft tissue infection; external genitalia and perineum

● **11005**   abdominal wall, with or without fascial closure

● **11006**   external genitalia, perineum and abdominal wall, with or without fascial closure

+● **11008** Removal of prosthetic material or mesh, abdominal wall for necrotizing soft tissue infection (List separately in addition to code for primary procedure)

▶(Use 11008 in conjunction with 11004-11006)◀

▶(Do not report 11008 in conjunction with 11000-11001, 11010-11044)◀

▶(Report skin grafts or flaps separately when performed for closure at the same session as 11004-11008)◀

▶(If orchiectomy is performed, use 54520)◀

▶(If testicular transplantation is performed, use 54680)◀

Rationale

Codes 11004-11006 were added to identify extensive debridement procedures necessary to treat necrotizing soft tissue infections, such as Fournier's gangrene. Generally, these debridement procedures are performed on high-risk patients. In addition to the risk and extensiveness involved in performance of the debridement procedure, transplantation or removal of organs (eg, testicular transplant, orchiectomy), hernia and/or intestinal repair, or fistula repair may be necessary. As indicated in the code descriptor language, these codes are used according to the specific area that receives treatment.

Add-on code 11008 has been established to identify concurrent removal of a mesh or prosthetic device.

Parenthetical notes have also been included to identify procedures that should be separately reported when performed in conjunction with the debridement; and to identify a list of exclusionary codes with which these codes should not be reported.

In addition, the exclusionary cross-reference following code 11044 was revised to include the new selective debridement codes (97597, 97598) which should not be reported together with the debridement codes in the Integumentary section (11040-11044).

Cross-references referring to the appropriate codes for reporting orchiectomy, testicular transplantation, and abdominal wall or genitalia debridement were also added.

Clinical Example (11004)

A 56-year-old diabetic male presents to the emergency room with a two-day history of increasing fever. On physical examination, he appears dehydrated with an elevated temperature. There are patchy areas of full thickness skin necrosis with surrounding erythema involving his scrotum, perineum and base of the penis. Laboratory examination reveals a white blood count of 18.6 and a blood sugar of 42. He is given fluid resuscitation and intravenous (IV) antibiotics. Since he has necrotizing soft tissue infection (Fournier's gangrene), he is taken to the operating room for immediate debridement.

Description of Procedure (11004)

The patient is taken to the operating room and placed in the supine position with the legs apart. Then the field is sterilized, prepared and draped. With the patient under anesthesia, the extent of the necrotic tissue is evaluated. Afterward, the patient's necrotic skin, subcutaneous tissue, fat and muscle are debrided back to healthy tissue. The penis and scrotum are debrided as necessary. Drains are placed and the wounds are packed open with gauze.

Clinical Example (11005)

A 43-year-old male is 10 days status post repair of a colon wound secondary to a shotgun injury to the abdomen. On physical examination, he appears dehydrated with an elevated temperature and toxic. Inspection of the partially opened abdominal midline wound reveal areas of full thickness skin necrosis with surrounding erythema and crepitus involving large areas of the abdominal wall skin, subcutaneous, abdominal wall fascia, and muscle. Laboratory examination demonstrates a white blood count of 25,000. He is given fluid resuscitation and IV antibiotics. Since he has fulminating necrotizing fasciitis, he is taken to the operating room for immediate debridement. Complete debridement of all involved skin, subcutaneous tissue, fascia, and muscle is carried out. The wounds are packed, dressed, and the fascia is partially reapproximated.

Description of Procedure (11005)

In the operating room, the patient's entire abdomen is prepped and draped. The skin is opened in its entirety, and the fascia opened along the necrotic portion. The necrotic skin, subcutaneous tissue, fascia, and underlying muscle of the rectus abdominus and external oblique are debrided by shard dissection. Multiple abscesses are entered and drained. The debridement is then carried cephalad, caudal, and lateral until healthy muscle and subcutaneous tissue is reached. All wound areas are irrigated with copious amounts of antibiotic solution. Multiple drains are placed in all wound sites and the wound beds are packed with gauze. The abdominal fascia is partially reapproximated with sutures. All wounds are dressed and the patient is taken to the recovery room.

Clinical Example (11006)

A 48-year-old leukemic male presents to the emergency room with a 24-hour history of fever and dehydration. On physical examination, he appears dehydrated with an elevated temperature. There are areas of full thickness skin necrosis with surrounding erythema and crepitus involving large areas of the scrotum, perineum, base of penis, upper thighs, and lower abdominal wall. Laboratory examination demonstrates an elevated white blood count and a creatinine of 2.8. He is given fluid resuscitation and IV antibiotics. Since he has fulminating necrotizing fascitus (Fournier's gangrene), he is taken to the operating room for immediate debridement of all these involved tissues.

Description of Procedure (11006)

In the operating room, the patient's scrotum, perineum, penis, lower abdomen, and thighs are prepped and draped. A catheter is inserted. Attention is first turned to the external genitalia. The necrotic skin, subcutaneous tissue, and underlying dartos muscle of the scrotum, perineum, and penis are debrided by sharp dissection down to the testes, corpora and urethra. Both testes are dissected free and appear healthy with no evidence of gross orchitis or necrosis. Multiple abscesses are entered and drained. The debridement is then carried cephalad onto the lower abdominal wall to the level of the umbilicus and caudal to the level of the upper thighs until healthy muscle and subcutaneous tissue is reached. Portions of skin, subcutaneous tissue, and fascia of the rectus abdominus and external oblique muscles are debrided until healthy tissue is encountered. A large abscess cavity with fistula tract is unroofed extending from the suprapubic solution. Multiple drains are placed in all wound sites and the wound beds are packed with saline soaked gauze. The abdominal fascia is partially reapproximated with monofilament sutures. The partially exposed testes are also covered with saline gauze and large scrotal dressings. All wounds are dressed and the patient is taken to the recovery room.

 Clinical Example (11008)

A 50-year-old male has had recurrent draining sinuses along and associated with a 12-month-old abdominal midline ventral hernia repair. He has had recurrent subcutaneous abscesses drained, with previously isolated gram-negative organisms. The repeated use of broad-spectrum antimicrobials and local wound care has failed to resolve the recurrent infections. He has infected polypropylene mesh in the hernia repair. The entire 6 by 4 inch section of mesh is removed by sharp dissection.

Description of Procedure (11008)

The mesh is completely exposed by sharp dissection. It is carefully dissected free circumferentially from the subcutaneous tissue, fascia and muscle. As it is removed, it is carefully and sharply dissected free from any underlying omentum and intestines. The mesh is completely removed. Any associated laparotomy, wound debridement, intestinal or fistula repair, or wound repair is reported separately.

11040   Debridement; skin, partial thickness

11041   skin, full thickness

11042   skin, and subcutaneous tissue

11043   skin, subcutaneous tissue, and muscle

11044   skin, subcutaneous tissue, muscle, and bone

(Do not report 11040-11044 in ►conjunction with 97597–◄97602)

Breast

EXCISION

►Excisional breast surgery includes certain biopsy procedures, the removal of cysts or other benign or malignant tumors or lesions, and the surgical treatment of breast and chest wall malignancies. Biopsy procedures may be percutaneous or open, and they involve the removal of differing amounts of tissue for diagnosis.◄

►Breast biopsies are reported using codes 19100-19103. The open excision of breast lesions (eg, lesions of the breast ducts, cysts, benign or malignant tumors), without specific attention to adequate surgical margins, with or without the preoperative placement of radiological markers, is reported using codes 19110-19126. Partial mastectomy procedures (eg, lumpectomy, tylectomy, quadrantectomy, or segmentectomy) describe open excisions of breast tissue with specific attention to adequate surgical margins.◄

►Partial mastectomy procedures are reported using codes 19160 or 19162 as appropriate. Documentation for partial mastectomy procedures includes attention to the removal of adequate surgical margins surrounding the breast mass or lesion.◄

►Total mastectomy procedures include simple mastectomy, complete mastectomy, subcutaneous mastectomy, modified radical mastectomy, radical mastectomy, and more extended procedures (eg, Urban type operation). Total mastectomy procedures are reported using codes 19180, 19182, 19200, 19220, or 19240 as appropriate.◄

►Excisions or resections of chest wall tumors including ribs, with or without reconstruction, with or without mediastinal lymphadenectomy, are reported using codes 19260, 19271, or 19272. Codes 19260-19272 are not restricted to breast tumors and are used to report resections of chest wall tumors originating from any chest wall component. (For excision of lung or pleura, see 32310 et seq.)◄

▲**19160**   Mastectomy, partial (eg, lumpectomy, tylectomy, quadrantectomy, segmentectomy);

19162   with axillary lymphadenectomy

►(For placement of radiotherapy afterloading balloon/brachytherapy catheters, see 19296-19298)◄

 Rationale

Code 19160 was revised to include alternative terms in the descriptor (eg, lumpectomy, tylectomy, quadrantectomy and segmentectomy) used for partial mastectomy. The inclusion of these terms in the descriptor language of code

19160 clarifies that they are interchangeable with the term partial mastectomy. New guidelines have been added at the beginning of the Breast Excision subsection to clarify appropriate reporting of breast biopsies, partial mastectomy, total mastectomy, and excision or resection of chest wall tumors. The appropriate code ranges are provided for each type of excisional breast surgery (ie, biopsy, mastectomy, excision/removal of chest wall tumors).

A cross-reference was added following code 19162 directing users to codes 19296 through 19298 for placement of radiotherapy afterloading balloon/brachytherapy catheters.

INTRODUCTION

●**19296**　Placement of radiotherapy afterloading balloon catheter into the breast for interstitial radioelement application following partial mastectomy, includes imaging guidance; on date separate from partial mastectomy

+●**19297**　　concurrent with partial mastectomy (List separately in addition to code for primary procedure)

▶(Use 19297 in conjunction with 19160 or 19162)◀

⊙●**19298**　Placement of radiotherapy afterloading brachytherapy catheters (multiple tube and button type) into the breast for interstitial radioelement application following (at the time of or subsequent to) partial mastectomy, includes imaging guidance

🖎 Rationale

Three codes were added to the Breast Introduction subsection to describe catheter placement and subsequent catheter removal for interstitial radioelement application in the breast following partial mastectomy. Additional codes should be separately reported for provision of the isodose plan (77326-77328) and the remote afterloading brachytherapy administration (77781-77784).

Code 19296 and add-on code 19297 describe interstitial radioelement application catheter placement for radiotherapy afterloading following a partial mastectomy. Code 19296 should be reported when the catheter is placed on a separate date from the partial mastectomy. Add-on code 19297 should be reported when the catheter is placed after the partial mastectomy during the same operative session (concurrent). A parenthetical note was added following code 19297 directing users to report code 19297 in conjunction with the concurrently performed partial mastectomy code (ie, 19160 or 19162). Code 19298 describes placement of catheters for radiotherapy afterloading brachytherapy following a partial mastectomy. Code 19298 is reported whether the catheters are placed at the time of or subsequent to the partial mastectomy.

🩺 Clinical Example (19296)

A 55-year-old female has recently undergone a lumpectomy for early stage (stage 0, I, or II) breast cancer. She had no prior history of breast cancer treated with a lumpectomy procedure and radiation in the same breast. At the conclusion of the patient's lumpectomy procedure, sutures were used to close the skin and subcutaneous tissue to maintain a skin spacing distance of 5-7 mm between the lumpectomy cavity and the skin surface for possible future placement of a radiotherapy afterloading balloon catheter. She now presents for placement of the balloon catheter into the breast, under imaging guidance, for interstitial radioelement application.

Description of Procedure (19296)

With the patient under appropriate anesthesia, the lumpectomy site and the remaining breast tissue are examined by the physician to ensure adequate tissue for the radiotherapy afterloading balloon catheter to be securely positioned. Then, the physician confirms that the site is appropriate (not too close to the sternum or in the axillary tail of the breast). Next, he/she confirms that the cavity has been kept open with only the subcutaneous and top skin layer closed. A skin spacing of 5-7 mm between the skin and lumpectomy cavity to protect the skin from radiation damage is confirmed. Using either a sterile ruler or imaging guidance, the size and shape of the lumpectomy cavity are evaluated to determine the appropriate technique for the implantation of the catheter. Prior to insertion, the selected balloon catheter is tested by inflating it with a saline solution. The symmetry and integrity of the balloon is assessed and the balloon is deflated. Next, a separate "stab-like" incision is made near the lumpectomy incision. Through this incision, a trocar is placed to create a separate pathway to the lumpectomy cavity. Fluid that may have accumulated in the cavity is drained. The catheter is then inserted into the lumpectomy cavity via this separate pathway. The balloon catheter is inflated with saline and contrast agent to allow the surrounding tissue to conform to the balloon element of the balloon. The surgeon monitors the amount of fluid during inflation to ensure that the balloon element is appropriately positioned in the lumpectomy cavity for the correct radiation dosimetry, previously supplied by the radiation oncologist. The 5-7 mm skin spacing between the cavity and skin is reconfirmed to ensure that it has remained intact. The surgeon confirms conformance of the cavity to balloon element of the radiotherapy afterloading balloon catheter. The surgeon verifies the placement and integrity of the radiotherapy afterloading balloon catheter after inflation with the saline and contrast agent. Having verified that the radiotherapy afterloading balloon element of the catheter is secure and appropriately placed, a stitch is placed on either side of the catheter, if the catheter was placed through the lumpectomy incision.

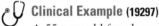 Clinical Example (19297)

A 55-year-old female presents as a candidate for a lumpectomy, followed by accelerated partial breast irradiation to treat a newly diagnosed, early stage (stage 0, I, or II) breast cancer. She has no prior history of breast cancer treated by lumpectomy and radiation in the same breast. At the conclusion of the patient's lumpectomy, surgical techniques are employed to maintain a skin spacing distance of 5-7 mm between the lumpectomy cavity and the skin surface. The surgeon's clinical judgment combined with immediate specimen evaluation indicated that the tissue margins surrounding the lumpectomy cavity were free of cancerous cells and a sentinel node biopsy or axillary dissection was negative in its findings. Using imaging guidance, a radiotherapy, afterloading, balloon catheter is placed into the breast for future interstitial radioelement application.

⊘ =Modifier 51 Exempt   ⊙ =Conscious Sedation   ✛ =Add-on Code

Description of Procedure (19297)

After excision of the cancer of the breast and pathology confirmation that the tissue margins surrounding the lumpectomy cavity were free of cancerous cells and that no positive lymph nodes were detected, the remaining breast tissue is examined to ensure adequate tissue for the radiotherapy, afterloading, balloon catheter to be securely positioned. A skin spacing of 5-7 mm between the skin and lumpectomy cavity to protect the skin from radiation damage is confirmed. Using either a sterile ruler or imaging guidance, the size and shape of the lumpectomy cavity are evaluated to determine the appropriate technique for the implantation of the catheter. Prior to insertion, the selected balloon catheter is tested by inflating it with a saline solution. The symmetry and integrity of the balloon is assessed and the balloon is deflated. Next, a separate "stab-like" incision is made near the lumpectomy incision. Through this incision, a trocar is placed to create a separate pathway to the lumpectomy cavity. The catheter is then inserted into the lumpectomy cavity via this separate pathway. The balloon catheter is inflated with saline and contrast agent to allow the surrounding tissue to conform to the balloon element of the balloon. The surgeon monitors the amount of fluid during inflation to ensure that the balloon element is appropriately positioned in the lumpectomy cavity for the correct radiation dosimetry, supplied by the radiation oncologist prior to surgery. The 5-7 mm skin spacing between the cavity and skin is reconfirmed to ensure that it has remained intact. The balloon catheter is deflated and withdrawn to allow closure of the lumpectomy site without compromising the integrity of the catheter. After the lumpectomy site is closed, the radiotherapy afterloading balloon catheter is re-advanced and re-inflated to the previously pre-determined volume. Placement and integrity of the catheter is verified after inflation with saline and contrast agent. Having verified that the radiotherapy afterloading balloon element of the catheter is secure and appropriately placed, a stitch is placed on either side of the catheter, if the catheter was placed through the lumpectomy incision.

 Clinical Example (19298)

A 55-year-old female is a candidate for a lumpectomy procedure followed by accelerated partial breast irradiation to treat a newly diagnosed, early stage (stage 0, I, or, II) breast cancer. Patient has no prior history of breast cancer treated with a lumpectomy procedure and radiation in the same breast. The surgical and radiation therapeutic alternatives have been fully discussed with the patient. After completion of the lumpectomy and pathological analysis of the surgical excisions specimen, it is determined that the patient is a candidate for interstitial tube and button type brachytherapy. The primary tumor margins are free of cancer cells and a sentinel node biopsy or axillary dissection indicates negative findings for cancer. The catheters are placed under imaging guidance. The brachytherapy applicator insertion is a separate procedure that may be performed immediately following the lumpectomy or delayed until a later date.

Description of Procedure (19298)

Once the distribution of catheters has been decided, the insertion process can begin. Hollow steel implant needles (or implant tubes with metal style) are used to insert the soft plastic catheters. The physician will use either a freehand or

---

template guided technique. In the freehand technique the physician determines the proper location and spacing of the brachytherapy catheters by sterile ruler measurements or with the template guide pattern. The entrance and exit sites are marked on the skin with a sterile marking pencil. For the template technique, the physician selects and marks the desired pattern on the template. The physician selects the correct length needle, for each puncture site, that corresponds to the tissue distance that must be traversed from the entrance to the exit site. The physician punctures the skin directly with the sterile, hollow, stainless steel, implant needles or a sharp blade may be needed to nick the skin to facilitate the entrance and exit. The physician then advances the needles through the skin and subcutaneous tissue as they are passed from the skin entrance to the exit site (usually tangential to the chest wall). The deep plane of the implant, located at the base of the excision cavity, is implanted first. The physician checks the catheter distribution and spacing through the open excision cavity to ensure full and complete coverage of the tissue. The most superficial plane is optimally 5 mm or more beneath the skin. The physician determines the number of catheters in each plane based upon the width of the region to be treated and the spacing interval between the catheters. The physician inserts the needles with clinical or image guidance or both. Once the needle or row of needles is in position the physician replaces them in the tissue with a series of brachytherapy tube catheters. The thin leader-end of the brachytherapy tube catheter is threaded through one end of the hollow needles and it exits at the opposite end, external to the patient. The physician pulls the needle and catheter assembly out as a unit so that the needle is removed and the brachytherapy tube catheter is left in situ. The catheter has a button-shaped or sphere end-piece that prevents it from being pulled through and out with the needle. After the catheter and end-piece are in position near the skin the physician threads a second fixing button or sphere over the opposite or leader end of the tube of the interstitial catheter, so that the apparatus is fixed in the breast tissue on both sides. The physician must check that individual buttons or spheres are placed snuggly, but not tightly onto the skin to allow for postoperative edema to avoid pressure injury of the skin. The physician inserts each catheter (typically 5-10 catheters per plane and 2-4 planes per implant) individually. A series of rows or planes must be created to give a 3-dimensional (3D) volume to the implanted region to achieve a proper treatment distribution that corresponds to the distribution of the disease and avoids important normal tissue structures. The inter-catheter and the inter-plane spacing must be monitored as the insertion proceeds. The brachytherapy tube and button catheters have some degree of rigidity to ensure that the radiation source passes smoothly and safely through the catheter array during treatment. The physician must check that each catheter is patent by passing a non-radioactive dummy cable through the length of the catheter. The physician confirms the position of the catheters within or around the target volume and the lumpectomy cavity by visual inspection, palpation, or by image guidance. The proximal or leader ends of the brachytherapy tube and button interstitial catheters project externally from the skin. The physician cuts them individually to length and the excess length is removed and discarded. The projecting catheter ends must be prepared to accept the high-dose-rate radiotherapy (HDR) afterloader connection tubing. In addition, the physician removes the internal stiffening-leader stripper device from the individual brachytherapy catheters. (These leaders are used to prevent the brachytherapy catheters from stretching during the pulling maneuver of the catheter insertion process.) After the catheters are correctly positioned, the dressing is applied. Care must be taken not to bend or kink the catheters, so special padding must be positioned by the physician. The cover sterile dressing is placed over the brachytherapy tube, button catheters and protection padding. After the brachytherapy devices insertion has been completed, the patient is moved to the recovery area.

Musculoskeletal System

Spine (Vertebral Column)

ARTHRODESIS

Arthrodesis may be performed in the ...

▶To report instrumentation procedures, see 22840-22855. (Codes 22840-22848, 22851 are reported in conjunction with code(s) for the definitive procedure(s) without modifier 51. When instrumentation reinsertion or removal is reported in conjunction with other definitive procedures including arthrodesis, decompression, and exploration of fusion, append modifier 51 to 22849, 22850, 22852, and 22855.) To report exploration of fusion, use 22830. (When exploration is reported in conjunction with other definitive procedures, including arthrodesis and decompression, append modifier 51 to 22830.) Do not append modifier 62 to spinal instrumentation codes 22840-22848 and 22850-22852.◀

EXPLORATION

▶To report instrumentation procedures, see 22840-22855. (Codes 22840-22848, 22851 are reported in conjunction with code(s) for the definitive procedure(s) without modifier 51. When instrumentation reinsertion or removal is reported in conjunction with other definitive procedures including arthrodesis, decompression, and exploration of fusion, append modifier 51 to 22849, 22850, 22852 and 22855.) To report exploration of fusion, see 22830. (When exploration is reported in conjunction with other definitive procedures, including arthrodesis and decompression, append modifier 51 to 22830.)◀

22830 Exploration of spinal fusion

SPINAL INSTRUMENTATION

▶List 22840-22855 separately, in conjunction with code(s) for fracture, dislocation, arthrodesis or exploration of fusion of the spine 22325-22328, 22548-22812, and 22830. Codes 22840-22848, 22851 are reported in conjunction with code(s) for the definitive procedure(s) without modifier 51. Codes 22849, 22850, 22852, and 22855 are subject to modifier 51 if reported with other definitive procedure(s), including arthrodesis, decompression, and exploration of fusion. Code 22849 should not be reported with 22850, 22852, and 22855 at the same spinal levels.◀

⊘ **22840** Posterior non-segmental instrumentation (eg, Harrington rod technique, pedicle fixation across one interspace, atlantoaxial transarticular screw fixation, sublaminar wiring at C1, facet screw fixation)

 Rationale

In order to clarify reporting for spinal procedures related to exploration of spinal fusion and revision of previously placed instrumentation, the introductory language of the Spinal Arthrodesis and Spinal Instrumentation subsections has been revised and expanded. Introductory language has been added to the Exploration subsection to instruct the appropriate method of reporting arthrodesis procedures which would be performed at the same session as the definitive spinal procedure. The introductory text revisions clarify that codes 22849, 22850, 22852, and 22855 for reporting revisions of previous instrumentation procedures are not designated to be exempt from modifier 51, and therefore are reported with modifier 51 when reported in addition to another definitive procedures (eg, arthrodesis, decompression, and exploration of fusion). The introductory text revisions further clarify that 22849 Reinsertion of spinal fixation device is not appropriately reported with instrumentation removal codes 22850, 22852, and 22855 when performed at the same spinal level. New text in each of the subsections clarifies that when exploration of spinal fusion (22830) is performed at the same session as definitive procedures for arthrodesis and decompression, 22830 should be reported separately with modifier 51.

Femur (Thigh Region) and Knee Joint

REPAIR, REVISION, AND/OR RECONSTRUCTION

● **27412** Autologous chondrocyte implantation, knee

▶(Do not report 27412 in conjunction with 20926, 27331, 27570)◀

▶(For harvesting of chondrocytes, use 29870)◀

 Rationale

In conjunction with the deletion of Category III codes 0012T, 0013T, and 0014T, five codes and nine cross-references were established to more accurately report techniques to provide hyaline or hyaline-like repair for articular knee defects. With the addition of these codes, two cross-references have been deleted following code 29870 which previously referred the user to the Category III codes for osteochondral grafting and meniscal transplantation. A cross-reference has been added following code 29871 to indicate that codes 27412, 27415, 29866 and 29867 should be reported for open and arthroscopic approach osteochondral graft implantation. A cross-reference has been added following code 29883 to indicate that code 29868 should be reported for arthroscopic medial or lateral knee meniscal transplantation.

Code 27412 was established to report performance of an open procedure of the knee for implantation of previously obtained autologous chondrocytes for treatment of diseased or injured articular cartilage. This procedure is typically performed for the repair of lesions of the femoral condyle, the patellofemoral joint,

⊘ =Modifier 51 Exempt   ⊙ =Conscious Sedation   ✚ =Add-on Code

and medial and lateral articular cartilage lesions of the distal femoral condyles or trochlea. Several weeks or months prior to this procedure, a biopsy specimen is taken first from the patient, and sent out for cellular expansion of the graft. At the time of the graft procedure, a bed is prepared at the defect to contain the graft, and a patch of periosteum is harvested from the femur or tibia. This patch is carefully sewn into place on the defect to maintain a watertight seal and the cultured chondrocyte material implanted. The remainder of the pocket is then sealed with fibrin glue to ensure that no leakage of the cells occurs. Since tissue graft, knee arthrotomy, exploration, removal of loose bodies, and manipulation of the knee joint and fixation are included in chondrocyte implantation, a new parenthetical note was added to indicate that code 27412 should not be reported in addition to codes 20926, 27331, and 27570 at the same session. Evaluation of the cells for implantation prior to the procedure is also inherent, and not separately reported.

 ### Clinical Example (27412)

A 27-year-old male presents with a history of traumatic injury to the knee causing him to have mechanical symptoms and significant pain. Radiographs showed no mal-alignment and little or no bony changes. A diagnostic arthroscopy and chondral biopsy confirmed a full thickness chondral defect. The patient continues to have pain despite conservative treatment. The size and/or location of the defect is not amenable to autograft tissue transfer or allograft tissue transplantation. At operation, he undergoes an autologous chondrocyte implantation.

Description of Procedure (27412)

With the patient under general anesthesia, an arthrotomy and excision of the diseased or injured articular cartilage, back to a stable rim, is performed. Care is taken not to disrupt the subchondral bone to avoid bleeding. A periosteal patch is harvested from the femur or tibia to cover the chondral defect. The patch is meticulously sewed into place to provide a watertight seal over the chondral defect. The previously obtained chondrocytes, which were cultured and prepared, are then re-implanted under the patch. The remainder of the patch is sealed with sutures and glue. Once the cells are properly introduced the arthrotomy is repaired and the patient is returned to the post-anesthesia recovery room and the floor for post-operative care.

●27415   Osteochondral allograft, knee, open

▶(For arthroscopic implant of osteochondral allograft, use 29867)◀

Rationale

Code 27415 was established to report open implantation of an osteochondral allograft in the knee performed for the treatment of moderate to large chondral or osteochondral knee defects. A cross-reference has been added to instruct that arthroscopic implantation of osteochondral allograft is reported with code 29867.

 ### Clinical Example (27415)

A 20-year-old male presents with a several-year history of pain and locking in his right knee. He states that he had previously injured the knee while playing sports and reports frequent knee pain with vigorous activities and weather changes, which is severe enough to limit his activities and requires non-steroidal anti-inflammatory drugs. He has had occasional giving-way episodes, locking with certain activities, and has had previous surgical treatment for a medial femoral condyle osteochondral injury. He has a large effusion with mild pain on palpation of the medial joint line. Range of motion of the knee is full, except in terminal flexion. Flexion and rotation cause pain over the medial joint line. There is normal stability and a normal weight bearing line. Imaging studies revealed intact menisci and ligamentous structures and an osteochondral defect of the medial femoral condyle. At operation, he undergoes resurfacing of the medial femoral osteochondral defect of his knee utilizing a fresh-frozen osteochondral allograft.

Description of Procedure (27415)
Under general anesthesia, a medial or lateral para-patellar arthrotomy is performed to allow exposure of the entire osteochondral defect. Appropriate debridement of the lesion is confirmed and/or completed. The defect is carefully sized and marked. The defect is then prepared for graft implantation (cylindrical lesions can be prepared with a dowel technique, whereas non-cylindrical lesions require manual recipient site preparation). The previously thawed osteochondral allograft is carefully prepared in a cylindrical or geographic shape. Multiple modifications of the allograft tissue are often required to obtain an appropriate fit to the articular surface defect. Once the graft is appropriately fashioned and placed, it is stabilized with resorbable or non-resorbable fixation. The knee is then brought through a range of motion to assure proper fixation and alignment of the osteochondral graft with the native medial femoral condyle.

Endoscopy/Arthroscopy

●**29866**   Arthroscopy, knee, surgical; osteochondral autograft(s) (eg, mosaicplasty) (includes harvesting of the autograft)

▶(Do not report 29866 in conjunction with 29870, 29871, 29874, 29875, 29877, 29884 when performed at the same session and/or 29879, 29885-29887 when performed in the same compartment)◀

●**29867**   osteochondral allograft (eg, mosaicplasty)

▶(Do not report 29867 in conjunction with 27570, 29870, 29871, 29874, 29875, 29877, 29884 when performed at the same session and/or 29879, 29885-29887 when performed in the same compartment)◀

▶(Do not report 29867 in conjunction with 27415)◀

●**29868**   meniscal transplantation (includes arthrotomy for meniscal insertion), medial or lateral

▶(Do not report 29868 in conjunction with 29870, 29871, 29874, 29875, 29880, 29883, 29884 when performed at the same session or 29881, 29882 when performed in the same compartment)◀

29870   Arthroscopy, knee, diagnostic, with or without synovial biopsy (separate procedure)

▶(For open autologous chondrocyte implantation of the knee, use 27412)◀

Ø=Modifier 51 Exempt   ⊙=Conscious Sedation   ✚=Add-on Code

29871   Arthroscopy, knee, surgical; for infection, lavage and drainage

▶(For implantation of osteochondral graft for treatment of articular surface defect, see 27412, 27415, 29866, 29867)◀

29873   with lateral release

29883   with meniscus repair (medial AND lateral)

▶(For meniscal transplantation, medial or lateral, knee, use 29868)◀

✐ Rationale

Two codes were established to report arthroscopic osteochondral mosaicplasty. Code 29866 was established to report arthroscopic osteochondral autograft harvest and implantation of femoral peripheral cartilage in the knee. As this procedure typically requires the placement of multiple grafts, code 29866 is reported one time per procedure, regardless of the number of grafts obtained and inserted. Harvest of the autograft is not reported separately in addition to 29866, as acquisition of the graft is inherent in arthroscopic osteochondral autograft implantation.

Two cross-references have been added to preclude the reporting of codes 29866 and 29867 in addition to procedures inherent in arthroscopic osteochondral autograft implantation. Codes 29870, 29871, 29874, 29875, 29877, 29884 are not reported separately in addition to code 29866 and 29867 when performed at the same session as arthroscopic implantation of osteochondral autografts since exploration, synovial biopsy, lavage, drainage, removal of loose bodies, synovectomy, shaving, or lysis of adhesions are inherent components of the procedure described by code 29866. The parenthetical note following code 29867 also includes code 27570 in the list of exclusionary codes. In addition, codes 29879, 29885-29887 are not reported separately in addition to 29866 and 29867 when performed in the same compartment as the arthroscopic implantation of osteochondral autografts as abrasion arthroplasty, drilling for osteochondritis dissecans are inherent components of the procedure described by codes 29866 and 29867.

Code 29867 was established to report performance of arthroscopic repair of lesions of the femoral condyle with placement of osteochondral allograft arthroscopic osteochondral allograft. An instructional note following 29867 also indicates that open code 27415 is not appropriately reported in addition to the arthroscopic procedure at the same session.

Mosaicplasty is a resurfacing technique which consists of the mosaic-like transplantation of multiple, small-sized cylindrical osteochondral grafts to provide a smooth resurfaced area. In the case of the autograft procedure, the grafts are harvested from the relatively less weight-bearing periphery of the patellofemoral joint and the donor sites are repaired by the natural healing process and results in filling of the tunnels with cancellous bone and coverage of the surface with reparative fibrocartilage. Insertion of the autografts and allografts is performed for the treatment of chondral and osteochondral defects of the weight-bearing surfaces to create hyaline or hyalinelike repair in the defect area, with the end result of transplanted hyaline cartilage with fibrocartilage filling the donor sites. Small, varying sized multiple cylindrical grafts provide almost complete coverage of the surface. If necessary, fibrocartilage grouting, stimulated by abrasion arthroplasty or sharp curettage at the base of the defect, may be performed to complete the new surface. In performance of the allograft and autograft procedures, conical recipient tunnels are created in the defect into which the graft material is delivered in a perpendicular fashion.

Code 29868 was established to report arthroscopic meniscal knee transplantation in the medial or lateral compartments. This procedure consists of preparation of the defect area with removal of the damaged portion of the meniscus, the crescent-shaped fibrocartilaginous structure of the tibial plateau of the knee. Tibial tunnels or a bone trough are then created as stabilizing structures for the implant. The meniscal graft is then inserted through an arthrotomy and secured to the stabilizing structures. Arthrotomy performed for meniscal insertion as an inherent component of the procedure should not be separately reported.

A cross-reference has been added to instruct that codes 29870, 29871, 29874, 29875, 29880, 29883, 29884 are not reported separately in addition to code 29868 when performed at the same session as arthroscopic meniscal knee transplantation, since joint exploration, synovial biopsy, lavage, drainage, removal of loose bodies, synovectomy, meniscectomy, medial and lateral meniscus repair and lysis of adhesions are inherent components of the procedure described by code 29868. In addition, codes 29881 and 29882 should not be reported separately in addition to 29868 when performed in the same compartment as arthroscopic meniscal knee transplantation, since meniscectomy, meniscal shaving and meniscal repair are inherent components of the procedure described by code 29868.

 Clinical Example (29866)

A 38-year-old female presents with medial right knee pain that began four months ago after a fall. She has pain that is worse with activity and associated with giving-way episodes. She denies locking, but has increased pain with stair climbing. She has been treated with non-steroidal anti-inflammatory drugs with only partial relief of her pain and no relief of her mechanical symptoms. Physical therapy has improved her pain with stair climbing, but has failed to return her knee to normal function. She has increased symptoms in flexion, which interferes with activities of daily living, and she can no longer exercise because of the pain. She has normal limb alignment, joint effusion, and some medial joint line tenderness. Her extension is full, but she flexes to only 115° with some pain on flexion and rotation. She has no evidence of instability. There is some patellofemoral crepitus, but no pain with compression of the patellofemoral joint. Imaging studies revealed an isolated osteochondral defect of the medial femoral condyle with an otherwise normal knee. Arthroscopically, she undergoes an autogenous osteochondral transplant to repair the 1.5 cm full thickness cartilage defect of the weight-bearing surface of the medial femoral condyle.

Description of Procedure (29866)

The index lesion is defined arthroscopically and the problemed area articular cartilage is resected until only normal articular cartilage remains. A measuring guide is used to determine the size of the articular cartilage lesion and the number of grafts necessary for the best fit into the articular cartilage defect. Multiple cylindrical grafts are then harvested from the far periphery of the femoral trochlea or the medial or lateral walls of the intercondylar notch. The grafts are harvested with a tubular chisel driven into the donor site at a precise right angle to the joint surface. Care must be taken during harvesting to ensure complete extraction of adequately sized cylindrical grafts with well-fixed cartilaginous caps. The grafts are delivered through a transfer tube with a guarded impaction device. A recipient tunnel is created with the appropriate sized drill guide. A dilator is used to create a conical tunnel. The graft is then inserted with a plunger to match the surface of the graft to the surrounding native articular cartilage. This step-by-step sequence is then repeated until the lesion is filled with autogenous grafts. The knee is then taken through a range of motion to reinsure stable graft placement. The knee is then drained and the portals and incisions are closed.

 Clinical Example (29867)

A 20-year-old male presents with a several year history of pain and locking in his right knee. He states that he had previously injured the knee while playing sports and reports frequent knee pain with vigorous activities and weather changes, severe enough to limit his activities and requiring non-steroidal anti-inflammatory drugs (NSAIDs). He has had occasional giving-way episodes, locking with certain activities, and has had previous surgical treatment for a medial, femoral, condyle osteochondral injury. He has a large effusion with mild pain on palpation of the medial joint line. Range of motion of the knee is full, except in terminal flexion. Flexion and rotation cause pain over the medial joint line. There is normal stability and a normal weight bearing line. Imaging studies revealed intact menisci and ligamentous structures and an osteochondral defect of the medial femoral condyle. Arthroscopically, he undergoes a resurfacing of the medial femoral osteochondral defect of his knee utilizing a fresh-frozen osteochondral allograft.

Description of Procedure (29867)

The articular lesion is often defined arthroscopically and a complete evaluation of the joint is performed to rule out associated pathology. Appropriate debridement of the lesion is confirmed and/or completed. The defect is carefully sized and marked. The defect is then prepared for graft implantation (cylindrical lesions can be prepared with a dowel technique, whereas non-cylindrical lesions require manual recipient site preparation). The previously thawed osteochondral allograft is carefully prepared in a cylindrical or geographic shape. Multiple modifications of the allograft tissue are often required to obtain an appropriate fit to the articular surface defect. Once the graft is appropriately fashioned and placed, it is stabilized with resorbable or non-resorbable fixation. The knee is then brought through a range of motion to assure proper fixation and alignment of the osteochondral graft with the native, medial, femoral condyle. The arthrotomy is repaired.

Clinical Example (29868)

A 24-year-old active male is status post meniscectomy with persistent activity-limiting knee pain and/or recurrent effusions. His pain is persistent despite ongoing conservative treatment including activity modification, physical therapy, and NSAIDs. He shows no significant malalignment or instability. At operation, he undergoes an arthroscopically aided meniscal transplantation.

Description of Procedure (29868)

The meniscal remnant is removed and the meniscal bed is prepared arthroscopically. Routinely, two tibial bone tunnels are created for a medial, meniscal transplant or a tibial trough is created for a lateral, meniscal transplant. This allows for maximal stabilization of the anterior and posterior horn attachments. The graft is carefully prepared to fit into the bone tunnels or trough. A mini-arthrotomy is made to introduce the meniscal allograft. Once the meniscus is positioned, it is secured to the tunnels or trough. The arthrotomy is repaired and the meniscus is arthroscopically sutured around its periphery to the meniscocapsular junction with multiple sutures. The meniscus is secured. The incisions are closed and the knee and portals are injected with marcaine with epinephrine.

Respiratory System

Larynx

ENDOSCOPY

●**31545** Laryngoscopy, direct, operative, with operating microscope or telescope, with submucosal removal of non-neoplastic lesion(s) of vocal cord; reconstruction with local tissue flap(s)

●**31546** reconstruction with graft(s) (includes obtaining autograft)

▶(Do not report 31546 in addition to 20926 for graft harvest)◀

▶(For reconstruction of vocal cord with allograft, use 31599)◀

▶(Do not report 31545 or 31546 in conjunction with 31540, 31541, 69990)◀

 Rationale

Codes 31545 and 31546 were added to the Larynx/Endoscopy subsection to describe direct operative laryngoscopy with removal of non-neoplastic lesion(s) of the vocal cord using the operating microscope or telescope. Code 31545 should be reported when reconstruction with local tissue flap(s) is performed. Code 31546 should be reported when reconstruction with graft(s) is performed. A parenthetical note was added to instruct that code 20926 should not be reported for harvesting of the graft, as code 31546 includes obtaining the graft. A cross-reference was added directing users to the unlisted code 31599 for reconstruction of the vocal cord with allograft. Another parenthetical note was added to instruct that codes 31545 or 31546 should not be reported in conjunction with codes 31540, 31541, or 69990.

⊘=Modifier 51 Exempt ⊙=Conscious Sedation ✚=Add-on Code

Clinical Example (31545)

A 34-year-old male presents with a six-month history of altered voice quality and a right vocal fold lesion demonstrating increased vascularity. Prior videostroboscopy revealed that the vibratory characteristics of the right vocal fold were significantly altered, while those on the left were within normal limits. During phonation, the larynx did not close completely due to the mass of the lesion. Medical therapy had not eliminated his hoarseness. He undergoes removal of lesions of the vocal cord and reconstruction with local tissue flaps.

Description of Procedure (31545)

A direct laryngoscope is used to examine the oral cavity, oropharynx, hypopharynx and larynx. Once it is ascertained that no additional lesions were present, the patient's vocal folds are visualized and the laryngoscope suspended. The larynx is examined with rigid optical telescopes so that the entire extent of the lesion could be determined. The operating microscope is used to view the larynx at high magnification. The affected vocal fold and lesion are palpated with microlaryngeal rigid probes and suction devices. A micro-sickle knife and micro-scissors are used to make an incision into the vocal fold lining. A micro-probe is used to microdissect within the lamina propria, so that the lesion is separated from the uninvolved lamina propria. A flap is developed that measures 5 mm in length, 4 mm from superior to inferior, and 400 μm in thickness. Sharp dissection is required to release the lesion from the surrounding normal tissues. Bimanual dissection is required throughout the dissection. Once the lesion is separated from adjacent tissue, it is removed. The preserved mucosal microflaps are then trimmed and repositioned so that, as much as possible, the defect over the medial surface of the vocal fold is closed primarily.

Clinical Example (31546)

A 27-year-old female presents with a three-year history of dysphonia. Two years prior, she was found to have vocal nodules, which subsequently were surgically excised. Her voice never returned to normal and she had significant difficulty fulfilling her vocal requirements at work. Recent videostroboscopy revealed that the middle portion of the left vocal fold was stiff and non-vibratory. Medical therapy has yielded no change in the vocal fold stiffness nor adequate improvement in voice quality. In an effort to reconstruct the vocal fold and improve the vibratory characteristics of the fold to improve her voice, she undergoes scar dissection and reconstruction with an autograft.

Description of Procedure (31546)

A direct laryngoscope is used to examine the oral cavity, oropharynx, hypopharynx, and larynx. Once it is ascertained that no additional lesions are present, the patient's vocal folds are visualized and the laryngoscope suspended. The larynx is examined with rigid optical telescopes so that the entire glottic region can be evaluated. The operating microscope is used to view the larynx at high magnification. The affected vocal fold is palpated with microlaryngeal rigid probes and suction devices, revealing that 50% of the vibratory portion of the left vocal fold is stiff and does not distract from the underlying structures. An incision is made in the overlying mucosa and a plane created between it and underlying structures. The surgical microdissection through scar tissue is meticulous. Caution is required to maintain the integrity of the delicate remaining vocal cord cover creating a microflap 700 μm in thickness. An autogenous fat tissue graft that had been separately harvested is placed in the region of the deficient lamina propria. Still under high magnification through the endoscope, the graft and mucosal flaps are fixed in place with microsutures.

Trachea and Bronchi

ENDOSCOPY

＋⊙●31620 Endobronchial ultrasound (EBUS) during bronchoscopic diagnostic or therapeutic intervention(s) (List separately in addition to code for primary procedure(s))

▶(Use 31620 in conjunction with 31622-31638)◀

⊙31622 Bronchoscopy, rigid or flexible, with or without fluoroscopic guidance; diagnostic, with or without cell washing (separate procedure)

▲31630 with tracheal/bronchial dilation or closed reduction of fracture

▲31631 with placement of tracheal stent(s) (includes tracheal/bronchial dilation as required)

▶(For placement of bronchial stent, see 31636, 31637)◀

▶(For revision of tracheal/bronchial stent, use 31638)◀

●31636 with placement of bronchial stent(s) (includes tracheal/bronchial dilation as required), initial bronchus

＋●31637 each additional major bronchus stented (List separately in addition to code for primary procedure)

▶(Use 31637 in conjunction with 31636)◀

●31638 with revision of tracheal or bronchial stent inserted at previous session (includes tracheal/bronchial dilation as required)

31640 with excision of tumor

✍ Rationale

Revisions to the bronchoscopy section have been made to distinguish among airway stents placed in the trachea versus the bronchus or bronchi. Code 31631 has been revised to describe placement of single or multiple tracheal stent(s), and a cross-reference directing the use of two new codes (31636, 31637) for insertion of bronchial stents has been added. Code 31636 was established to report stenting of the first or initial mainstem bronchus, and code 31637 was established as an add-on code, to be reported when a second stent is placed in a different or more distal bronchus.

Patients with non-resectable airway obstruction from benign or malignant diseases or bronchial anastomotic stenosis following lung transplantation are eligible for

⊘=Modifier 51 Exempt   ⊙=Conscious Sedation   ＋=Add-on Code

tracheobronchial stent therapy. In the second case of anastomotic stenosis following transplantation, granulation tissue (often associated with ischemia or prior infection) at the anastomotic site is removed, and a stent is inserted to maintain airway patency and maximal luminal diameter. Prior to the development of endobronchial stent therapy, chemotherapy and/or radiation to reduce tumor size and open the obstructed airway was the only therapeutic option available.

Code 31638 has been added for revision or adjustment of tracheal or bronchial stents placed at a previous session. Dilation is inherent in all the tracheobronchial stent procedure codes, and should not be reported separately. Dilation peformed without further therapeutic intervention is described by code 31630.

Lastly, add-on code 31620 has been added under the Trachea and Bronchi subsection to describe endobronchial ultrasound to be reported in conjunction with primary bronchoscopic procedures (ie, 31622-31638). Additional bronchoscopy procedures with which code 31620 may be reported include the procedures described by codes 31640, 31641, 31643, 31645, and 31646. Endobronchial ultrasound is designed to enhance visualization (eg, differentiating vascular from non-vascular structures), provide guidance (eg, transbronchial needle guidance), assist in assessments (eg, tumor volume) and is useful in other interventions (eg, airway recanalization).

Clinical Example (31620)

A patient has a 1.0 cm nodule identified on chest computed tomography (CT) scan. The nodule appears to abut the left, upper lobe bronchus. At bronchoscopy, a decision is made to perform an endobronchial ultrasound to determine if the nodule invades the bronchial wall.

Description of Procedure (31620)

The physician inserts the flexible bronchoscope with a biopsy channel of at least 2.8 mm and inspects the left upper lobe bronchus. No abnormality is identified. Then a miniaturized ultrasound catheter probe bearing a mechanical transducer at its tip that rotates 360° is inserted. To ensure complete contact with the tracheobronchial wall, the catheter has a balloon at the tip that, after being filled with water, provides complete circular contact. Once inside the airways, the balloon is inflated until complete circular contact with the left upper lobe bronchus is achieved, and the airway wall, adjacent lung parenchyma, and the surrounding mediastinum become visible. To add the longitudinal dimension to the cross-sectional image, the probe is moved along the axis of the airways, attempting to localize and examine the ultrasound characteristics of the lesion. An ultrasound picture is taken for the patient's record, even if the lesion is not identified.

Clinical Example (31630)

A 50-year-old female presents with shortness of breath 6 months after prolonged hospitaliztion for sepsis, during which she required a tracheostomy. The tracheostomy tube was removed 5 months previously. Plain radiographs and CT scans confirm the presence of a focal stenosis in the mid-trachea. It was elected to proceed with a bronchoscopy and tracheal dilation and, if necessary, placement of a stent. After successful dilation, no residual stenosis exists; hence no stent is necessary.

Description of Procedure (31630)

A rigid bronchoscope is advanced to the stenotic area. A dilation catheter is placed through the bronchoscope into the opening of the focal stenosis and under fluoroscopy is threaded distally to just beyond the focal stenosis.

 Clinical Example (31631)

A patient is evaluated for dyspnea and stridor and is found to have squamous cell carcinoma extensively involving the distal trachea. At bronchoscopy, the markedly narrow lumen is dilated, and a tracheal stent is placed.

Description of Procedure (31631)

A rigid bronchoscope is advanced to the stenotic area. A dilation catheter is placed through the bronchoscope into the small opening in the tumor mass and threaded through the tumor mass under fluoroscopy. The dilating catheter is removed, and a guidewire is inserted through the bronchoscope into the now patent trachea. The bronchoscope is removed, leaving the guidewire in place, and the stent catheter is manipulated over the guidewire into the previously stenotic area. The bronchoscope is again inserted and the area is visualized both through the bronchoscope and by fluoroscopy.

 Clinical Example (31636)

A patient with Stage IV (metastatic) adenocarcinoma of the left, lower lobe develops shortness of breath, and left lower lobe atelectasis from progressive endobronchial tumor growth, seen on serial computed tomography (CT) scans. At bronchoscopy, following dilation a stent is placed in the left lower lobe bronchus.

Description of Procedure (31636)

A rigid bronchoscope is advanced to the stenotic area. A dilation catheter is placed through the bronchoscope into the small opening in the tumor mass and is threaded distally to just beyond the tumor mass under fluoroscopy. The dilating catheter is removed, and a guidewire is inserted through the bronchoscope into the now patent trachea. The bronchoscope is removed, leaving the guidewire in place, and the stent catheter is manipulated over the guidewire into the previously stenotic area. The bronchoscope is again inserted and the area is visualized both through the bronchoscope and by fluoroscopy. Two metal markers are taped to the external chest wall under fluoroscopy. The stent is then deployed, using both of the markers for fluoroscopic guides and under direct vision by the physician using the bronchoscope.

 Clinical Example (31637)

A patient with Stage IV (metastatic) adenocarcinoma of the left lower lobe develops shortness of breath and left lower lobe atelectasis from progressive endobronchial tumor growth, seen on serial chest CT scans. It was elected to proceed with bronchoscopy with dilation and stenting of the left lower lobe bronchus. At bronchoscopy, it becomes evident that the right main bronchus is circumferentially involved and nearly obstructed by tumor; therefore, a decision was made to dilate and stent also the right main bronchus.

Description of Procedure (31637)

The computed tomography (CT) scan is re-reviewed to pre-measure and ascertain the size of the stent to be deployed. Proper stent sizing is critical. The stent length should exceed the length of the lesion to some degree to ensure patency. If the stent is too small in diameter, it may migrate; conversely, if it is too large, it may not open upon deployment or may cause stress on the airway wall. Following removal of the bronchoscope after deploying the first stent, the bronchoscope is inserted into the right main bronchus and is advanced to the obstruction in the right bronchus, where bulky tumor is visualized both through the bronchoscope and by fluoroscopy extending down to where a small opening is seen through a tumor mass into the right main bronchus. A dilation catheter is placed through the bronchoscope into the small opening in the tumor mass, and threaded through the tumor mass into the right, lower lobe bronchus under fluoroscopic guidance. Then, under fluoroscopic guidance, the obstructed endobronchial area is dilated. The dilating catheter is removed and repositioned more proximally in the right mainstem where a repeat dilation is performed under fluoroscopy. Next, a guidewire is inserted through the bronchoscope into the now patent right lower lobe. Then, the bronchoscope is removed, leaving the guidewire in place, and the stent catheter is manipulated over the guidewire into the right, lower lobe bronchus. Two metal markers (eg, paper clips) are taped to the external chest wall under fluoroscopy. The stent is then deployed, using both of the markers for fluoroscopic guides and under direct vision by the physician using the bronchoscope. The two metal markers are repositioned and taped to the external chest wall under fluoroscopy to mark the carina and left mainstem bronchus. Care must be taken to ensure overlap between the distal end of the proximal stent and the proximal end of the distal stent.

 ### Clinical Example (31638)

A 45-year-old female is seen for dyspnea, cough, and fever two months after placement of a bronchial stent for narrowing of the bronchial anastamosis after a single right lung transplant. Diagnostic studies indicate that the stent has migrated distally in the airway to partially obstruct the middle and lower lobe bronchi. Therefore, a decision is made to perform a bronchoscopy and reposition the stent to obtain optimum results.

Description of Procedure (31638)

A rigid bronchoscope is advanced to the focal stenotic area. Under fluoroscopic guidance and direct visualization through the bronchoscope, the migrated stent is located. Using forceps, the physician removes any necrotic tissue and, finally, the stent. The bronchoscope is removed and reinserted. A dilation catheter is placed through the bronchoscope into the small opening of the focal stenosis and under fluoroscopy is threaded distally to just beyond the focal stenosis. The dilating catheter is removed, and a guidewire is inserted through the bronchoscope into the now patent bronchi. The bronchoscope is removed, leaving the guidewire in place, and the stent catheter is manipulated over the guidewire into the previously stenotic area. The bronchoscope is again inserted and the area is visualized both through the bronchoscope and by fluoroscopy. Two metal markers are taped to the external chest wall under fluoroscopy. The stent is then deployed, using both of the markers for fluoroscopic guides and under direct vision by the physician using the bronchoscope.

Lungs and Pleura

INCISION

 32019   Insertion of indwelling tunneled pleural catheter with cuff

▶(Do not report 32019 in conjunction with 32000-32005, 32020, 36000, 36410, 62318, 62319, 64450, 64470, 64475)◀

▶(If imaging guidance is performed, use 75989)◀

Rationale
Code 32019 was established to report insertion of a tunneled catheter into the pleural space for drainage and management of pleural effusions. The technique of insertion and management of this pleural catheter with a cuff requires multiple incisions and subcutaneous tunneling of the indwelling pleural catheter through multiple incisions in the thorax into the pleural space, with perioperative management. This procedure is commonly performed for the management of malignant pleural effusion (MPE). The technique of subcutaneous tunneling is intended to accommodate the long-term placement of the catheter, and drainage of the pleural effusion over a prolonged period (typically greater than 4 weeks).

An exclusionary parenthetical note has been added to identify procedure codes inherent to code 32019, which should not be separately reported.

A cross-reference has been added to instruct reporting code 75989 if imaging guidance is required.

Existing code 32020 is distinguished from the procedure described by code 32019, as it describes a procedure most commonly performed at the bedside, consisting of a single chest wall puncture and insertion of a chest tube into the pleural space for drainage. The chest tube inserted and reported with code 32020 is generally left in for only a short period (usually less than 7 days).

Clinical Example (32019)
A 68-year-old female presents with breast cancer. She has undergone a mastectomy with post-operative chemotherapy presents six months later with chronic, malignant, pleural effusion.

Description of Procedure (32019)
The patient is taken to the operating room or clean procedure room and placed in a semi-Fowler position with the arm extended. After placement of appropriate intravenous catheters, nasal oxygen, and monitoring equipment, the right chest is prepped and draped in the usual sterile fashion. Patient is given moderate sedation

⊘=Modifier 51 Exempt   ⊙=Conscious Sedation   ✚=Add-on Code

intravenously. Local anesthesia is used. Using the Seldinger technique, the free-flowing pleural fluid is located and a wire is inserted into the pleural space along the right axillary line. Local anesthetic is used to allow for painless 1 cm incision over the wire. A second (counter) incision is made lower and medial to the first incision, under local anesthesia, and placed approximately 5-10 cm away. The subcutaneous space between the two incisions is anesthetized with the local anesthetic solution. A tunneling device is then utilized to pass the chronic indwelling catheter with cuff through the lower incision through the subcutaneous tissue, and then into and exiting from the upper incision. Care is taken to place the cuff in a subcutaneous position just lateral (within 1 cm) of the lower incision (just under the skin incision). An obturator/dilator with a peel-away sheath is then used to tunnel through the intercostal space, through the parietal pleura, and into the pleural space while guided by the previously placed wire. The obturator/dilator is removed, and the catheter is fed through the peel-away sheath, through the pleural defect, and into the pleural cavity. The peel-away sheath is removed as the catheter is positioned without twists or bends, to allow easy egress of the pleural fluid. The upper incision is then closed in two layers. A suction bottle is attached to the external portion of the catheter to drain the effusion. The catheter is secured into position at the lower, medial incision. Sterile dressings are applied.

LUNG TRANSPLANTATION

►Lung allotransplantation involves three distinct components of physician work:◄

   ►1) *Cadaver donor pneumonectomy(s)*, which include(s) harvesting the allograft and cold preservation of the allograft (perfusing with cold preservation solution and cold maintenance) (use 32850).◄

   ►2) *Backbench work*:◄

      ►Preparation of a cadaver donor single lung allograft prior to transplantation, including dissection of the allograft from surrounding soft tissues to prepare the pulmonary venous/atrial cuff, pulmonary artery, and bronchus unilaterally (use 32855).◄

      ►Preparation of a cadaver donor double lung allograft prior to transplantation, including dissection of the allograft from surrounding soft tissues to prepare the pulmonary venous/atrial cuff, pulmonary artery, and bronchus bilaterally (use 32856).◄

   ►3) *Recipient lung allotransplantation*, which includes transplantation of a single or double lung allograft and care of the recipient (see 32851-32854).◄

▲ **32850**   Donor pneumonectomy(ies) (including cold preservation), from cadaver donor

32851   Lung transplant, single; without cardiopulmonary bypass

32852   with cardiopulmonary bypass

32853   Lung transplant, double (bilateral sequential or en bloc); without cardiopulmonary bypass

32854   with cardiopulmonary bypass

● **32855**   Backbench standard preparation of cadaver donor lung allograft prior to transplantation, including dissection of allograft from surrounding soft tissues to prepare pulmonary venous/atrial cuff, pulmonary artery, and bronchus; unilateral

● **32856**   bilateral

▶(For repair or resection procedures on the donor lung, see 32491, 32500, 35216, or 35276)◀

Rationale

Codes 32855 and 32856 were added to the Lung Transplantation subsection of the Respiratory section to describe backbench preparation of a cadaver donor lung allograft prior to lung transplantation. Code 32855 is reported for a unilateral procedure, and code 32856 is reported for a bilateral procedure. Code 32850 was revised to no longer include preparation and maintenance of cadaver allograft, since this work is now separately reportable with the two new backbench preparation codes (32855, 32856). A cross-reference was added following code 32856 directing users to codes 32491, 32500, 35216, or 35276 for repair or resection procedures on the donor lung. New guidelines were added at the beginning of the Lung Transplantation section describing the three components of physician work involved in lung allotransplantation, which are cadaver donor pneumonectomy, backbench work, and recipient lung allotransplantation.

Clinical Example (32850)

An 18-year-old male sustained a severe closed head injury in a motor vehicle accident and was declared brain dead the following day. At thoracotomy, the great vessels and trachea are dissected and cardioplegia and pulmonoplegia are administered. The heart and lung block is removed, dividing the superior and inferior vena cava, the aorta and the trachea. The heart is then separated from the heart-lung block and the lungs are separated from each other, preserving the appropriate tissue with each organ. The organs are packed separately for transportation.

Clinical Example (32855)

A cadaver donor single lung allograft that has been procured with cold preservation and maintained cold is received at the transplant recipient site of service. Standard backbench preparation, including dissection of the allograft from surrounding soft tissues to prepare the pulmonary venous/atrial cuff, pulmonary artery, and bronchus, unilaterally, is performed.

Description of Procedure (32855)

The single lung graft is received in a sterile container and is maintained in cold preservation solution. The surgeon requests and confirms that a sterile backbench is set up in the operating room, with appropriate instruments for the backbench dissection. An appropriate recipient has been identified. The correct identification process is carried out to make sure that the single lung graft is being allocated to the right recipient. The surgeon must make the appropriate arrangements with the operating room and staff to allow for sterile dissection of the organ in coordination with the recipient procedure. The surgeon scrubs and gowns. The single lung is removed from the sterile container and placed on a sterile table, on ice, while bathing in cold preservation solution. The single lung graft is inspected to be certain that it is grossly intact and that its appearance is acceptable.

On ice, with continuous bathing in cold preservation solution, the external surface is examined for blebs, nodules, contusions, hematomas or lacerations (repair or resection, if necessary, is reported separately). The pulmonary venous orifices and surrounding left atrial cuff are inspected, checking length and for the presence of surgical injuries. The pulmonary artery is inspected, checking for length and the presence of surgical injuries. Attached pericardium is identified and excised. The pulmonary artery is inspected and any thrombus that may have formed as a result of the placement of a Swan-Ganz catheter is removed and sent for culture. The pulmonary artery is dissected free of surrounding tissue. The bronchial staple line is removed and any secretions present in the airway are sent for cultures and Gram stain. The bronchus is trimmed to desired length of one to two cartilaginous rings prior to bifurcation. The bronchial and lobar orifices are suctioned clean, as necessary, using saline irrigation.

The lung is then wrapped in an iced laparotomy pad and placed in a basin with the bronchus anterior and open to air and the lung bathed in cold saline prior to beginning the transplantation. If necessary, the lung allograft is repackaged in a sterile fashion and maintained cold prior to transplantation.

 Clinical Example (32856)

A cadaver donor double lung allograft that has been procured with cold preservation and maintained cold is received at the transplant recipient site of service. Standard backbench preparation, including dissection of the allograft from surrounding soft tissues to prepare the pulmonary venous/atrial cuff, pulmonary artery, and bronchus, bilaterally, is performed.

Description of Procedure (32856)

The double lung graft is received in a sterile container and is maintained in cold preservation solution. The surgeon requests and confirms that a sterile backbench is set up in the operating room, with appropriate instruments for the backbench dissection. An appropriate recipient has been identified. The correct identification process is carried out to make sure that the double lung graft is being allocated to the right recipient. The surgeon must make the appropriate arrangements with the operating room and staff to allow for sterile dissection of the organ in coordination with the recipient procedure. The surgeon scrubs and gowns. The double lung is removed from the sterile container and placed on a sterile table, on ice, while bathing in cold preservation solution. The double lung graft is inspected to be certain that it is grossly intact and that its appearance is acceptable.

On ice, with continuous bathing in cold preservation solution, the external surface is examined for blebs, nodules, contusions, hematomas, or lacerations (repair or resection, if necessary, is reported separately). The left and right main pulmonary arteries are divided at the bifurcation. Each pulmonary artery is inspected, trimmed, and checked for the presence of surgical injuries. Attached pericardium is identified and excised. Each pulmonary artery is internally inspected and any thrombus that may have formed as a result of the placement of a Swan-Ganz catheter is removed and sent for culture. Each pulmonary artery is dissected free of surrounding tissue. The internal aspect of the left atrium is inspected and the posterior wall of the left atrium is divided midway between the left and right pulmonary veins. The pulmonary venous orifices and surrounding bilateral atrial cuffs are inspected, trimmed, and checked for the presence of surgical injuries. The carina and proximal aspects of both main stem bronchi are dissected free of surrounding tissue. Using a non-vascular stapler, a staple line is delivered at the bronchial-carinal junction on the side of the first lung to be transplanted and the main bronchus is divided distal to the staple line. The lung that is to be implanted second is kept inflated, surrounded by cold preservation solution, re-packaged in a sterile fashion, and placed in ice prior to transplantation.

Next, attention is focused on the lung that will be implanted first. Any secretions present in the bronchus are sent for cultures and Gram stain. The bronchus is trimmed to desired length of one to two cartilaginous rings prior to bifurcation. The bronchial and lobar orifices are suctioned clean, if necessary, using saline irrigation. This lung is then wrapped in an iced laparotomy pad and placed in a basin with the bronchus anterior and open to air and the lung bathed in cold saline prior to beginning the implantation.

While the first lung is being implanted, the bronchial staple line on the second lung is removed and any secretions present in the airway are sent for cultures and Gram stain. The bronchus is trimmed to desired length of one to two cartilaginous rings prior to bifurcation. The bronchial and lobar orifices are suctioned clean, as necessary, using saline irrigation.

This second lung allograft is then wrapped in an iced laparotomy pad and placed in a basin with the bronchus anterior and open to air and the lung bathed in cold saline prior to beginning the transplantation. If necessary, the allograft is repackaged in a sterile fashion and maintained cold prior to transplantation.

Cardiovascular System

Heart and Pericardium

HEART/LUNG TRANSPLANTATION

▶Heart with or without lung allotransplantation involves three distinct components of physician work:◀

▶1) **Cadaver donor cardiectomy with or without pneumonectomy**, which includes harvesting the allograft and cold preservation of the allograft (perfusing with cold preservation solution and cold maintenance) (see 33930, 33940).◀

▶2) **Backbench work**:◀

►Preparation of a cadaver donor heart and lung allograft prior to transplantation, including dissection of the allograft from surrounding soft tissues to prepare the aorta, superior vena cava, inferior vena cava, and trachea for implantation (use 33933).◄

►Preparation of a cadaver donor heart allograft prior to transplantation, including dissection of the allograft from surrounding soft tissues to prepare aorta, superior vena cava, inferior vena cava, pulmonary artery, and left atrium for implantation (use 33944).◄

►3) *Recipient heart with or without lung allotransplantation*, which includes transplantation of allograft and care of the recipient (see 33935, 33945).◄

▲ **33930** Donor cardiectomy-pneumonectomy (including cold preservation)

● **33933** Backbench standard preparation of cadaver donor heart/lung allograft prior to transplantation, including dissection of allograft from surrounding soft tissues to prepare aorta, superior vena cava, inferior vena cava, and trachea for implantation

33935 Heart-lung transplant with recipient cardiectomy-pneumonectomy

▲ **33940** Donor cardiectomy (including cold preservation)

● **33944** Backbench standard preparation of cadaver donor heart allograft prior to transplantation, including dissection of allograft from surrounding soft tissues to prepare aorta, superior vena cava, inferior vena cava, pulmonary artery, and left atrium for implantation

►(For repair or resection procedures on the donor heart, see 33300, 33310, 33320, 33400, 33463, 33464, 33510, 33641, 35216, 35276 or 35685)◄

33945 Heart transplant, with or without recipient cardiectomy

Rationale

Codes 33933 and 33944 were added to the Heart and Pericardium Heart/Lung Transplantation subsection of the Cardiovascular System section to describe backbench preparation of cadaver donor heart/lung allograft prior to transplantation. Code 33933 is reported for backbench preparation of heart/lung allograft, and code 33944 is reported for backbench preparation of heart allograft. Codes 33930 and 33940 were revised to include cold preservation and to eliminate inclusion of preparation and maintenance of the allograft. A cross-reference was added following code 33944 directing users to the appropriate codes for repair or resection procedures on the donor heart. New guidelines were added at the beginning of the Heart/Lung Transplantation subsection describing the three distinct components of transplantation involved in the physician work, which are donor cardiectomy with or without a pneumonectomy, backbench work, and allotransplantation.

Clinical Example (33930)

A 35-year-old male is involved in a motor vehicle accident and undergoes brain death. The family gives permission for organ donation and the organ procurement organization contacts a potential recipient center and reports the following information: patient history and physical examination, electrocardiogram, echocardiogram, chest x-ray, appropriate virology titers, arterial blood gases, myocardial enzymes, and the patient's clinical condition emphasizing hemodynamics. The donor's family history and extensive social history is also reported. Arrangements are then made to transport the procurement team to the donor hospital via car, ambulance, helicopter, or airplane. The procurement team assembles, checks equipment, and proceeds to the donor hospital. Upon arrival, coordination takes place with the renal, pancreas, and liver procurement teams. The chart is inspected and the donor is examined. A bronchoscopy is performed to examine the airways and cultures are obtained. At operation, inspection and palpation of the organs document the lack of any significant abnormalities. Once all of the preliminary dissection is performed and the various procurement teams are satisfied with the organs, separate perfusion of the pulmonary artery and aorta is initiated with cold crystalloid solutions to initiate the preservation process. The heart and both lungs are removed and placed in sterile plastic bags, which are then placed in a container surrounded by ice, to maintain hypothermia. The organs are then transported to the recipient hospital.

Description of Procedure (33930)

A bronchoscopy is performed. The patient is positioned, prepped and draped. A midline sternotomy incision with midline abdominal extension is performed. The organs are inspected and palpated. Preliminary dissection of both lungs and the heart, and placement of a perfusion cannulae in the pulmonary artery and ascending aorta are performed. Aortic cross-clamping and perfusion with application of topical cold (4°C) saline were initiated. The heart and both lungs were removed and placed in sterile plastic bags followed by placement in containers surrounded by ice. Preparations were made for transportation of the team and organ to the recipient hospital.

Clinical Example (33933)

A cadaver donor heart/lung allograft that has been procured with cold preservation and maintained cold is received at the transplant recipient site of service. Standard backbench preparation, including dissection of the allograft from surrounding soft tissues to prepare the aorta, superior vena cava, inferior vena cava, and trachea for implantation, is performed.

Description of Procedure (33933)

The heart/lung graft is received in a sterile container and is maintained in cold preservation solution. The surgeon requests and confirms that a sterile backbench is set up in the operating room, with appropriate instruments for the backbench dissection. An appropriate recipient has been identified. The correct identification process is carried out to make sure that the heart/lung graft is being allocated to the right recipient. The surgeon must make the appropriate arrangements with the operating room and staff to allow for sterile dissection of the organ in coordination with the recipient procedure. The surgeon scrubs and gowns. The heart/lung is removed from the sterile container and placed on a sterile table, on ice, while bathing in cold preservation solution. The heart/lung graft is inspected to be certain that it is grossly intact and that its appearance is acceptable.

Ⓢ =Modifier 51 Exempt   ⊙ =Conscious Sedation   ✚=Add-on Code

On ice, with continuous bathing in cold preservation solution, the external surface of the heart is examined for unexpected hematomas or lacerations, and the coronary arteries are inspected and palpated (repair, if necessary, is reported separately). The aorta is inspected for a cardioplegia site. If a cardioplegia site is identified, it is excised or over sewn, depending on the length of the aorta. The superior vena cava is inspected, checking the length and for the presence of the azygous vein orifice. If present, the azygous vein orifice is excised or over sewn depending on the length of the superior vena cava. The lumen is inspected and any thrombus that may have formed as a result of the placement of a central venous catheter is removed and sent for culture. The inferior vena cava is inspected and the distance between the division of the vein and the coronary sinus is assessed. The atrial septum is inspected (defect closure, if necessary, is reported separately). The aorta is trimmed. The left atrial appendage is inspected, and if partially amputated, it is over sewn. The heart may then be perfused with cardioplegia solution, depending on the cold ischemic time.

Next, attention is focused on the lungs. The external surface of the lungs is examined for unexpected blebs, nodules, contusions, hematomas, or lacerations (repair or resection, if necessary, is reported separately). Attached pericardium is identified and excised. The tracheal staple line is removed and any secretions present in the airway are sent for cultures and Gram stain. The trachea is trimmed to desired length of one to two cartilaginous rings prior to the carina. The right and left bronchial orifices are suctioned clean, as necessary, using saline irrigation.

The heart/lung allograft is wrapped in an iced laparotomy pad and placed in a basin with the trachea anterior and open to air and the heart/lung allograft bathed in cold saline prior to beginning the transplantation. If necessary, the heart/lung allograft is repackaged in a sterile fashion and maintained cold prior to transplantation.

Clinical Example (33940)

A 37-year-old male involved in a motor vehicle accident undergoes brain death. The family gives permission for organ donation and the organ procurement organization contacts a potential recipient center and reports the following information: patient history and physical examination, electrocardiogram, chest x-ray, appropriate virology titers, arterial blood gases, myocardial enzymes, and the patient's clinical condition, emphasizing hemodynamics. The donor's family history and extensive social history are also reported. Arrangements are then made to transport the procurement team to the donor hospital via car, ambulance, helicopter, or airplane. The procurement team is assembled, equipment checked, and it proceeds to the donor hospital. Upon arrival, coordination takes place with the renal, pancreas, lung, and liver procurement teams. The chart is inspected and the donor is examined. At operation, inspection and palpation of the heart document the lack of any significant abnormalities. Once all of the preliminary dissection is performed and the various procurement teams are satisfied with the organs, perfusion of the aorta is initiated with cold crystalloid solution to initiate the preservation process. The heart is removed and placed in a sterile plastic bag, which is then placed in a container surrounded by ice, to maintain hypothermia. The heart is then transported to the recipient hospital.

Description of Procedure (33940)

A bronchoscopy is performed. The patient is positioned, prepped and draped. A midline sternotomy incision with midline abdominal extension is performed. The organs are inspected and palpated. Preliminary dissection of both lungs and the heart, and placement of a perfusion cannulae in the pulmonary artery and ascending aorta are performed. Aortic cross-clamping and perfusion with application of topical cold (4°C) saline were initiated. The hart and both lungs were removed and placed in sterile plastic bags followed by placement in containers surrounded by ice. Preparations were made for transportation of the team and organ to the recipient hospital.

Clinical Example (33944)

A cadaver donor heart allograft that has been procured with cold preservation and maintained cold is received at the transplant recipient site of service. Standard backbench preparation, including dissection of the allograft from surrounding soft tissues to prepare the aorta, superior vena cava, inferior vena cava, pulmonary artery, and left atrium for implantation, is performed.

Description of Procedure (33944)

The heart graft is received in a sterile container and is maintained in cold preservation solution. The surgeon requests and confirms that a sterile backbench is set up in the operating room, with appropriate instruments for the backbench dissection. An appropriate recipient has been identified. The correct identification process is carried out to make sure that the heart graft is being allocated to the right recipient. The surgeon must make the appropriate arrangements with the operating room and staff to allow for sterile dissection of the organ in coordination with the recipient procedure. The surgeon scrubs and gowns. The heart is removed from the sterile container and placed on a sterile table, on ice, while bathing in cold preservation solution. The heart graft is inspected to be certain that it is grossly intact and that its appearance is acceptable.

On ice, with continuous bathing in cold preservation solution, the external surface is examined for unexpected hematomas or lacerations, and the coronary arteries are inspected and palpated (repair, if necessary, is reported separately). The aorta is inspected for a cardioplegia site. If a cardioplegia site is identified, it is excised or over sewn, depending on the length of the aorta. The superior vena cava is inspected, checking length and for the presence of the azygous vein orifice. If present, the azygous vein orifice is excised or over sewn depending on the length of the superior vena cava. The lumen is inspected and any thrombus that may have formed as a result of the placement of a central venous catheter is removed and sent for culture. The inferior vena cava is inspected and the distance between the division of the vein and the coronary sinus is assessed. The pulmonary artery is separated from the aorta utilizing electrocautery. The pulmonic valve is inspected. The pulmonary vein orifices are joined creating a wide opening into the left atrium. The mitral valve is inspected. The atrial septum is inspected (defect closure, if necessary, is reported separately). Excess left atrial tissue is then trimmed to create the left atrial cuff. The pulmonary artery is trimmed. The aorta is trimmed. The aortic valve is inspected. The left atrial appendage is inspected, and if partially amputated, it is over sewn. The heart may then be perfused with cardioplegia solution, depending on the cold ischemic time.

The heart allograft is wrapped in an iced laparotomy pad and kept cold in anticipation of transplantation. If necessary, the heart allograft is repackaged in a sterile fashion and maintained cold prior to transplantation.

Arteries and Veins

ENDOVASCULAR REPAIR OF ABDOMINAL AORTIC ANEURYSM

34800   Endovascular repair of infrarenal abdominal aortic aneurysm or dissection; using aorto-aortic tube prosthesis

34802   using modular bifurcated prosthesis (one docking limb)

● **34803**   using modular bifurcated prosthesis (two docking limbs)

►(For endovascular repair of abdominal aortic aneurysm or dissection involving visceral vessels using a fenestrated modular bifurcated prosthesis (two docking limbs), use Category III codes 0078T, 0079T)◄

+34808   Endovascular placement of iliac artery occlusion device (List separately in addition to code for primary procedure)

(Use 34808 in conjunction with 34800, 34805, 34813, 34825, 34826)

(For radiological supervision and interpretation, use 75952 in conjunction with ►34800-34808◄)

(For open arterial exposure, report 34812, 34820, 34833, 34834 as appropriate, in addition to ►34800-34808◄)

(For radiological supervision and interpretation, use 75953)

✍️ Rationale

Category III code 0001T has been deleted and converted to Category I code 34803 to report endovascular abdominal aortic aneurysm repair using a modular bifurcated two-docking limb device. Cross-references following codes 34802 and 34808 have been revised to accommodate the Category I conversion.

Code 34803 is similar to the other prosthesis placement codes 34800, 34802, 34804, and 34805 found in this endovascular family of codes. Each of these codes is used to report the placement of the primary prosthesis for endovascular repair of an infrarenal aortic aneurysm. The main difference between these codes is the device shape and number of components. Code 34800 describes a tubular-shaped prosthesis that lies only within the abdominal aorta. Code 34803 describes an inverted-Y shaped three-piece modular prosthesis which spans the infrarenal abdominal aorta with the limbs extending into each iliac artery. The proximal ends of the limbs are joined to the main prosthesis component in a modular fashion after the main body component of the prosthesis is deployed within the aneurysm during the procedure. The distal ends of each limb are extended into the iliac arteries. The clinical choice between these procedures depends on the distal extent of the aortic aneurysm. In some abdominal aortic aneurysms

(AAAs), the dilated aneurysmal segment terminates high enough above the aortic bifurcation to allow a suitable seal between the distal portion of a tubular endoprosthesis and the distal aorta. That configuration would be amenable to reporting with code 34800. Code 34803 would be more appropriately reported for treatment where the aneurysmal dilation extends to the aortic bifurcation or into the common iliac arteries.

In the comparison of the procedures described by 34802 and 34803, both procedures employ modular components that attain an inverted-Y shape following complete deployment. The primary difference between the procedures in codes 34802 and 34803 is the number of modular components that make up the device. The prosthesis procedure repair described by code 34802 has two separate pieces that are joined inside the patient's body during placement, with the main body prosthesis component extending into the ipsilateral iliac artery and creating a distal seal; while code 34803 has three components that are joined inside the patient during the procedure.

Comparing codes 34803 and 34804, again both procedures describe placement of a prosthesis for endovascular aortic aneurysm repair. The primary differences between the procedures described are the configuration, length, and shape of the prosthesis required for effective aneurysm treatment. The prosthesis procedure repair described by code 34804 is a one-piece design with an inverted-Y shape in which one of the limbs is extended into each iliac artery during deployment. The prosthesis procedure repair described by code 34803 employs a three-piece modular prosthesis, as described above. The clinical choice between the device insertion/repairs described by codes 34802, 34803, and 34804 depends on the exact diameter and shape of the infrarenal aortic neck, the iliac artery landing zones, and physician preference. Some patients will be candidates for repair using the device described by one code, but not suitable for the others.

A directional cross-reference has been added following code 34803 to direct the use of codes 0078T-0079T for endovascular repair of abdominal aortic aneurysm or dissection involving visceral vessels using fenestrated modular bifurcated prostheses.

Open femoral or iliac artery exposure, arterial catheterization, and radiologic supervision and interpretation are separately reportable in addition to endovascular aortic aneurysm repair. As with the other prosthesis placement codes, angioplasty within the target zone is included and not separately reported. Placement of stent(s) within the target zone, which are occasionally required within the prosthesis to seal endoleaks or to treat kinks, is not separately reportable. However, as with the other prosthesis placement codes, placement of proximal or distal extension prostheses to treat endoleak is/are separately reportable using code 34825 for the initial vessel treated with one or more extension prostheses, and code 34826 for each additional vessel treated with one or more extension prostheses.

Radiological supervision and interpretation (S&I) code 75952 should be reported separately for the imaging work associated with endovascular repair of infrarenal abdominal aortic aneurysm or dissection prosthesis placement in conjunction with codes 34800-34808. Radiological S&I code 75953 should be additionally reported in conjunction with imaging services for each vessel treated with extension prosthesis placement.

 Clinical Example (34803)

A 67-year-old male with coronary artery disease status post myocardial infarction (MI) and chronic obstructive pulmonary disease (COPD) was found to have a 5.8 cm diameter abdominal aortic aneurysm (AAA) by abdominal exam and subsequent ultrasound. Risks and benefits of open surgical repair, endovascular repair, and watchful waiting are discussed with the patient, and he opts for repair. History, physical examination, and perioperative risk evaluation including cardiac workup are performed to determine the patient's suitability for surgery. Imaging studies (typically a combination of computed tomography [CT] scan, magnetic resonance imaging [MRI], and/or angiography) indicate that the aneurysm is infrarenal in nature with an adequate neck of normal diameter aorta below the renal artery origins to allow successful deployment of endovascular prosthesis.

Description of Procedure (34803)

After each groin is accessed by open femoral or iliac artery exposure or percutaneously and catheters and/or sheaths are positioned into the aorta from each side, the physician performs an aortogram to reconfirm anatomy of the aorta and iliac arteries to confirm previously planned endorepair. (Note: Code 75952 includes all imaging work associated with endovascular repair of infrarenal abdominal aortic aneurysm or dissection.) A final examination is conducted of endovascular components for correct models, sizing, etc. Next, soft J-wires are exchanged for superstiff exchange wires. Reconfirming that the appropriate device has been chosen, the physician unpackages the main-body component and prepares the device for insertion. The patient's blood is then anticoagulated with IV heparin. Then, the main-body component is loaded onto the ipsilateral superstiff wire and advanced to the femoral artery. The tip of the main device is introduced into arteriotomy. The physician opens the proximal vascular clamp and advances the tip of the device into the artery, using rubber constrictors to limit blood loss as necessary. Under fluoroscopic guidance, the main-body device is advanced through the iliac arteries, and then into the aorta. The physician pushes the device through AAA carefully so the proximal edge lies below the renal arteries. The arteriography is repeated as needed to confirm the renal origin locations. Deployment is begun. Adjustments are made to align the top of the graft just below the renal origins. The main-body device is deployed with constant attention to exact positioning, watching both the renal arteries proximally and checking distally to determine that the position above the aortic bifurcation is correct. The main-body device is deployed to the point of opening the contralateral, docking port. The physician next cannulates the contralateral, docking port using a selective catheter/guidewire combination, and advances the catheter into the main body of the graft to the level of the proximal anastomosis. Contrast material is injected and an image of the graft is taken to confirm placement of the catheter within the graft. Aortic angiography is performed to confirm position of the proximal anastomosis, and any final adjustments needed are made to position of the proximal anastomosis at the level of the renals. Once this final position is confirmed, the suprarenal fixation portion of the main-body component is deployed. The contralateral superstiff wire is advanced into the suprarenal aorta. Through a contralateral sheath, angiography of the contralateral iliac bifurcation is performed to roadmap the position for the distal anastomosis. Once the appropriate length and diameter of the contralateral limb is confirmed, the physician unpackages the limb and prepares the device to be introduced. Then the contralateral limb is loaded onto the contralateral superstiff wire and advanced to the femoral artery. The contralateral limb device is advanced through the arteriotomy, and under fluoroscopy is advanced through the iliac artery into docking position. Next, the physician confirms the appropriate overlap of the contralateral limb with the main body device, and confirms the appropriate position of the distal anastomosis above the internal iliac origin. Then the contralateral docking limb is deployed. Afterward, he/she finishes deployment of the main-body component by deploying of the ipsilateral, docking port. The proximal portion of the delivery device is recaptured above the suprarenal fixation portion of the device, and the delivery device is removed from the main-body component and from the patient. Angiography is performed through the sheath to confirm position of ipsilateral common iliac bifurcation. Then the physician confirms the appropriate length and diameter of the ipsilateral limb and opens and prepares the device for insertion into the patient. The ipsilateral limb device is loaded onto superstiff wire, advanced to the ipsilateral femoral artery, and introduced through an arteriotomy. The physician observes fluoroscopically, as the ipsilateral limb is advanced through the iliac arteries into docking position. He or she then confirms the appropriate overlap of the limb with the main-body device, and the appropriate position of the distal anastomosis above the internal iliac origin. He/she then deploys the ipsilateral limb. The introducer devices are removed from the bilateral iliac limbs, using fluoroscopic guidance to prevent disruption of the graft position. The physician uses angioplasty on all 5 anastomoses to seat the graft, and angioplasty of any or all graft components as needed for complete expansion. The physician repositions the flush catheter to the level of the proximal anastomosis, and performs the completion arteriogram. Any areas of Type I endoleak or incomplete graft opening are re-ballooned as needed. If needed, stents are deployed within the body of the prosthesis to seal endoleaks or treat kinks or areas of incomplete opening. The physician performs the final completion arteriogram and completion pressure measurements. Finally, he/she removes catheters/wires/sheaths using fluoroscopic guidance.The arteriotomies are closed appropriately for the type of arteriotomy used.

DIRECT REPAIR OF ANEURYSM OR EXCISION (PARTIAL OR TOTAL) AND GRAFT INSERTION FOR ANEURYSM, PSEUDOANEURYSM, RUPTURED ANEURYSM, AND ASSOCIATED OCCLUSIVE DISEASE

Procedures 35001-▶35152◀ include preparation of artery for anastomosis including endarterectomy.

▶(35161, 35162 have been deleted. To report, use 37799)◀

Rationale

Codes 35161 and 35162 have been deleted due to infrequent use. A parenthetical note has been added to instruct that code 37799 should be reported for direct aneurysm repair of other arteries, not otherwise specified.

BYPASS GRAFT

In-Situ Vein

▶(35582 has been deleted)◀

35583   In-situ vein bypass; femoral popliteal

▶ (To report aortobifemoral bypass using synthetic conduit, and femoral-popliteal bypass with vein conduit in-situ, use 35646 and 35583. To report aorto(uni)femoral bypass with synthetic conduit, and femoral-popliteal bypass with vein conduit in-situ, use 35647 and 35583. To report aortofemoral bypass using vein conduit, and femoral-popliteal bypass with vein conduit in-situ, use 35546 and 35583)◀

Rationale

Code 35582 has been deleted, as this code presents a confusing redundancy with respect to other more recently established CPT codes. Code 35583 has been editorially revised to accommodate this deletion. Parenthetical notes have been added to indicate code 35582 has been deleted, and to explain proper reporting of codes 35546, 35583, 35646, and 35647 for various combinations of aorto-femoral bypass procedures.

VENOUS

●**36475**   Endovenous ablation therapy of incompetent vein, extremity, inclusive of all imaging guidance and monitoring, percutaneous, radiofrequency; first vein treated

+●**36476**   second and subsequent veins treated in a single extremity, each through separate access sites (List separately in addition to code for primary procedure)

▶(Use 36476 in conjunction with 36475)◀

▶(Do not report 36475, 36476 in conjunction with 36000-36005, 36410, 36425, 36478, 36479, 37204, 75894, 76000-76003, 76937, 76942, 93970, 93971)◀

●**36478**   Endovenous ablation therapy of incompetent vein, extremity, inclusive of all imaging guidance and monitoring, percutaneous, laser; first vein treated

+●**36479**   second and subsequent veins treated in a single extremity, each through separate access sites (List separately in addition to code for primary procedure)

▶(Use 36479 in conjunction with 36478)◀

▶(Do not report 36478, 36479 in conjunction with 36000-36005, 36410, 36425, 36475, 36476, 37204, 75894, 76000-76003, 76937, 76942, 93970, 93971)◀

✍ Rationale

Four codes have been established to report endovenous ablation therapy for incompetent veins. These codes are distinguished by the energy modalities and describe thermally induced ablation of incompetent veins for venous insufficiency, extremity venous reflux and varicose veins via laser and radiofrequency technology. Endovenous obliteration of the vein consists of percutaneous insertion of a catheter into the vein, and is appropriately reported for obliteration of the longer veins of the upper and lower extremities. When performed in the lower extremity, the point of incision is typically at the ankle level of the leg. The procedure, via either radiofrequency or laser modality, results in shrinkage of the diameter of the vein by destroying the intima and shrinking the vein wall to achieve complete elimination and obliteration of the lumen of the vein.

An add-on code to each of the initial codes is intended to report performance of ablation for each additional vein after the first vein. Instructional parenthetical notes indicate that the add-on code should be reported in addition to the initial code. Exclusionary parenthetical notes instruct that these codes are not appropriately reported in addition to the needle or catheter introduction codes (36000-36005); endovenous ablation procedures of a different modality (36475-36479); venipuncture (36410, 36425); percutaneous transcatheter occlusion code (37204); duplex extremity venous study codes (93970-93971) and ultrasound and fluoroscopic imaging codes 75894, 76000-76003, 76937, 76942, as the endovenous ablation procedure codes include all imaging guidance and monitoring. Endovenous ablation therapy requires imaging to direct this therapy. These codes include ultrasound for access, ultrasound for guidance and monitoring, and in some cases fluoroscopy for negotiating the venous structures. Codes 93970 and 93971 are not appropriately reported in addition to codes 36475, 36476, 36478, and 36479 when performed at the same session to ensure proper occlusion of the vein. However, codes 93970-93971 may be reported separately when performed as an independent diagnostic study on the same date of service. Endovenous ablation therapy is performed on patients with symptomatic venous insufficiency and/or vein reflux for the treatment of varicose veins of the extremities with ulcer and inflammation, venous (peripheral) insufficiency, venous embolism and/or thrombosis of other specified veins and superficial thrombophlebitis.

Although percutaneous access is specified in the descriptor, the vein is occasionally accessed by way of a small cut down. A small cut down, if performed to achieve access, is also included in the procedure and would not be separately reported. Modifier 50 should be appended to the procedure code when the procedure is performed in both legs at the same session.

Clinical Example (36475)

The patient is a 50-year-old, gravida 2, para 2, female with painful, unilateral leg swelling that increases during the course of the day while she is at her job that requires standing for a significant portion of the day. She has been diagnosed with great saphenous vein insufficiency with resultant superficial varicosities by way of history, physical examination, and non-invasive ultrasound testing, all of which were performed during a previous outpatient office visit. At that time, various treatment options were discussed and the patient has decided to undergo percutaneous endovenous radiofrequency ablation therapy of the insufficient saphenous vein. If it is necessary for endovenous ablation therapy to be coupled with stab phlebectomy and/or sclerotherapy, these services are separately reportable using existing codes.

Description of Procedure (36475)

The physician sets up the operating field and then attaches a pressurized, heparin, saline drip to the sterile radiofrequency ablation catheter. He/she then tests actuation, temperature, and impedance to ensure that all components are connected and operating properly. Next, ultrasound guidance is used to find the targeted greater saphenous vein (GSV) access site. Again using ultrasound guidance, the physician maps and marks the entire length of the targeted vein, noting the vein depth and diameter, and vein tributaries. Local anesthetic is given at the access site. The skin over the GSV access site is incised and a venotomy is performed. The physician uses the Seldinger technique to introduce the guidewire next and then advances the dilator over the guidewire. The exchange of the dilator for the sheath of the appropriate size occurs. The sheath is secured in place by suture, the guidewire is removed and the sheath flushed. Next the radiofrequency (RF) probe is placed through the sheath and advanced to the saphenofemoral junction using ultrasound guidance. The tip of the probe just below the superficial epigastric tributary vein is located. Then the RF probe's position is verified by ultrasound. Continuing the use of ultrasound guidance, the physician infiltrates tumescent anesthesic into the perivenous space to create a "halo" of fluid around the GSV from the entry site to the saphenofemoral junction. With the patient in the Trendelenburg position, he/she verifies that the target parameters are within acceptable range. Afterward, the RF position is reconfirmed with ultrasound imaging. Next, RF energy is applied. The physician carefully withdraws the probe, maintaining the target vein wall temperature by varying the pullback rate and/or applying compression over the limb. The physician continues to monitor impedance, power, and vein wall temperature throughout the procedure. Finally, he/she records the total RF application time and repeats the ultrasound of the saphenous vein to confirm successful ablation.

Clinical Example (36476)

The patient is a 50-year-old, gravida 2, para 2, female with painful, unilateral leg swelling that increases during the course of the day while at her job that requires that she is standing for a significant portion of the day. She has been diagnosed with great and small saphenous vein insufficiency with resultant superficial varicosities by way of history, physical examination, and non-invasive ultrasound testing, all of which were performed during a previous outpatient office visit. At that time various treatment options were discussed and the patient has decided to undergo percutaneous endovenous radiofrequency ablation therapy of the insufficient great and small saphenous veins. If it is necessary for endovenous ablation therapy to be coupled with stab phlebectomy and/or sclerotherapy, these services are separately reportable using existing codes.

Description of Procedure (36476)

The physician retests actuation, temperature, and impedance to ensure that all components are connected and operating properly. Next, he/she uses ultrasound guidance to find the targeted secondary vein access site. Again using ultrasound guidance, he/she maps and marks the entire length of the targeted vein, noting vein depth and diameter and maps vein tributaries. Local anesthesic is given at the new access site. Then skin is incised over the new access site. A venotomy is performed. The physician uses the Seldinger technique to introduce the guidewire next. Then he/she advances the dilator over the guidewire. The exchange of the dilator for the sheath of the appropriate size occurs. Then the sheath is secured in place by suture, the guidewire is removed, and the sheath flushed. Next the RF probe is placed through the sheath and advanced to the targeted endpoint using ultrasound guidance. The RF probe position is verified by ultrasound. Continuing the use of ultrasound guidance, the physician infiltrates tumescent anesthetic into the perivenous space to create a "halo" of fluid around the targeted vein from the entry site to the endpoint. With the patient in the Trendelenburg position, he/she verifies that the target parameters are within acceptable range. Afterward, the RF position is reconfirmed with ultrasound imaging. Next, RF energy is applied. The physician carefully withdraws the probe, maintaining the target vein wall temperature by varying pullback rate and/or applying compression over the limb. The physician continues to monitor impedance, power and vein wall temperature throughout the procedure. Finally, he/she records the total RF application time and repeats the ultrasound of the saphenous vein to confirm successful ablation.

 ### Clinical Example (36478)

The patient is a 50-year-old, gravida 2, para 2, female with painful, unilateral leg swelling that increases during the course of the day while she is at her job that requires standing for a significant portion of the day. She has been diagnosed with great saphenous vein insufficiency with resultant superficial varicosities by way of history, physical examination, and non-invasive, ultrasound testing, all of which were performed during a previous, outpatient, office visit. At that time, various treatment options were discussed and the patient has decided to undergo percutaneous, endovenous, laser, ablation therapy of the insufficient saphenous vein. If it is necessary for endovenous, ablation therapy to be coupled with stab phlebectomy and/or sclerotherapy, these services are separately reportable using existing codes.

Description of Procedure (36478)

The physician sets up the operating field and then attaches a pressurized, heparin, saline drip to the sterile, laser, ablation catheter. He/she then tests actuation, temperature, and impedance to ensure that all components are connected and operating properly. Next, he/she uses ultrasound guidance to find the targeted greater saphenous vein (GSV) access site. Again using ultrasound guidance, he/she maps and marks the entire length of the targeted vein, noting vein depth and diameter and maps vein tributaries. Local anesthetic is given at the access site. Then skin over the GSV access site is incised. A venotomy is performed. The physician uses the Seldinger technique to introduce the guidewire next. Then

Ⓢ=Modifier 51 Exempt   ☉=Conscious Sedation   ✚=Add-on Code

he/she advances the dilator over the guidewire. The exchange of the dilator for the sheath of the appropriate size occurs. Then the sheath is secured in place by suture, the guidewire is removed and the sheath flushed. Next the laser fiber is advanced through the sheath and advanced to the saphenofemoral junction using ultrasound guidance. The tip of the fiber just below the superficial epigastric tributary vein is located. Then the fiber position is verified by ultrasound. Continuing the use of ultrasound guidance, the physician infiltrates tumescent anesthetic into the perivenous space to create a "halo" of fluid around the GSV from the entry site to the saphenofemoral junction. With the patient in the Trendelenburg position, he/she verifies that the target parameters are within acceptable range. Afterward, the laser fiber position is reconfirmed with ultrasound imaging. Next laser energy is applied. The physician carefully withdraws the probe, maintaining the target vein wall temperature by varying the pullback rate and/or applying compression over the limb. The physician continues to monitor impedance, power and vein wall temperature throughout the procedure. Finally, he/she records the total laser application time and repeats the ultrasound of the saphenous vein to confirm successful ablation.

 Clinical Example (36479)

The patient is a 50-year-old, gravida 2, para 2, female with painful, unilateral leg swelling that increases during the course of the day while she is at her job that requires standing for a significant portion of the day. She has been diagnosed with great and small saphenous vein insufficiency with resultant superficial varicosities by way of history, physical examination, and non-invasive ultrasound testing, all of which were performed during a previous, outpatient, office visit. At that time, various treatment options were discussed and the patient has decided to undergo percutaneous, endovenous, laser, ablation therapy of the insufficient great and small saphenous veins. If it is necessary for endovenous, ablation therapy to be coupled with stab phlebectomy and/or sclerotherapy, these services are separately reportable using existing codes.

Description of Procedure (36479)

The physician uses ultrasound guidance to find the targeted secondary vein access site. Again using ultrasound guidance, he/she maps and marks the entire length of the targeted vein, noting the vein depth and diameter, and maps vein tributaries. Local anesthetic is given at the new access site. Then skin over the new access site is incised. A venotomy is performed. The physician uses the Seldinger technique to introduce the guidewire next. Then he/she advances the dilator over the guidewire. The exchange of the dilator for the sheath of the appropriate size occurs. Then the sheath is secured in place by suture, the guidewire is removed and the sheath flushed. Next the laser fiber is placed through the sheath and advanced to target endpoint using ultrasound guidance. The laser fiber position is verified by ultrasound. Again using ultrasound guidance, the physician infiltrates tumescent anesthetic into the perivenous space to create a "halo" of fluid around the target vein from the entry site to the endpoint. With the patient in the Trendelenburg position, he/she verifies that the target parameters are within acceptable range. Afterward, the laser fiber position is reconfirmed with ultrasound imaging. Laser energy is applied. The physician carefully withdraws the laser fiber, maintaining target vein wall temperature by varying the pullback rate and/or applying compression over the limb. The physician continues to monitor impedance, power and vein wall temperature throughout the procedure. Finally, he/she records the total laser application time and repeats the ultrasound of the saphenous vein to confirm successful ablation.

HEMODIALYSIS ACCESS, INTERVASCULAR CANNULATION FOR EXTRACORPOREAL CIRCULATION, OR SHUNT INSERTION

● **36818** Arteriovenous anastomosis, open; by upper arm cephalic vein transposition

▶(Do not report 36818 in conjunction with 36819, 36820, 36821, 36830 during a unilateral upper extremity procedure. For bilateral upper extremity open arteriovenous anastomoses performed at the same operative session, use modifier 50 or 59 as appropriate)◀

36819 by upper arm basilic vein transposition

▶(Do not report 36819 in conjunction with 36818, 36820, 36821, 36830 during a unilateral upper extremity procedure. For bilateral upper extremity open arteriovenous anastomoses performed at the same operative session, use modifier 50 or 59 as appropriate)◀

36820 by forearm vein transposition

36821 direct, any site (eg, Cimino type) (separate procedure)

✍ Rationale

Code 36818 was added to the series of codes for permanent native hemodialysis access to report performance of open upper arm cephalic vein transposition to include tunneling for brachiocephalic anastomosis.

This code describes a procedure which requires two upper arm incisions, one medial over the brachial artery, the other lateral to expose the vein. A tunnel is created between the incisions, and complete dissection of a substantial portion of the cephalic vein is required to allow it to be moved to a more superficial location and pulled through the tunnel for anastomosis with the brachial artery on the medial aspect of the upper arm. This approach is often performed in patients with large or obese arms.

Code 36818 differs from existing code 36819 in that the procedure described by code 36819 consists of the basilic vein transposition for brachiobasilic anastomosis. Code 36818 differs from existing code 36820 in that the procedure described by code 36820 consists of forearm vein transposition performed in the lower arm between the elbow and the wrist. Code 36818 differs from existing code 36830 in that the procedure described by code 36830 is the most commonly performed hemodialysis access operation, and is used to report placement of a synthetic subcutaneous tube graft in which one end is anastomosed to the brachial artery and the other to a large vein. This is most often performed when patients do not have large, visible wrist veins for performance of a native Cimino fistula (36821).

⊘=Modifier 51 Exempt   ⊙=Conscious Sedation   ✛=Add-on Code

An instructional parenthetical note was added following code 36819 to indicate that basilic vein transposition, forearm vein transposition, direct arteriovenous anastomosis, and creation of a fistula using non-autogenous graft, reported with codes 36819, 36820, 36821 and 36830, are mutually exclusive from 36818 if performed on the same arm, at the same operative session. Two procedures would not be performed in the same patient, same limb, during same encounter. Under unusual situations a patient might undergo 36818 on one upper extremity and a procedure described by code 36819, 36820, 36821 or 36830 on the contralateral upper extremity. This circumstance would be reported by adding modifier 59 for the second side. One indication for the unusual pair of simultaneous operations would be in a procedure setting in which hemodialysis access is needed in the immediate future, but caregivers hope to avoid a catheter. A permanent native fistula could be placed in one arm (36818) while a prosthetic hemodialysis graft is placed in other arm (36830). The shorter-lived prosthetic graft would then be immediately available for hemodialysis (useable in less than a week if necessary) while allowing 6-8 weeks for the native fistula to mature.

To accommodate placement of code 36818, code 36819 was editorially revised for placement as an indented code below code 36818. An instructional parenthetical note was added to indicate that cephalic vein transposition, forearm vein transposition, direct arteriovenous anastomosis, and creation of a fistula using non-autogenous graft, reported with codes 36818, 36820, 36821 and 36830, are mutually exclusive from 36819 if performed on the same arm, at the same operative session. Two procedures would not be performed in the same patient, same limb, during same encounter. Under unusual situations a patient might undergo a procedure described by code 36819 on one upper extremity and a procedure described by code 36818, 36820, 36821 or 36830 on the contralateral upper extremity. This circumstance would be reported by reporting modifier 59 for the second procedure.

Clinical Example (36818)

A 38-year-old, obese, diabetic female requires hemodialysis for chronic renal failure. On physical exam, she has no visible superficial veins on either side at the wrist, forearm, antecubital fossa or upper arm. Duplex ultrasound identifies a normal diameter cephalic vein 1 cm under the skin on the lateral aspect of her upper arm. To create an autogenous, hemodialysis access, the vein must be rerouted through a superficial tunnel to reach the brachial artery on the medial aspect of her arm, just above the elbow. A cephalic vein transposition is recommended.

Description of Procedure (36818)

The physician makes a skin incision over the approximate location of the cephalic vein from the elbow towards the shoulder for distance that is long enough to accomplish transposition. Then the subcutaneous tissue is dissected until the vein is located. Next, he/she ligates and divides all vein branches. The vein is dissected entirely from the surrounding tissue with careful attention to avoid venous injury. The physician makes separate small incisions over the brachial artery just proximal to the antecubital crease. Then, he/she dissects brachial veins and adjacent soft tissue from the artery. Small branches of the artery are encircled with silk ties. The physician then creates a superficial, subcutaneous tunnel that is long enough for adequate hemodialysis access and appropriate to allow the vein to reach across the arm to the brachial artery. Intravenous anticoagulant is administered. The physician ligates and divides the cephalic vein near the antecubital area. The physician then inserts the cannula into the transected end of the vein and gently distends the vein. Next, he/she searches for any venous leaks and sutures them if found. The physician marks a stripe on the vein longitudinally with a tissue marking pen to avoid twisting on its passage through the tunnel. The end of the cephalic is clamped and pulled through the tunnel. The brachial artery is occluded with vascular clamps. Next, the brachial artery is incised to create a 7 mm longitudinal arteriotomy. The end of the cephalic vein is trimmed to match the arteriotomy. The physician performs a cobra-head-shaped anastomosis end-of-vein to side-of-artery with suture. The proximal and distal artery are vented to flush air and debris out of the anastomosis. Then the anastomotic suture is tied and the physician checks for thrill in the vein. The vein is inspected in the tunnel to ensure no leaks or kinks exist. The wounds are irrigated and hemostasis is achieved. The physician closes the subcutaneous tissue of both incisions. He/she then closes the skin of both incisions. Finally, the wrist pulse and hand are checked to ensure adequate perfusion.

TRANSCATHETER PROCEDURES

▲**37205** Transcatheter placement of an intravascular stent(s), (except coronary, carotid, and vertebral vessel), percutaneous; initial vessel

(For radiological supervision and interpretation, use 75960)

▶(For coronary stent placement, see 92980, 92981)◀

+**37206** each additional vessel (List separately in addition to code for primary procedure)

(Use 37206 in conjunction with 37205)

(For transcatheter placement of ▶intravascular cervical carotid◀ artery stent(s), see ▶37215, 37216F)

▶(For transcatheter placement of extracranial vertebral or intrathoracic carotid artery stent(s), see Category III codes 0075T, 0076T)◀

⊙●**37215** Transcatheter placement of intravascular stent(s), cervical carotid artery, percutaneous; with distal embolic protection

⊙●**37216** without distal embolic protection

▶(37215 and 37216 include all ipsilateral selective carotid catheterization, all diagnostic imaging for ipsilateral, cervical and cerebral carotid arteriography, and all related radiological supervision and interpretation. When ipsilateral carotid arteriogram (including imaging and selective catheterization) confirms the need for carotid stenting, 37215 and 37216 are inclusive of these services. If carotid stenting is not indicated, then the appropriate codes for carotid catheterization and imaging should be reported in lieu of 37215 and 37216)◀

▶(Do not report 37215, 37216 in conjunction with 75671, 75680)◀

►(For transcatheter placement of extracranial vertebral or intrathoracic carotid artery stent(s), see Category III codes 0075T, 0076T)◄

►(For percutaneous transcatheter placement of intravascular stents other than coronary, carotid, or vertebral, see 37205, 37206)◄

✐ Rationale

Two codes, 37215 and 37216, have been established for reporting percutaneous stent placement in the cervical portion of the extracranial carotid artery. The codes are further distinguished by the use of or lack of employment of an embolic protection system. As these procedures are inclusive of all associated radiologic supervision and interpretation, a parenthetical note has been added to indicate that codes 75671 and 75680 would not be separately reported in addition to codes 37215 and 37216. A cross-reference has also been added to instruct that the appropriate codes for reporting carotid catheterization and imaging only are reported for those circumstances in which the carotid catheterization and imaging have been performed, and stent placement is not indicated for treatment. This cross-reference also instructs that all arteriographic imaging of the ipsilateral cervical and cerebral carotid arteries is included and not separately reported. Therefore, codes 37215 and 37216 include selective carotid access, all diagnostic imaging for ipsilateral common carotid bifurcation and cerebral vessels, plus all radiological supervision and interpretation. When the physician work of the initial ipsilateral carotid arteriogram (including imaging and access) confirms the need for carotid stenting, codes 37215 and 37216 are inclusive of these services. If carotid stenting is not indicated, then the appropriate codes for carotid catheterization and imaging would be reported in lieu of codes 37215 and 37216.

Carotid stenting and the associated radiologic services were previously encompassed within Category III codes 0005T and 0007T. To accommodate the addition of codes 37215 and 37216, Category III codes 0005T and 0007T have been revised and renumbered, with Category III code 0006T to continue to represent the services previously reported with these codes, other than transcatheter intravascular stent placement in the cervical carotid artery. A cross-reference following codes 37215 and 37216 instructs that Category III codes 0075T and 0076T would be reported for transcatheter placement of extracranial vertebral or intrathoracic carotid artery stents. The cross-reference following code 37206 has been revised to instruct appropriate reporting for transcatheter intravascular stent placement in the cervical carotid artery, and a second cross-reference added to instruct that Category III codes 0075T and 0076T would be reported for transcatheter placement of extracranial vertebral or intrathoracic carotid artery stents.

In a departure from the previous structure of the Category III codes which described these services (0005T-0007T), codes 37215 and 37216 currently describe transcatheter intravascular stent placement in the cervical carotid artery, distinguished by the use or lack of use of embolic protection (a screen, filter, or basket deployed beyond the stent target site with the intent to capture any particles that break loose, while simultaneously allowing uninterrupted blood flow to the brain to prevent peri-procedural embolization to the brain). While it is expected that the use of embolic protection would be reported in the majority of cases, in some circumstances, use of these devices would not be indicated. An example of this would be during treatment for early post-carotid endarterectomy intimal hyperplasia. This hyperplastic tissue is rubbery and not at all friable, with little probability of embolism. In such cases, the complexity of using the embolic protection device would not be justified.

The term "cervical" has replaced "extracranial" in the new carotid stent codes to clarify the intended site at or near the carotid bifurcation in the neck. In addition, this modification clarifies that Category III code 0075T is reported for placement of a stent in the common carotid artery in the chest. A small number of patients undergoing stenting of the carotid bifurcation in the neck will require simultaneous stent placement at the origin of the common carotid artery in the chest. This work is distinct and different from the carotid bifurcation stent, and would be separately reported with Category III code 0075T. The "each additional vessel" approach would not work well because the carotid bifurcation stent already will have one end in the common carotid, so this would not be an additional vessel.

An "each additional vessel" add-on code was not established for the cervical carotid artery system to mirror the structure of the Category III code 0006T. Since the typical carotid stent application results in deployment with one end of the stent in the common carotid and the other end in the internal carotid with the stent spanning the external carotid origin, there is no "additional vessel" in the cervical carotid system that could be treated. Occasionally, a patient will require an additional stent in the more distal internal carotid artery. In this unusual circumstance, this rarely required additional work is inherent within the scope of a single carotid stent code. In the equally unusual situation where bilateral carotid stents are deployed at the same session, the procedure can be reported with modifier 50.

 Clinical Example (37215)

A 66-year-old male has recurrent episodes of transient, right hemiparesis while on aspirin. Neurologic evaluation reveals no fixed neurological deficit. Carotid ultrasound demonstrates an 80-99% stenosis of his left internal carotid artery. Diagnostic cervico-cerebral arteriography confirms an 80% focal left internal carotid stenosis (NASCET measurement method). The patient is 10 years post coronary bypass surgery. He had a subendocardial myocardial infarction (MI) two months ago with subsequent cath showing diffuse distal disease, and an ejection fraction of 30%. He has angina at low levels of exercise. Discussion with a surgeon who performs carotid endarterectomy leads to agreement that the patient is at high risk for open carotid surgery. Carotid stent placement with embolic protection is therefore recommended.

Description of Procedure (37215)

Initial Arterial Access and Monitoring
The physician ensures electrocardiogram (ECG) and hemodynamic monitors are in place and functioning. All the following steps are performed under fluoroscopic

guidance. The common femoral artery is punctured for inserting the sheath. The physician directs the technical personnel throughout the procedure. He/she also interprets the imaging of the vessel being treated, including complete intracranial and extracranial views of the target vessel in all views necessary. Accurate radiological views, exposures, shielding, image size, injection sequences, radiation protection and management for patient and staff is ensured. He/she performs real-time analysis of all imaging during the procedure, including pre-treatment imaging, fluoroscopic and angiographic imaging throughout the procedure as required to perform the procedure, and post-procedure fluoroscopic and angiographic imaging. This includes all imaging to manipulate the wires, catheters, devices into position as well as correct positioning and deployment of embolic protection system (EPS), stable positioning of EPS throughout procedure, correct positioning and deployment of stent, opening balloon, assessing post-op success and complications, complete intra- and extracranial study post-stent, recapture of protection device, and removal of catheters. The physician performs quantitative measurement of the lesion, target vessel and distal EPS landing zone to determine appropriate balloon, stent and EPS sizes. Continuous fluoroscopic imaging is conducted during all catheter/stent manipulations to assess proper EPS position and adequate EPS performance throughout the procedure.

Baseline Cervical and Cerebral Angiography and Quantitative Measurements
The physician advances a standard guidewire into the aortic arch at the base of the great vessels. He/she advances the carotid configuration catheter to the aortic arch and roadmaps the common carotid artery origin and proximal segment. Then the standard wire is removed and replaced with a hydrophilic wire. The carotid-selective, reverse, curve catheter is inserted into the sheath over the hydrophilic wire. Intravenous(IV) anticoagulant is administered. Next the physician reforms the shape of the carotid-selective catheter in the aortic arch. Then the carotid catheter is used to selectively catheterize the origin of the common carotid artery. The contrast material is injected to perform the initial roadmap arteriogram of the common carotid artery and bifurcation. Afterward, the cervical carotid angiography is performed in anteroposterior (AP) and lateral views. The physician performs quantitative measurements of the vessels including the area of stenosis and area of EPS landing zone. Cerebral angiography is performed including, at minimum, lateral and AP views. The catheter is placed to continuously flush heparin.

Selection of Appropriate Stent and Embolic Protection System
The physician chooses equipment based on the results of the quantitative measurements. He/she connects the side-arm of the long guiding sheath to the arterial pressure transducer. Next, he/she performs a focused arteriogram of bifurcation and distal internal carotid through the guiding sheath.

Prepare Distal Embolic Protection System (EPS)
The physician prepares the wire on the back table and ensures the filter is completely air-free. Then the delivery system is assembled and he/she assures it is air-free. Afterward, the retrieval system is assembled and the physician also assures it is air-free.

Exchange for Guiding Catheter/Sheath
The hydrophilic wire is advanced under the roadmap into the external carotid artery. Next, the physician advances the catheter into the external carotid artery. He/she removes the hydrophilic wire and then inserts the stiff exchange-length wire. The long guiding sheath/catheter is exchanged into the common carotid artery. Then the wire is removed and next the carotid-selective catheter. Finally, the physician checks the activated clotting time (ACT) to ensure adequate anticoagulation.

Placement of Distal Embolic Protection System
The wire/EPS/delivery system is loaded and advanced into the common carotid artery. The physician performs a high-magnification pre-deployment arteriogram of the carotid bifurcation. Then, he/she checks the patient's neurological status now and throughout the case at intervals. He/she advances and maneuvers the wire/EPS across the lesion into the distal extracranial internal carotid artery with careful positioning, using confirmatory angiography and road-mapping. Next, the EPS is activated by opening the filter umbrella in the distal internal carotid artery. The EPS deployment catheter is removed. The deployed EPS position is confirmed with an angiogram to ensure good flow and filter/wall apposition. The physician repositions the EPS and repeats as necessary until the proper position is attained.

Pre-Stent Carotid Angioplasty
The physician prepares an angioplasty balloon to be air-free. He/she advances the low-profile balloon across the lesion and checks the position. Next, the balloon is insufflated to pre-dilate the lesion. Finally, the balloon is removed.

Carotid Stent Placement
The stent delivery system is prepared to be air-free. Then the appropriately sized self-expanding stent is loaded into the guiding catheter. Next, the stent delivery catheter is advanced very carefully across the lesion. The physician performs the final angiographic check to ensure exact positioning. He/she deploys the stent and removes the stent delivery device. The balloon is loaded and advanced. The balloon is positioned within the stent and inflated for post dilatation. The physician checks the ECG for bradycardia or other arrhythmia, and provides treatment as needed with IV medications.

EPS Removal
The EPS retrieval system is advanced through the stent to the distal EPS position. Then the EPS is deactivated, and the wire/EPS is removed.

Final Carotid and Cerebral Angiography
The physician performs the completion bifurcation arteriogram. He/she then checks carefully for residual stenosis, dissection, or vasospasm. The above are treated if present (eg, nitroglycerin is used for treating vasospasm). The completion intra-cerebral arteriogram is performed in anteroposterior (AP), lateral, and Towne views. The cerebral images are reviewed in detail for emboli, vasospasm, cross-filling, etc. The soft-tip guidewire is inserted into the long

guiding sheath/catheter. Then the guiding sheath/catheter is removed from the common carotid artery. The physician removes the guiding sheath and guidewire from the puncture site and attains hemostasis. The final neurological check is performed prior to transferring the patient to the recovery area.

 Clinical Example (37216)

A 66-year-old male underwent a left carotid endarterectomy one year ago. An initial postoperative duplex exam at 1 month demonstrated a widely patent carotid bifurcation, but follow-up at 6 months revealed early recurrent stenosis in the 50-79% range. When the duplex scanning was repeated at 12 months, progression was identified to 80-99% diameter reduction. The diagnosis is intimal hyperplasia at the endarterectomy site causing a severe to critical recurrent stenosis. The patient is 10 years post coronary bypass surgery. He developed recurrent angina recently and suffered a myocardial infarction 1 month ago. Cardiac catheterization revealed diffuse distal disease and an ejection fraction of 30%. He has angina at low levels of exercise. Discussion with a surgeon who performs carotid endarterectomy leads to agreement that the patient is at high risk for open surgery. Carotid stent placement is therefore recommended.

Description of Procedure (37216)

The physician directs technical personnel throughout the procedure. He/she interprets the imaging of the vessel being treated, including complete intracranial and extracranial views of the targeted vessel in all views necessary. Accurate radiological views, exposures, shielding, image size, injection sequences, radiation protection and management for patient and staff are ensured. He/she performs real-time analysis of all imaging during the procedure, including pre-treatment imaging, fluoroscopic and angiographic imaging throughout the procedure as required to perform the procedure, and post-procedure fluoroscopic and angiographic imaging. This includes all imaging to manipulate the wires, catheters, and devices into position, plus correct positioning and deployment of the stent and opening the balloon. In addition, the physician assesses post-operative success and complications, completes intra- and extracranial study post-stent, and removes the catheters. The physician also takes quantitative measurements of the lesion and targeted vessel to determine the appropriate balloon and stent sizes.

Initial Arterial Access and Monitoring
The physician ensures that the electrocardiograph (ECG) and hemodynamic monitors are in place and functioning. All the following steps are performed under fluoroscopic guidance. He/she punctures the common femoral artery for insertion of the sheath.

Baseline Cervical and Cerebral Angiography and Quantitative Measurement
The standard guidewire is advanced into the aortic arch at the base of the great vessels. Next, the carotid-configuration catheter is advanced to the aortic arch. Then the roadmap is created of the common carotid artery origin and proximal segment. The standard wire is removed and replaced with hydrophilic wire. The carotid-selective, reverse-curve catheter is inserted into the guiding sheath over

the hydrophilic wire. Intravenous (IV) anticoagulant is administered. The physician reforms the shape of the carotid-selective catheter in the aortic arch. Then the carotid catheter is used to selectively catheterize the origin of the common carotid artery. The contrast material is injected to perform the initial roadmap arteriogram of the common carotid artery and bifurcation. The physician performs cervical carotid angiography in AP and lateral views. Then quantitative measurements are taken of the vessels including the area of stenosis. Cerebral angiography including lateral and AP views is performed. Finally, the catheter is placed to continuous heparin flush.

Selection of Appropriate Stent
The physician chooses equipment based on the results of the quantitative measurements. He/she then connects the side-arm of the long guiding sheath to the arterial pressure transducer. Then the physician performs a focused arteriogram of bifurcation and the distal internal carotid artery through the guiding sheath.

Exchange for Guiding Catheter/Sheath
The hydrophilic wire is advanced under roadmap into the external carotid. The catheter is advanced into the external carotid artery. Then the physician removes the hydrophilic wire and inserts the stiff wire. The long guiding sheath is exchanged into the common carotid, over the carotid-selective catheter. The wire is removed and then the carotid-selective catheter is also removed. Finally, the physician checks the ACT to ensure adequate anticoagulation.

Placement of Small Diameter Wire Across Lesion
The wire is loaded and advanced into the common carotid artery. Then the high-magnification pre-deployment arteriogram of carotid bifurcation is performed. Next the patient's neurological status is checked now and throughout the case at intervals. The wire is advanced and maneuvered across the lesion into the distal, extracranial, internal, carotid artery with careful positioning using confirming angiography and roadmapping.

Pre-Stent Carotid Angioplasty
The physician prepares the angioplasty balloon to be air-free. Then the low-profile balloon is advanced across the lesion and the position is checked. Atropine is administered. The balloon is insufflated to pre-dilate the lesion. Finally, the balloon is removed.

Carotid Stent Placement
The physician prepares the stent delivery system to be air-free. Then the appropriately sized self-expanding stent is loaded into the guiding catheter. Next, the stent delivery catheter is advanced very carefully across the lesion. The final angiographic check is then performed to ensure exact positioning. The stent is deployed. Afterward, the stent delivery device is removed. The balloon is loaded and advanced. Then the balloon is positioned within the stent and inflated for post dilatation. The ECG is checked for bradycardia or other arrhythmia, and the patient is treated as needed with IV medications.

Final Carotid and Cerebral Angiography

The completion bifurcation arteriogram is performed. The physician checks carefully for residual stenosis, dissection, or vasospasm. He/she provides treatment for any of the above if present (eg, nitroglycerin is used to treat vasospasm). The completion intra-cerebral arteriogram is performed in lateral and Towne views. Then the cerebral images are reviewed in detail for emboli, vasospasm, cross-filling, etc. The wire is exchanged for guidewire through the guiding sheath. Afterward the guiding sheath/catheter is removed from the common carotid artery. The guiding sheath and guidewire are removed from the puncture site.

Groin Management

The physician removes the sheath and attains hemostasis.

Neurologic Assesment

The physician performs a final neurological check.

Hemic and Lymphatic Systems

General

BONE MARROW OR STEM CELL SERVICES/PROCEDURES

(Do not report 38207-38215 in conjunction with ▶88182, 88184-88189◀)

Rationale

The cross-reference following code 38215 has been revised in conjunction with the deletion of code 88180 and the addition of codes 88184-88189 to instruct the appropriate reporting for flow cytometric testing.

Digestive System

Esophagus

ENDOSCOPY

⊙ **43235** Upper gastrointestinal endoscopy including esophagus, stomach, and either the duodenum and/or jejunum as appropriate; diagnostic, with or without collection of specimen(s) by brushing or washing (separate procedure)

⊙● **43257** with delivery of thermal energy to the muscle of lower esophageal sphincter and/or gastric cardia, for treatment of gastroesophageal reflux disease

Rationale

Category III code 0057T has been deleted and converted to Category I code 43257 to report thermal treatment of the esophagus by endoscopy.

Code 43257 is intended to be reported for the treatment of gastroesophageal reflux disease (GERD). This procedure consists of the delivery of endoscopically guided radiofrequency thermal energy via electrodes to electrosurgically coagulate the muscle of the distal portion of the lower esophageal sphincter and/or gastric cardia for the treatment of GERD. The coagulation of the muscle of the lower esophageal sphincter, via a series of deliveries of thermal energy via endoscopically introduced needle electrodes, results in increased lower esophageal sphincter pressure (LESP) and augmentation of the anti-reflux barrier, thus improving the barrier to reflux during the postprandial period.

Clinical Example (43257)

A 66-year-old female presents for surgery with a history of chronic heartburn and regurgitation symptoms three times or more per week that has not responded to lifestyle management strategies and intensive daily pharmacologic therapy. She has peak esophageal peristaltic amplitude > 30 mm Hg, LESP > 5 mm Hg, complete LES relaxation in response to swallow, a DeMeester score >14.7, Hetzel grade 1 esophagitis, and no hiatal hernia > 2 cm. Under conscious sedation, an upper GI endoscopy, with delivery of radiofrequency thermal energy to the muscle of the lower esophageal sphincter and/or gastric cardia, is performed.

Description of Procedure (43257)

After intravenous access is obtained and conscious sedation administered, an esophagogastroduodenoscopy (EGD) is performed to confirm the absence of pathology that would represent a contraindication to the performance of the proposed procedure. The upper endoscope is then positioned in the gastric antrum, and a guidewire is passed through the endoscope into the duodenum or gastric antrum. The endoscope is withdrawn while noting the distance from the incisors to the gastroesophageal junction. The thermal catheter is passed over the guidewire and positioned 1 cm proximal to the squamocolumnar junction. The thermal catheter balloon is inflated to 2.5 psi, needle electrodes (4) deployed, and radiofrequency (RF) energy delivery commenced. This treatment is repeated after rotating the catheter 45 degrees and then again by advancing it 5 mm (4 treatments thus far). The catheter is then advanced into the stomach. An endoscope is re-introduced per-oral and passed alongside the catheter to confirm accurate positioning of the first 2 rings. The endoscope is then withdrawn. Third and fourth rings, comprised of eight lesions per ring, are then placed in 5 mm increments distal to the second ring, adjusting the measurements according to the endoscopic findings. The catheter is then advanced into the stomach, fully inflated to 25 cc of air, and withdrawn into the gastric cardia. Three such deployments and lesion sets are created, totaling 12 lesions in the distal cardia. This is repeated with a balloon inflated to 22 cc, creating 12 lesions in the proximal cardia. A third EGD is performed to confirm lesion placement. The catheter is then withdrawn.

⊘=Modifier 51 Exempt   ☉=Conscious Sedation   ✛=Add-on Code

Stomach

LAPAROSCOPY

● **43644**   Laparoscopy, surgical, gastric restrictive procedure; with gastric bypass and Roux-en-Y gastroenterostomy (roux limb 150 cm or less)

▶(Do not report 43644 in conjunction with 43846, 49320)◀

▶(Esophagogastroduodenoscopy (EGD) performed for a separate condition should be reported with modifier 59)◀

● **43645**   with gastric bypass and small intestine reconstruction to limit absorption

▶(Do not report 43645 in conjunction with 49320, 43847)◀

OTHER PROCEDURES

● **43845**   Gastric restrictive procedure with partial gastrectomy, pylorus-preserving duodenoileostomy and ileoileostomy (50 to 100 cm common channel) to limit absorption (biliopancreatic diversion with duodenal switch)

▶(Do not report 43845 in conjunction with 43633, 43847, 44130, 49000)◀

▲ **43846**   Gastric restrictive procedure, with gastric bypass for morbid obesity; with short limb (150 cm or less) Roux-en-Y gastroenterostomy

▶(For greater than 150 cm, use 43847)◀

▶(For laparoscopic procedure, use 43644)◀

✐ Rationale

Several new gastric restrictive surgery codes were added to reflect the rapidly expanding field of bariatric surgery.

Codes 43644 and 43645 employ laparoscopic techniques to perform gastric restrictive procedures for morbid obesity including Roux-en-Y gastric bypass and small bowel reconstruction to limit absorption.

Code 43845 was added to describe a biliopancreatic diversion with duodenal switch, a surgical treatment for morbid obesity that combines moderate gastric restriction with a mechanism that promotes fat malabsorption, and includes duodenal division and pylorus preservation with two reconstructive anastomoses.

For consistency, an editorial revision was made to the existing open Roux-en-Y code 43846 to designate short limb to be 150 cm as specified in the laparoscopic Roux-en-Y gastroentrostomy code 43644.

Code 43846 was revised to more accurately describe the location of the division of the section of small intestine and to reflect the typical current practice for this procedure, in which it has become the standard of care to perform a longer Roux-en-Y gastroenterostomy (limbs up to 150 cm). This procedure has evolved in order to provide more effective treatment for patients with greater obesity (ie, 225% of ideal body weight or greater). In these patients, a 150 cm proximal Roux-en-Y procedure (long-limb gastric bypass (GBP)) has been found to increase weight loss to two thirds of excess weight without causing an increase in nutritional complications.

Clinical Example (43644)

A 44-year-old male, who stands 5 feet 11 inches tall, weighs 390 pounds for a body mass index (BMI) of 55 kg/m², presents with a history of Type II diabetes controlled with three oral hypoglycemic medications, and hypertension controlled with two medications. A recent sleep study showed severe, obstructive sleep apnea for which he was placed on continuous positive airway pressure (CPAP) with subjective improvement, but complaints of poor tolerance of the mask. His gastroesophageal reflux is controlled with an H2-blocker, but his mobility is compromised due to severe arthritis of his lower back and right knee. Family and diet history confirm morbid obesity began at age nine. The patient underwent multiple weight-loss programs, losing up to 75 pounds three times. However, the weight loss was never maintained for more than six months and each weight regain was more than what was originally lost. Weight loss programs utilized included very low calorie diets, a popular commercial program, exercise, appetite suppressants, and meal replacements. At operation, he undergoes a laparoscopic gastric restrictive procedure with gastric bypass and Roux-en Y gastroenterostomy.

Description of Procedure (43644)

Under general anesthesia, the abdomen is entered under direct vision or using a Veress needle technique to obtain access for pneumoperitoneum. Carbon dioxide is pumped into the abdominal cavity, through tubing connected to an insufflator, to expand the abdominal cavity. A laparoscopic camera is introduced into the abdomen to allow visualization of the internal organs. Four to six trocar ports are placed in the anterior abdominal wall above the umbilicus. The liver is retracted to expose the upper stomach. (Because the liver is typically fatty, it must be handled with extra care to avoid tearing, puncture or cracking.) The gastroesophageal junction is identified and a small incision is made in the gastrohepatic ligament along the edge of the lesser curve between the first and second vessel caudad to the gastroesophageal junction. Using blunt and ultrasonic dissection, a retrogastric tunnel is made cephalad, toward the angle of His. A small (15-20 cc) gastric pouch is made after the stomach is transected with repeated firings of an endoscopic linear stapler. An orogastric tube may be used to calibrate the size of the pouch. Minor bleeding from the staple lines is controlled using hemoclips. The ligament of Treitz is identified, and the small intestine measured distally for a short distance and transected with a linear stapler. The distal limb is brought up to the proximal gastric pouch; either anterior to the transverse colon (ante-colic) or posterior to the transverse colon (retro-colic). The omentum may be divided longitudinally with an ultrasonic scalpel or endoscopic stapler, to allow for decreased tension for passage of the Roux limb in an ante-colic position. The transverse mesocolon is incised to create a tunnel for a

⊘ =Modifier 51 Exempt   ⊙ =Conscious Sedation   ✚ =Add-on Code

retro-colic Roux limb position, as indicated. Care must be taken to avoid twisting of the Roux limb to avoid obstruction or ischemia of the intestine. The mesenteric defect is closed to prevent internal herniation. A gastrojejunal anastomosis is performed between the Roux limb and the gastric pouch, by using either hand-sewn technique, stapled technique or a combination of both. The Roux limb is then measured up to 150 cm distal from the gastrojejunal anastomosis and marked. A jejunojejunostomy is performed between the bypassed biliopancreatic limb and the marked segment of the Roux limb. This anastomosis is performed by using either hand-sewn technique, stapled technique, or combination of both. Intra-operative testing for anastomotic leak may be performed as clinically indicated, utilizing air, intra-operative endoscopy or methylene blue. Drains(s) are placed and/or distal gastrostomy performed as indicated. Finally, the fascia and skin are closed.

Clinical Example (43645)

A 44-year-old male, who stands 5 feet 11 inches tall, weighs 420 pounds for a body mass index (BMI) of 60 kg/m^2, presents with a history of Type II diabetes controlled with three oral hypoglycemic medications and hypertension controlled with two medications. A recent sleep study showed severe obstructive sleep apnea for which he was placed on continuous positive airway pressure (CPAP) with subjective improvement, but complaints of poor tolerance of the mask. His gastroesophageal reflux is controlled with an H2-blocker, but his mobility is compromised due to severe arthritis of his lower back and right knee. Family and diet history confirm morbid obesity began at age nine. The patient underwent multiple weight-loss programs, losing up to 75 pounds three times. However, the weight loss was never maintained for more than six months and each weight regain was more than what was originally lost. Weight loss programs utilized included very low calorie diets, a popular commercial program, exercise, appetite suppressants, and meal replacements. At operation, he undergoes a laparoscopic, gastric, restrictive procedure with gastric bypass and small intestine reconstruction to limit absorption.

Description of Procedure (43645)

Under general anesthesia, the abdomen is entered under direct vision or using a Veress needle technique to obtain access for pneumoperitoneum. Carbon dioxide is pumped into the abdominal cavity through tubing connected to an insufflator to expand the abdominal cavity. A laparoscopic camera is introduced into the abdomen to allow visualization of the internal organs. Four to six trocar ports are placed in the anterior abdominal wall above the umbilicus. The liver is retracted to expose the upper stomach. (Because the liver is typically fatty, it must be handled with extra care to avoid tearing, puncture or cracking.) The gastroesophageal junction is identified and a 2 cm incision is made in the gastrohepatic ligament along the edge of the lesser curve between the first and second vessel caudad to the gastroesophageal junction. Using blunt and ultrasonic dissection, a retrogastric tunnel is made cephalad, toward the angle of His. A small (15-20 cc) gastric pouch is made after the stomach is transected with repeated firings of an endoscopic linear stapler. An orogastric tube may be used to calibrate the size of the pouch. Minor bleeding from the staple lines is controlled using hemoclips. The small bowel is transected using a specialized endoscopic linear stapler at a measured distance from the ligament of Treitz or the ileocecal valve. The distal limb is brought up to the proximal gastric pouch, either anterior to the transverse colon (ante-colic) or posterior to the transverse colon (retro-colic). The omentum may be divided longitudinally using an ultrasonic scalpel or endoscopic stapler, to allow for decreased tension for passage of the Roux limb in an ante-colic position. The transverse mesocolon is incised to create a tunnel for a retro-colic Roux limb position, if indicated. Care must be taken to avoid twisting of the Roux limb to avoid obstruction or ischemia of the intestine. The mesenteric defect is closed to prevent internal herniation. A gastrojejunal anastomosis is performed between the Roux limb and the gastric pouch by using either hand-sewn technique, stapled technique, or a combination of both. The Roux limb is then measured greater than 150 cm distal from the gastrojejunal anastomosis and marked. An enteroenterostomy is performed between the bypassed biliopancreatic limb and the marked segment of the Roux limb. This anastomosis is performed by using either hand-sewn technique, stapled technique, or a combination of both. The length of the biliopancreatic limb and the Roux limb may vary in order to produce malabsorption of variable nutrients. The variations may include: (1) a short biliopancreatic limb measuring 20 to 90 cm with a very long Roux limb measuring 150 to 250 cm from the gastrojejunostomy; or (2) transection of the small intestine at a point 250 to 360 cm proximal to the ileocecal valve, to create a 151 to 250 cm Roux limb, with a distal enteroenterostomy anastomosis at a point 50 to 150 cm proximal to the ileocecal valve. Both techniques result in fat malabsorption. Intra-operative testing for anastomotic leak may be performed as clinically indicated, utilizing air, intra-operative endoscopy or methylene blue. Drains(s) are placed and/or distal gastrostomy performed as indicated. Finally, the fascia and skin are closed.

Clinical Example (43845)

The patient is a 44-year-old male who stands 5 feet 11 inches tall, weighs 390 pounds (210 pounds overweight) for a body mass index (BMI) of 55 kg/m². He has a history of Type II diabetes mellitus, which was diagnosed 4 years ago and is presently controlled with 3 oral hypoglycemics, as well as hypertension for which he takes 2 medications. In addition, a recent sleep study showed severe obstructive sleep apnea, for which he was placed on continuous positive airway pressure (CPAP) with subjective improvement, but complains of poor tolerance of the mask. His gastroesophageal reflux is controlled with H2-blocker, but his mobility is severely compromised due to severe arthritis of his lower back and right knee. Family history and diet history confirm morbid obesity, with obesity beginning since age 9. The patient underwent multiple weight loss programs resulting in weight losses of up to 75 pounds three times. However, the weight loss was never maintained for more than 6 months, and each weight regain was more than what was originally lost. Weight loss programs utilized included very low calorie diets, support groups, exercise, appetite suppressants, and meal replacements.

⊘ =Modifier 51 Exempt   ⊙ =Conscious Sedation   ✚ =Add-on Code

Description of Procedure (43845)

The patient is positioned, prepped, and draped with special attention to positioning to prevent neuropraxias and pressure necrosis of skin. Under general anesthesia, generally a midline incision is employed with lysis of adhesions as needed. Starting from the lateral mid antrum, the stomach is divided longitudinally with a staple division technique to the top of the gastric fundus lateral to the gastroesophageal junction at the angle of His. The gastric pouch may be sized with a bougie placed in the stomach, to make a longitudinal 150-200 cc pouch. The lateral gastric specimen is discarded. The first portion of the duodenum is mobilized and transected with a stapler approximately 3 to 5 cm distal to the pylorus. The small bowel is transected with a stapler approximately 250 cm from the ileocecal valve. The distal end (alimentary limb) is anastomosed to the proximally divided duodenal limb. The proximal transected small bowel (biliopancreactic limb) is anastomosed 50 to 100 cm proximal to the ileocecal valve on the distal previously divided small bowel. Close fascia and skin. Drain, as indicated by clinical situation.

Clinical Example (43846)

The patient is a 40-year-old male who weighs 390 pounds (210 pounds overweight), is hypertensive on two medications without good control, has severe gastroesophageal reflux, and near disabling arthritis of his lower back and right knee. In addition, a recent sleep study showed severe obstructive sleep apnea and he has been placed on continous positive airway pressure (CPAP) with some limited improvement, but continued dependent edema suggestive of right heart failure. Family history and diet history confirm morbid obesity with obesity since childhood and multiple weight losses of up to 75 pounds in the past with no significant weight maintenance and rapid recent weight gain since sleep apnea symptoms have been present. Preoperatively, the surgeon re-evaluates history, laboratory, and physical findings and finalizes extensive informed consent. At laparotomy, a gastric bypass procedure with a measured 30 cc pouch and 45 cm Roux-en-Y gastrojejunostomy is fashioned and the small gastic pouch is divided from the remainder of the stomach. A gastrostomy tube is placed and the wound is drained. Postoperatively, the patient is stabilized in the intensive care unit (ICU) with careful monitoring of ventilation, hemodynamics, fluid balance, and also with nightly recorded oximetry with alteration of CPAP pressure and oxygen volumes as needed. Vigorous pulmonary re-inflation measures are pressed due to the marked intra-abdominal obesity. Special bed with trapezes is used. Mini-dose heparin, drains and tube losses are monitored with wound checks and dressing changes. Drains and tubes are removed appropriately and oral fluids are begun on the 4th postoperative day and advanced. The patient is discharged on the 7th to 9th postoperative day with extensive instructions concerning the dramatically altered gastric physiology, including inability to take food and liquids simultaneously with avoidance of true solids for several weeks. Techniques of taking vitamins and medications orally are stressed. Arrangements are made for continued CPAP and oxygen postoperatively.

Description of Procedure (43846)

Special positioning of the patient with a footboard, taping of the ankles and strapping of the knees in preparation for a 50% tilt of the table. The patient was prepped, draped and set up with mechanical, table-mounted retractors. The gastric bypass procedure is performed with total division of the pressure/volume-measured 30 mL pouch from the remainder of the stomach with a 45 cm Roux limb and a 10 mm gastrojejunostomy. A gastrostomy is performed in the distal stomach, the wound drained and closed in layers. A medication block is placed to aid postoperative pulmonary mechanics. The wound and tubes are dressed.

Intestines (Except Rectum)

EXCISION

▶Intestinal allotransplantation involves three distinct components of physician work:◀

▶1) *Cadaver donor enterectomy*, which includes harvesting the intestine graft and cold preservation of the graft (perfusing with cold preservation solution and cold maintenance) (use 44132). *Living donor enterectomy*, which includes harvesting the intestine graft, cold preservation of the graft (perfusing with cold preservation solution and cold maintenance), and care of the donor (use 44133).◀

▶2) *Backbench work*:◀

▶Standard preparation of an intestine allograft prior to transplantation includes mobilization and fashioning of the superior mesenteric artery and vein (see 44715).◀

▶Additional reconstruction of an intestine allograft prior to transplantation may include venous and/or arterial anastomosis(es) (see 44720-44721).◀

▶3) *Recipient intestinal allotransplantation with or without recipient enterectomy*, which includes transplantation of allograft and care of the recipient (see 44135, 44136).◀

▲ **44132**   Donor enterectomy (including cold preservation), open; from cadaver donor

   44133   partial, from living donor

▶(For backbench intestinal graft preparation or reconstruction, see 44715, 44720, 44721)◀

● **44137**   Removal of transplanted intestinal allograft, complete

▶(For partial removal of transplant allograft, see 44120, 44121, 44140)◀

OTHER PROCEDURES

● **44715**   Backbench standard preparation of cadaver or living donor intestine allograft prior to transplantation, including mobilization and fashioning of the superior mesenteric artery and vein

● **44720**   Backbench reconstruction of cadaver or living donor intestine allograft prior to transplantation; venous anastomosis, each

● **44721**   arterial anastomosis, each

⊘=Modifier 51 Exempt   ⊙=Conscious Sedation   ✚=Add-on Code

✍️ Rationale

New guidelines have been added at the beginning of the Intestines Excision subsection to clarify the three components of physician work involved in intestinal allotransplantation, which are cadaver or living donor enterectomy, backbench work, and recipient intestinal allotransplantation.

Code 44137 was added to the Intestine Excision subsection of the Digestive System section to describe complete removal of transplanted intestinal allograft. In the Intestine Other Procedures subsection, code 44715 was added to describe backbench preparation of cadaver or living donor intestine allograft including mobilization and fashioning of the superior mesenteric artery and vein prior to transplantation. Codes 44720 and 44721 were added to describe backbench reconstruction of cadaver or living donor intestine allograft prior to transplantation. Code 44720 should be reported for each venous anastomosis and code 44721 should be reported for each arterial anastomosis. Code 44132 was revised to include cold preservation and not to include preparation and maintenance of the allograft, since new codes 44715, 44720 and 44721 now describe the preparation and maintenance services. A cross-reference was added below code 44133 directing users to codes 44715, 44720 and 44721 for backbench intestinal graft preparation or reconstruction.

🩺 Clinical Example (44137)

A 22-year-old male with a history of multiple abdominal surgeries and recurrent episodes of line infection, thrombosis of the major central veins, significant elevation of liver enzymes, and histopathologic evidence of portal fibrosis required small bowel transplantation. Following the transplantation, he experienced acute and chronic rejection that resulted in chronic graft dysfunction and repeated episodes of bacterial translocation. He now requires surgical removal of the entire intestinal allograft with reinstitution of total parenteral nutrition (TPN) therapy.

Description of Procedure (44137)

Pre-operative orders for peri-operative medications are written. Next, a review of pre-operative work-up is performed with particular attention to pathology reports and films. The physician changes into scrub clothes, and checks with lab making certain that blood and/or x-match is available. A review of the surgical procedure and expected outcome(s) is detailed for the patient and family, including a review of expectations for post-operative recovery both in and out of the hospital. The physician answers questions for both the patient and the family and obtains informed consent. A review of the length and type of anesthesia by the anesthesiologist is provided. The physician reviews the planned procedure and positioning and draping of patient, verifying that all necessary surgical instruments and supplies are readily available in the operative suite. The physician will also monitor the patient's positioning and draping and assist with positioning as needed.

An extended midline skin incision is made and anterior abdominal wall is carefully divided. The peritoneal cavity is entered and the bowel protected. A self-retaining retractor is inserted to facilitate exposure. Adhesions are lysed, freeing the small intestine. After full mobilization of the bowel, the intestinal loops on the left side are retracted medially and the aorta is exposed. The infrarenal aortic graft that was constructed at the time of transplantation is dissected from the intestinal loops and encircled with a vessel loop. This same technique is applied to the venous graft that connects the superior mesenteric vein of the intestine to the recipient native portal vein. After clamping and transecting both the aortic and venous grafts, both the proximal and distal bowel anastomoses are identified and a stapler is applied to each limb and fired, dividing the transplanted bowel from the native remaining intestine both proximally and distally. The allograft intestine is removed en-bloc and the remnant stumps of both the aortic and vein graft are oversewn with prolene sutures. The enterectomy specimen is sent for full histopathologic examination. The distal stump of the native residual large bowel, if present, is oversewn with non-absorbable sutures. The proximal end of the remaining native small intestine is exteriorized as an end stoma. A gastrostomy tube is placed and anchored to the abdominal wall. Hemostasis is carried out through the entire operation using the Argon beam and suture ligature. The abdominal cavity is checked meticulously for bleeding and irrigated. Multiple drains are applied and the abdominal wall is closed in a single layer using semi-absorbable material. The abdominal wall is closed using interrupted sutures. The skin is closed using non-absorbable monofilament interrupted sutures.

Clinical Example (44715)

An intestine allograft that has been procured with cold preservation and maintained cold is received at the transplant recipient site of service and requires preparation prior to transplantation. Standard backbench preparation, including mobilization and fashioning of the superior mesenteric artery and vein, is performed.

Description of Procedure (44715)

The intestine allograft is received in a sterile container and is maintained in cold preservation solution. The surgeon requests and confirms that a sterile backbench is set up in the operating room (OR), with appropriate instruments for the backbench dissection. An appropriate recipient has been identified. The correct identification process is carried out to make sure that the intestine allograft is being allocated to the right recipient. The surgeon must make the appropriate arrangements with the operating room and staff to allow for sterile dissection of the allograft in coordination with the recipient procedure. The surgeon scrubs and gowns. The allograft is removed from the sterile container and placed on a sterile table, on ice, while bathing in cold preservation solution. The intestine allograft is inspected to be certain that it is grossly intact and that its appearance is acceptable.

With continuous bathing in cold preservation solution, dissection and removal of surrounding soft tissues are carried out. The superior mesenteric artery and vein are identified and evaluated to ensure that their integrity is not violated and that they have been mobilized to an adequate length and are otherwise fashioned appropriately to perform anastomoses with the intended recipient vessels.

The intestine allograft is kept cold in anticipation of transplantation. If necessary, the intestine allograft is repackaged in a sterile fashion prior to transplantation.

 ### Clinical Example (44720)

A vein of an intestine allograft is too short or is damaged in such a way that it is not suitable for anastomosis with the intended transplant recipient artery. Using a vein graft procured from the donor (or properly preserved vein graft procured from another ABO compatible donor allograft), a backbench venous anastomosis is performed on the allograft to create an extension graft.

Description of Procedure (44720)

On ice, with continuous bathing in cold preservation solution, a vein graft is procured from the donor (or properly preserved vein graft procured from another ABO compatible donor). The ends of the extension graft and the superior mesenteric vein are brought in close apposition. Using 5-0 or 6-0 prolene suture, the two vessels are sewn together end-to-end to create an extension graft. (Alternatively, if no vein graft is available, a comparably sized arterial graft obtained from the donor, the recipient, or another ABO compatible donor may be used.)

 ### Clinical Example (44721)

An artery of an intestine allograft is too short or is damaged in such a way that it is not suitable for anastomosis with the intended transplant recipient artery. Using an arterial graft procured from the donor (or properly preserved arterial graft procured from another ABO-compatible donor allograft), a backbench, arterial anastomosis is performed on the allograft to create an extension graft.

Description of Procedure (44721)

On ice, with continuous bathing in cold preservation solution, an arterial graft is procured from the donor (or properly preserved arterial graft procured from another ABO-compatible donor). The ends of the extension graft and the superior mesenteric artery are brought in close apposition. Using 6-0 or 7-0 prolene suture, the two vessels are sewn together end-to-end to create an extension graft. (Alternatively, if no arterial graft is available, a comparably sized vein graft obtained from the donor, the recipient, or another ABO-compatible donor may be used.)

Rectum

ENDOSCOPY

⊙ **45378** Colonoscopy, flexible, proximal to splenic flexure; diagnostic, with or without collection of specimen(s) by brushing or washing, with or without colon decompression (separate procedure)

⊙● **45391** with endoscopic ultrasound examination

▶(Do not report 45391 in conjunction with 45330, 45341, 45342, 45378, 76872)◀

⊙●45392 with transendoscopic ultrasound guided intramural or transmural fine needle aspiration/biopsy(s)

▶(Do not report 45392 in conjunction with 45330, 45341, 45342, 45378, 76872)◀

✍ Rationale

Codes 45391 and 45392 have been added to the Rectum Endoscopy subsection of the Digestive System section to describe proximal to splenic flexure flexible colonoscopy with endoscopic ultrasound examination and with transendoscopic ultrasound guided intramural or transmural fine needle aspiration/biopsy(s). Prior to 2005, there were no CPT codes that described colonoscopy with endoscopic ultrasound of the entire colon. Colonoscopy and endoscopic ultrasound evaluation of a detected abnormality with or without transendoscopic ultrasound guided fine needle aspiration/biopsy(s) during the same procedure may eliminate the need for subsequent procedures.

Code 45391 describes the proximal to splenic flexure flexible colonoscopy with endoscopic ultrasound examination. Code 45392 describes the proximal to splenic flexure flexible colonoscopy with transendoscopic ultrasound guided intramural or transmural fine needle aspiration/biopsy(s). Exclusionary notes were added following codes 45391 and 45392 instructing the user not to report codes 45391 and 45392 in conjunction with codes 45330, 45341, 45342, 45378, or 76872.

 ## Clinical Example (45391)

Physical examination in a 52-year-old female reveals guaiac positive stools and a rectal mass identified on digital rectal examination. A computed tomography (CT) scan reveals rectal wall thickening but no metastatic disease. Colonoscopy with endoscopic ultrasound is requested to evaluate and further stage the suspected tumor, and to assess the remainder of the colon for additional lesions.

Description of Procedure (45391)

A standard colonoscope is inserted into the rectum and advanced through the colon to the cecum. The colonic mucosa appears normal except for an ulcerated 2 cm lesion which is seen in the lower rectum. A dedicated echoendoscope is prepared with a balloon placed over the transducer housing. The echoendoscope is inserted into the rectum and advanced under direct visualization. In the area of the mucosal lesion, the balloon is filled with water to achieve acoustic coupling. Continuous imaging with ultrasound is performed and visualization of the lesion, the colonic wall layers, and the peri-colonic structures is procured. No regional lymph node enlargement is identified. The echoendoscope is withdrawn.

 ## Clinical Example (45392)

A 72-year-old male presents with left flank pain. He underwent gastrectomy for gastric cancer two years earlier. An abdominal CT scan demonstrates a 2 cm mass adjacent to the sigmoid colon. Colonoscopy with endoscopic ultrasound and a possible transendoscopic, ultrasound-guided biopsy are requested.

Description of Procedure (45392)

A standard colonoscope is inserted into the rectum and advanced through the colon to the cecum. The colonoscope is withdrawn and the mucosa carefully

⊘=Modifier 51 Exempt   ⊙=Conscious Sedation   ✚=Add-on Code

examined. In the sigmoid colon, there is a smooth, extrinsic appearing compression of the colonic lumen without obvious mucosal abnormalities. The remainder of the procedure is unremarkable. A dedicated echoendoscope is prepared with a balloon placed over the transducer housing. The echoendoscope is inserted into the rectum and advanced through the colon under direct visualization. In the area of the suspected lesion, the acoustic coupling balloon is filled with water. Continuous imaging with ultrasound is performed and visualization of the lesion, the colonic wall layers and the peri-colonic structures is procured. An extracolonic mass is seen adjacent to the sigmoid colon. As the identified abnormality may represent recurrent disease, fine needle aspiration biopsy is undertaken. Intravenous antibiotics are administered to the patient. The first echoendoscope is withdrawn. A linear scanning echoendoscope is prepared for the exam. The linear scanning echoendoscope is introduced into the rectum and advanced to the sigmoid colon under direct visualization. A needle biopsy catheter is advanced through the linear scanning echoendoscope and directed under ultrasound guidance into the lesion of interest. Multiple biopsies are taken until an adequate sample is procured. The echoendoscope is withdrawn.

Anus

EXCISION

46260   Hemorrhoidectomy, internal and external, complex or extensive;

46261   with fissurectomy

46262   with fistulectomy, with or without fissurectomy

▶(For injection of hemorrhoids, use 46500; for destruction, see 46934-46936; for ligation, see 46945, 46946; for hemorrhoidopexy, use 46947)◀

INTRODUCTION

▶(For excision of hemorrhoids, see 46250-46262; for destruction, see 46934-46936; for ligation, see 46945, 46946; for hemorrhoidopexy, use 46947)◀

46500   Injection of sclerosing solution, hemorrhoids

DESTRUCTION

46934   Destruction of hemorrhoids, any method; internal

46935   external

46936   internal and external

▶(For excision of hemorrhoids, see 46250-46262; for injection, use 46500; for ligation, see 46945, 46946; for hemorrhoidopexy, use 46947)◀

SUTURE

 ●46947 Hemorrhoidopexy (eg, for prolapsing internal hemorrhoids) by stapling

▶(For excision of hemorrhoids, see 46250-46262; for injection, use 46500; for destruction, see 46934-46936)◀

 Rationale

Code 46947 was established to allow a method for coding repair of a hemorrhoidal prolapse utilizing a stapling technique. This procedure is different than other internal hemorrhoidectomy codes, which involve either excision and suture ligation or rubber band ligation of hemorrhoidal tissue. Use of the anoscope is included as part of the procedure. Cross-references were added following the Introduction heading and codes 46462, 46936, 46947 and preceding code 46500 referring to the appropriate codes for other procedures which may be performed for treatment of hemorrhoids.

Clinical Example (46947)

A 36-year-old female presents with grade III, prolapsing, internal hemorrhoids that have failed non-operative management. After the decision is made to operate, the surgeon reviews all the previous laboratory and endoscopic studies, and informed consent is obtained. At operation, she undergoes a stapled hemorrhoidopexy. Postoperative visits are conducted as necessary during the 90-day global period to assure normal recovery and the absence of complications.

Description of Procedure (46947)

A progressive anal dilation is performed, and a circular anoscope is inserted into the anus. A purse-string suture anoscope is inserted through the circular anoscope. A circumferential purse-string suture is placed into the mucosa and submucosa only. A digital vaginal examination is performed to confirm that the posterior vaginal wall is not incorporated into the purse-string suture. Once the vaginal exam is completed, the purse-string suture is gently tightened to draw the redundant rectal mucosa into the lumen of the rectum. An opened stapler is inserted through the circular anoscope, and the anvil is passed through the purse-string suture. The purse-string suture is tied around the shaft of the stapler. The suture threader is used to pull the free ends of the suture through lateral channels of the stapler housing. The stapler is tightened. The vagina is once again examined to confirm that the posterior vaginal wall is not incorporated into the stapler. The stapler is fired and held closed for one minute to assist hemostasis. The head of the stapler is opened, and the stapler and circular anoscope are removed together. The specimen is removed from the stapler and inspected by the surgeon to verify that a complete circumferential excision of tissue was obtained. A digital examination confirms that the staple line is circumferential. The purse-string anoscope or a retractor is then inserted into the anus to inspect for bleeding at the staple line. Local anesthetic may be injected for post-operative analgesia.

Liver

▶LIVER TRANSPLANTATION◀

▶Liver allotransplantation involves three distinct components of physician work:◀

▶1) ***Cadaver donor hepatectomy***, which includes harvesting the graft and cold preservation of the graft (perfusing with cold preservation solution and cold maintenance) (use 47133). ***Living donor hepatectomy***, which includes harvesting the graft, cold preservation of the graft (perfusing with cold preservation solution and cold maintenance), and care of the donor (see 47140-47142).◀

▶2) ***Backbench work***:◀

▶Standard preparation of the whole liver graft will include one of the following:◀

▶Preparation of whole liver graft (including cholecystectomy, if necessary, and dissection and removal of surrounding soft tissues to prepare vena cava, portal vein, hepatic artery, and common bile duct for implantation) (use 47143).◀

▶Preparation as described for whole liver graft, plus trisegment split into two partial grafts (use 47144).◀

▶Preparation as described for whole liver graft, plus lobe split into two partial grafts (use 47145).◀

▶Additional reconstruction of the liver graft may include venous and/or arterial anastomosis(es) (see 47146, 47147).◀

▶3) ***Recipient liver allotransplantation***, which includes recipient hepatectomy (partial or whole), transplantation of the allograft (partial or whole), and care of the recipient (see 47135, 47136).◀

▲**47133**   Donor hepatectomy (including cold preservation), from cadaver donor

▲**47140**   Donor hepatectomy (including cold preservation), from living donor; left lateral segment only (segments II and III)

●**47143**   Backbench standard preparation of cadaver donor whole liver graft prior to allotransplantation, including cholecystectomy, if necessary, and dissection and removal of surrounding soft tissues to prepare the vena cava, portal vein, hepatic artery, and common bile duct for implantation; without trisegment or lobe split

●**47144**   with trisegment split of whole liver graft into two partial liver grafts (ie, left lateral segment (segments II and III) and right trisegment (segments I and IV through VIII))

●**47145**   with lobe split of whole liver graft into two partial liver grafts (ie, left lobe (segments II, III, and IV) and right lobe (segments I and V through VIII))

●**47146**   Backbench reconstruction of cadaver or living donor liver graft prior to allotransplantation; venous anastomosis, each

●**47147**   arterial anastomosis, each

▶(Do not report 47143-47147 in conjunction with 47120-47125, 47600, 47610)◀

✍ Rationale

A new heading, new guidelines and five new codes have been added to the Liver subsection of the Digestive System section to describe liver allotransplantation services. Codes 47133 and 47140 have been revised to include cold preservation and to not include preparation and maintenance of allograft. An exclusionary note has been added following code 47147 instructing the user not to report codes 47143 through 47147 in conjunction with codes 47120-47125, 47600 or 47610.

The new guidelines clarify the three distinct components of physician work involved in liver allotransplantation, which are donor hepatectomy, backbench work, and recipient liver allotransplantation.

Codes 47143, 47144, and 47145 describe backbench preparation of cadaver donor whole liver graft, including cholecystectomy, if necessary, and dissection and removal of surrounding soft tissues to prepare the vena cava, portal vein, hepatic artery, and common bile duct for implantation. Code 47143 is reported when the procedure is performed without a trisegment. Code 47144 is reported when the procedure is performed with a trisegment split of a whole liver graft into two partial liver grafts. Code 41745 is reported when the procedure is performed with a lobe split of a whole liver graft into two partial liver grafts.

Codes 47146 and 47147 describe backbench preparation of a cadaver or living donor liver graft prior to allotransplantation. Code 47146 is reported when the procedure includes venous anastomosis. Code 47147 is reported when the procedure includes arterial anastomosis.

🩺 Clinical Example (47133)

In a previously healthy 30-year-old, non-obese, brain-dead, automobile accident victim, who had a moderate elevation of blood alcohol level on admission, the retrieval surgeon assesses the liver visually, by palpation, and decides to biopsy, which is satisfactory. Coordination between the other organ teams is provided for. The dissection of the hilum, the coronary ligaments, and preservation of an accessary left gastric artery are done. The biliary tract is flushed. The inferior epigastric/portal vein and the aorta are dissected and prepared for flushing. Cannulation and flushing with vena cava venting are carried out. The hilum dissection is completed with care to avoid damage to accessory arteries. The remaining attachments with the cava are cut, and the liver is removed and packaged.

After the trip back to the transplanting hospital, on the back table the vena cavae are dissected and tested for leaks. The protal vein is dissected, cannulated for later flushing, and tested for leaks. The artery is dissected, with care to preserve the accessory left.

Description of Procedure (47133)

The brain-dead, ventilated donor is positioned, prepped, and drapped. Exploration of the abdomen through a midline incision extending cephalad from the pubis through the sternum and diaphragming is performed as necessary, and manual palpation of intra-abdominal viscera is done to rule out unanticipated masses,

⊘=Modifier 51 Exempt   ⊙=Conscious Sedation   ✚=Add-on Code

abcesses, etc. Dissection is performed of all attachments to the liver so that the liver is fully mobilized and attached only by the suprahepatic vena cava, infrahepatic vena cava, portal vein and celiac artery trunk (look for accessory or anomalous hepatic arteries). The common hepatic duct is dissected to the head of the pancreas; heparinize the patient and cannulate the infrarenal aorta and cannulate the inferior mesenteric vein; apply occluding vascular clamps to the suprahepatic aorta and flush both cannulas with cold preservation solution while applying cold topical rinse solution; divide the portal vein, hepatic artery, common bile duct, and inferior vena cava above and below the liver; remove the common iliac artery and its bifurcation branches and a segment of external iliac vein for possible use in reconstructing the liver's vasculature; reexamine the liver on the back table and package it in sterile fashion with vessels in preservation solution in ice for transport and procure additional lymph nodes from small bowel mesentery as needed for completion of crossmatching.

Clinical Example (47140)

A willing volunteer living-donor has been identified for this infant. In this particular case, it is a parent whose blood type is compatible, who has been evaluated and been found not to have any medical or psychosocial conditions that would contraindicate living donation, is free from coercion, and has been given every opportunity to decline the procedure. The anatomical data on the donor liver reveals no vascular or biliary anatomical variance that would preclude the use of the left lateral segment (Couinaud segments II and III). The volume of the left lateral segment is measured radiologically as 120 cc 3, equivalent roughly to 120 gm of liver tissue [graft to body weight ratio (GBWR) is 1.2%—must exceed 0.8%]. Therefore, the left lateral segment is considered to be the graft of choice for the recipient. No hepatic steatosis is identified. To the best of the transplant team's knowledge, there is no financial compensation planned and the risks of the procedure have been thoroughly covered by the transplant team.

Once a decision has been made to proceed, the surgeon reviews laboratory and x-ray/imaging studies to plan the operative approach, discusses the procedure with the patient and his/her family, and obtains informed consent. At operation, the liver is mobilized appropriately and a careful examination is made of the entire abdomen and liver to rule out any pathology that might contraindicate living donation. A donor hepatectomy, with preparation and maintenance of allograft, left lateral segment only (segments II and III) is performed. Postoperative care of the donor includes all necessary hospital and office visits through the 90-day global period.

Description of Procedure (47140)

A skin incision is made consisting of bilateral subcostal incisions extended to the xiphoid in the midline. The anterior abdominal wall is carefully divided. The peritoneum is entered. The round and falciform ligaments are divided. The self-retaining mechanical retractor is secured to the operating room table and the various attachments are utilized and exposure obtained for the hepatic mobilization and resection. A thorough exploration of the area around the liver is undertaken, including palpation and visualization of the left lateral segment. The abdominal contents are examined for any evidence of pathology. The left triangular ligament is taken down, exposing the left hepatic vein. Any adhesions present are taken down by sharp and blunt dissection. The porta hepatis is isolated and encircled with a Penrose drain. The left hepatic artery is identified within the porta hepatis and is dissected free of the surrounding tissues and looped with a vessel loop.

The gastrohepatic ligament is taken down and great care is taken to identify any potential aberrant left hepatic arteries within the ligament. If an artery is found, the aberrant left hepatic artery is meticulously dissected back to the junction with the left gastric artery. The left lateral segment is reflected anteriorly and the ligamentum venosum is transected. The round ligament is carefully dissected away from segment IV of the liver in the recess of Rex and all comeback vessels and bile ducts are transected in this plane. Dissection is carried down to the left portal vein as the falciform remnant enters the portal vein. The left portal vein is dissected and encircled and great care is taken not to injure the portal bifurcation. Short caudate branches of the left portal vein are divided. The left bile duct is identified within the liver parenchyma, preferably after the segment IV duct has entered. The left hepatic duct is transected sharply within the liver parenchyma. There are often multiple bile ducts and these need to be carefully identified and transected within the liver parenchyma aiming to preserve vascular supply to the bile duct and great care is taken not to injure the remaining bile duct. The left hepatic vein is carefully dissected and, if possible, encircled within the liver parenchyma. Intraoperative ultrasound is undertaken to locate the junction of the left and middle hepatic veins. The ultrasound dissector is then grasped and the presumed area for resection is marked with a cautery. The ultrasound dissector is then used to outline the area for dissection. Individual vessels and bile ducts are identified in the depths of the ultrasonic dissection and ligated carefully with suture and divided. Hemostasis within the liver is secured, and suture is used as necessary to repair vessels which one wishes to preserve. The harmonic scalpel may be used in thin areas of the liver. Hemostasis is secured in both raw surfaces making certain that there are no bile leaks.

The argon beam coagulator may be utilized continuously on the raw surface of the liver to stop minimal oozing in an effort to prevent blood transfusion in an otherwise healthy donor, thus achieving meticulous hemostasis while taking care not to coagulate bile ducts. Once the parenchymal transection is completed and in coordination with the recipient's procedure, appropriate vascular clamps are applied to the left portal vein, left hepatic artery, and left hepatic vein and the left lateral segment is removed. This previous step requires two additional assistants who will prepare and preserve the left lateral segment organ donation, including perfusion with cold preservation solution while the vascular and biliary stumps are carefully oversewn by the primary surgeon in the donor. The left portal vein, left hepatic artery and left hepatic veins, and left bile duct(s) is(are) oversewn with suture in turn. The artery is doubly ligated with suture. A careful check of the raw surface is carried out, assuring hemostasis and the absence of new bile leaks. The abdominal cavity is copiously irrigated with antibiotic-laden solution. One closed-suction drain is placed in the immediate vicinity of the resection towards the cut edge of the liver. The position of the nasogastric tube is checked. Perioperative antibiotics are given preoperatively, and are repeated as necessary. Wound towels and the retractor are removed. The abdominal wall is closed in layered fashion. The skin is closed in the usual fashion.

 Clinical Example (47143)

A cadaver whole liver graft that has been procured with cold preservation and maintained cold is received at the transplant recipient site of service and requires preparation prior to transplantation. Standard backbench preparation, including a cholecystectomy and dissection of surrounding soft tissues to prepare the vena cava, portal vein, hepatic artery, and common bile duct for implantation, is performed.

Description of Procedure (47143)

The whole liver graft is received in a sterile container and is maintained in cold preservation solution. The surgeon requests and confirms that a sterile backbench is set up in the operating room, with appropriate instruments for the backbench dissection. An appropriate recipient has been identified. The correct identification process is carried out to make sure that the liver graft is being allocated to the right recipient. The surgeon must make the appropriate arrangements with the operating room and staff to allow for sterile dissection of the organ in coordination with the recipient procedure. The surgeon scrubs and gowns. The liver is removed from the sterile container and placed on a sterile table, on ice, while bathing in cold preservation solution. The liver graft is inspected to be certain that it is grossly intact and that its appearance is acceptable.

With continuous bathing in cold preservation solution, dissection and removal of surrounding soft tissues are carried out. The retrohepatic vena cava is identified and stay sutures are placed in both the supra- and infra-hepatic aspects of the cava to allow for appropriate dissection. The left triangular ligament, as well as the remaining coronary ligaments, are dissected free of the supra hepatic cava. Phrenic veins are identified and suture-ligated as necessary on both the right and left sides. The dissection is continued caudad and the adrenal vein is identified and ligated. The adrenal gland is then freed from the bare area and this dissection is continued by dividing the right triangular ligament. At this point, the cava is tested for leaks by placing a vascular clamp at both the upper and lower ends in sequence and injecting preservation solution into the cava under pressure. Once the cava is prepared for implantation, if a "piggy-back" caval anastomosis is planned, the posterior surface of the cephalad end of the donor cava is cleared adequately to allow sufficient cava to sew to on either side of a longitudinal posterior caval slit. This caval slit is created by dividing the posterior aspect of the cava from the suprahepatic caval orifice caudad for 3-4 cm to allow an adequate orifice for a triangulated anastomosis with the recipient cava.

Attention is now focused on the porta hepatis. The celiac axis is identified and, using meticulous dissection, the splenic, left gastric and gastroduodenal arteries are identified and ligated. Next, the portal vein is dissected free of surrounding soft tissues, inspected for holes and prepared for implantation. The common bile duct is then identified and dissected away from surrounding soft tissues taking care not to devascularize the duct. A cholecystectomy is performed by identifying and ligating the cystic artery and the cystic duct, and dissecting the gallbladder away from the gallbladder fossa using sharp dissection.

The liver graft is kept cold in anticipation of transplantation. If necessary, the liver graft is repackaged in a sterile fashion and maintained cold prior to transplantation.

Clinical Example (47144)

A cadaver whole liver graft that has been procured with cold preservation and maintained cold is received at the transplant recipient site of service and requires preparation prior to transplantation. There are two transplant recipients scheduled to receive partial graft transplants. Standard backbench preparation, including a cholecystectomy and dissection of surrounding soft tissues to prepare the vena cava, portal vein, hepatic artery, and common bile duct for implantation, is performed. Additionally, an ex vivo trisegment split is performed on the whole liver graft to prepare a left lateral segment graft (segments II and III) and a right trisegment graft (segments I and IV through VIII) for transplantation into two recipients.

Description of Procedure (47144)

The whole liver graft is received in a sterile container and is maintained in cold preservation solution. The surgeon requests and confirms that a sterile backbench is set up in the operating room, with appropriate instruments for the backbench dissection. Appropriate recipients have been identified. The correct identification process is carried out to make sure that the liver graft is being allocated to the correct recipients. The surgeon must make the appropriate arrangements with the operating room staff to allow for sterile dissection of the organ in coordination with both recipient procedures. The surgeon scrubs and gowns. The whole liver is removed from the sterile container and placed on a sterile table, on ice, while bathing in cold preservation solution. The liver graft is inspected to be certain that it is grossly intact and that its appearance is acceptable.

With continuous bathing in cold preservation solution, dissection and removal of surrounding soft tissues are carried out. The retrohepatic vena cava is identified and stay sutures are placed in both the supra- and infra-hepatic aspects of the cava to allow for appropriate dissection. The left triangular ligament, as well as the remaining coronary ligaments, are dissected free of the supra hepatic cava. Phrenic veins are identified and suture-ligated as necessary on both the right and left sides. The dissection is continued caudad and the adrenal vein is identified and ligated. The adrenal gland is then freed from the bare area and this dissection is continued by dividing the right triangular ligament. At this point, the cava is tested for leaks by placing a vascular clamp at both the upper and lower ends in sequence and injecting preservation solution into the cava under pressure. Once the cava is prepared for implantation, if a "piggy-back" caval anastomosis is planned, the posterior surface of the cephalad end of the donor cava is cleared adequately to allow sufficient cava to sew to on either side of a longitudinal posterior caval slit. This caval slit is created by dividing the posterior aspect of the cava from the suprahepatic caval orifice caudad for 3-4 cm to allow an adequate

⊘ =Modifier 51 Exempt   ⊙ =Conscious Sedation   ✚ =Add-on Code

orifice for a triangulated anastomosis with the recipient cava.

Attention is now focused on the porta hepatis. The celiac axis is identified and using meticulous dissection, the splenic, left gastric and gastroduodenal arteries are identified and ligated. Next, the portal vein is dissected free of surrounding soft tissues, inspected for holes and prepared for implantation. The common bile duct is then identified and dissected away from surrounding soft tissues taking care not to devascularize the duct. A cholecystectomy is performed by identifying and ligating the cystic artery and the cystic duct, and dissecting the gallbladder away from the gallbladder fossa using sharp dissection.

Next, attention is turned to splitting the whole graft into two partial grafts. The left hepatic vein is dissected free of the liver at its origin and transected sharply. The defect in the cava is repaired with a layer of fine (6-0) monofilament suture. The left portal structures are inspected and identified. The left hepatic artery is transected either beyond the bifurcation with the right hepatic artery or beyond a significant branch to segment IV, depending on the existing arterial anatomy. The arterial stump is oversewn in the main hepatic artery with a layer of fine (6-0) monofilament suture, making sure not to compromise the lumen of the main hepatic artery. Alternatively, the right hepatic artery is cut at the bifurcation with the left, and the stump of the right hepatic artery is oversewn, leaving the celiac trunk with the left lateral segment. The round ligament is identified and the "come-back" vessels to segment IV are meticulously divided between ligatures until the left portal vein is identified. The left portal vein is dissected free from the surrounding soft tissues, ligating and dividing caudate branches as necessary. The left portal vein is transected at the bifurcation and the stump is oversewn with fine (6-0) monofilament suture. Alternatively, the right portal vein is transected and its stump oversewn, leaving the main portal vein with the left lateral segment. A small probe is inserted into the main bile duct and the location of the right and left ducts is determined. If necessary, a cholangiogram is obtained using fluoroscopy. The left duct is transected at the desired level (alternatively, the right duct is transected) and the stump oversewn with fine (6-0) Prolene. The parenchyma of the liver is now dissected along the plane of the falciform ligament aiming towards the Rex fissure, ligating all visible tubular structures encountered with silk ligatures until the left lateral segment (segments II and III) is completely separated (split) from the remaining liver (segments I and IV through VIII—right trisegment).

Both grafts are perfused with cold preservation solution looking for obvious leaks in the parenchyma which are oversewn where necessary. The two grafts are packaged separately in cold preservation solution and kept cold in anticipation of transplantation. If necessary, the liver grafts are repackaged in a sterile fashion and maintained cold prior to transplantation.

 Clinical Example (47145)

A cadaver whole liver graft that has been procured with cold preservation and maintained cold is received at the transplant recipient site of service and requires preparation prior to transplantation. There are two transplant recipients scheduled to receive partial graft transplants. Standard backbench preparation, including a cholecystectomy and dissection of surrounding soft tissues to prepare the vena cava, portal vein, hepatic artery, and common bile duct for implantation, is performed. Additionally, a backbench lobe split is performed on the whole liver graft to prepare a left lobe graft (segments II, III, and IV) and a right lobe graft (segments I and V through VIII) for transplantation into two recipients.

Description of Procedure (47145)

The whole liver graft is received in a sterile container and is maintained in cold preservation solution. The surgeon requests and confirms that a sterile backbench is set up in the operating room, with appropriate instruments for the backbench dissection. Appropriate recipients have been identified. The correct identification process is carried out to make sure that the liver graft is being allocated to the correct recipients. The surgeon must make the appropriate arrangements with the operating room staff to allow for sterile dissection of the organ in coordination with both recipient procedures. The surgeon scrubs and gowns. The whole liver is removed from the sterile container and placed on a sterile table, on ice, while bathing in cold preservation solution. The liver graft is inspected to be certain that it is grossly intact and that its appearance is acceptable.

With continuous bathing in cold preservation solution, dissection and removal of surrounding soft tissues are carried out. The retrohepatic vena cava is identified and stay sutures are placed in both the supra- and infra-hepatic aspects of the cava to allow for appropriate dissection. The left triangular ligament, as well as the remaining coronary ligaments, are dissected free of the supra hepatic cava. Phrenic veins are identified and suture-ligated as necessary on both the right and left sides. The dissection is continued caudad and the adrenal vein is identified and ligated. The adrenal gland is then freed from the bare area and this dissection is continued by dividing the right triangular ligament. At this point, the cava is tested for leaks by placing a vascular clamp at both the upper and lower ends in sequence and injecting preservation solution into the cava under pressure. Once the cava is prepared for implantation, if a "piggy-back" caval anastomosis is planned, the posterior surface of the cephalad end of the donor cava is cleared adequately to allow sufficient cava to sew to on either side of a longitudinal posterior caval slit. This caval slit is created by dividing the posterior aspect of the cava from the suprahepatic caval orifice caudad for 3-4 cm to allow an adequate orifice for a triangulated anastomosis with the recipient cava.

Attention is now focused on the porta hepatis. The celiac axis is identified, and using meticulous dissection, the splenic, left gastric, and gastroduodenal arteries are identified and ligated. Next, the portal vein is dissected free of surrounding soft tissues, inspected for holes and prepared for implantation. The common bile duct is then identified and dissected away from surrounding soft tissues taking care not to devascularize the duct. A cholecystectomy is performed by identifying and ligating the cystic artery and the cystic duct, and dissecting the gallbladder away from the gallbladder fossa using sharp dissection.

Next, attention is turned to splitting the whole graft into two partial grafts. The left and middle hepatic veins will be dissected free of the liver at their origin and will be transected sharply. The defect in the cava will be repaired with a layer of fine monofilament suture. Next, the left portal structures will be inspected and identified. The left hepatic artery is transected beyond the bifurcation with the right hepatic. The arterial stump will be oversewn in the main hepatic artery with a layer of fine monofilament suture, making sure not to compromise the lumen of the main hepatic artery. Alternatively, the right hepatic artery is cut at the bifurcation with the left, and the stump of the right hepatic artery is oversewn, leaving the celiac trunk with the left lobe. The left portal vein is dissected free from the surrounding soft tissues, ligating and dividing caudate branches as necessary. The left portal vein is transected at the bifurcation and the stump is oversewn with fine monofilament suture. Alternatively, the right portal vein is transected and its stump oversewn, leaving the main portal vein with the left lobe. A small probe is inserted into the main bile duct and the location of the right and left ducts is determined. If necessary, a back table cholangiogram is obtained using fluoroscopy. The left duct is transected at the desired level (alternatively, the right duct is transected) and the stump oversewn with fine suture material. The parenchyma of the liver is now dissected along Cantlie's line (major fissure), ligating all visible tubular structures encountered with silk ligatures until the left lobe (segments II, III, and IV) is completely separated (split) from the right lobe (segments I and V through VIII).

Both grafts are perfused with cold preservation solution looking for obvious leaks in the parenchyma which are oversewn where necessary. The two grafts are packaged separately in cold preservation solution and kept cold in anticipation of transplantation. If necessary, the liver grafts are repackaged in a sterile fashion and maintained cold prior to transplantation.

Clinical Example (47146)

The patient is a liver graft recipient whose portal vein is thrombosed (non-usable) and a venous extension is necessary on the donor, liver, allograft, portal vein. Under loupe magnification, an anastomosis between a conduit (either the common or external iliac arteries) and the portal vein is performed on the donor allograft.

Description of Procedure (47146)

In the case of portal vein thrombosis in the recipient, a venous extension may be needed on the donor portal vein. On ice, with continuous bathing in cold preservation solution, a segment of donor iliac vein with matching diameter to the portal vein (either common or external iliac vein) is anastomosed end-to-end to the portal vein. This anastomosis is performed with fine monofilament suture. The liver graft is kept cold in anticipation of transplantation. If necessary, the liver graft is repackaged in a sterile fashion and maintained cold prior to transplantation.

Clinical Example (47147)

The right, hepatic artery of a liver allograft is aberrant or injured (lacerated) and continuity between the celiac axis and the vessel is necessary. Under loupe magnification, an arterial anastomosis is performed on the patient to reconstruct the right hepatic artery on the donor allograft.

Description of Procedure (47147)

On ice, with continuous bathing in cold preservation solution, an end-to-end or end-to-side arterial anastomoses between the right hepatic artery and the celiac axis is performed using either running or interrupted, fine monofilament suture under loupe magnification between either the superior mesenteric artery or the replaced (or injured) right, hepatic artery, and either the splenic artery stump, or the gastroduodenal artery stump. Depending on the anatomy of the donor, other techniques for arterial reconstruction may be applied. The liver graft is kept cold in anticipation of transplantation. If necessary, the liver graft is repackaged in a sterile fashion and maintained cold prior to transplantation.

Pancreas

PANCREAS TRANSPLANTATION

▶Pancreas allotransplantation involves three distinct components of physician work:◀

▶1) *Cadaver donor pancreatectomy*, which includes harvesting the pancreas graft, with or without duodenal segment, and cold preservation of the graft (perfusing with cold preservation solution and cold maintenance) (use 48550).◀

▶2) *Backbench work*:◀

▶Standard preparation of a cadaver donor pancreas allograft prior to transplantation includes dissection of the allograft from surrounding soft tissues, splenectomy, duodenotomy, ligation of bile duct, ligation of mesenteric vessels, and Y-graft arterial anastomoses from the iliac artery to the superior mesenteric artery and to the splenic artery (use 48551).◀

▶Additional reconstruction of a cadaver donor pancreas allograft prior to transplantation may include venous anastomosis(es) (use 48552).◀

▶3) *Recipient pancreas allotransplantation*, which includes transplantation of allograft, and care of the recipient (use 48554).◀

▲ 48550 Donor pancreatectomy (including cold preservation), with or without duodenal segment for transplantation

● 48551 Backbench standard preparation of cadaver donor pancreas allograft prior to transplantation, including dissection of allograft from surrounding soft tissues, splenectomy, duodenotomy, ligation of bile duct, ligation of mesenteric vessels, and Y-graft arterial anastomoses from iliac artery to superior mesenteric artery and to splenic artery

● 48552 Backbench reconstruction of cadaver donor pancreas allograft prior to transplantation, venous anastomosis, each

▶(Do not report 48551 and 48552 in conjunction with 35531, 35563, 35685, 38100-38102, 44010, 44820, 44850, 47460, 47505-47525, 47550-47556, 48100-48120, 48545)◀

✍ Rationale

New guidelines were added at the beginning of the Pancreas Transplantation subsection of the Digestive System section to clarify the three components of physician work involved in pancreas allotransplantation, which are cadaver donor pancreatectomy, backbench work, and recipient pancreas allotransplantation.

Codes 48551and 48552 were added to describe backbench preparation of a cadaver donor pancreas allograft prior to transplantation. Code 48551 is reported when dissection of the allograft from surrounding soft tissues, splenectomy, duodenotomy, ligation of bile duct, ligation of mesenteric vessels, and Y-graft arterial anastomosis from the iliac artery to the superior mesenteric artery and to the splenic artery are performed. Code 48552 is reported when venous anastomosis is performed.

Code 48550 was revised to include cold preservation and to not include preparation and maintenance of the allograft from the cadaver donor. An exclusionary note was added following code 48552 instructing the user not to report codes 48551 and 48552 in conjunction with 35531, 35563, 35685, 38100-38102, 44010, 44820, 44850, 47460, 47505-47525, 47550-47556, 48100-48120, and 48545.

 Clinical Example (48550)

The patient is brain-dead and on life support, and is to be used as a multiple organ donor, including a heart, lung, and liver and kidneys in addition to the pancreas. A cruciate incision, extending from the sternal notch to the pubis and from the right to the left flank, is used to expose all organs. The pancreas and liver are mobilized together as the initial maneuvers. The portal vein, hepatic artery and bile duct are dissected in the porta-hepatis and the gastro-duodenal artery ligated. The hepatic artery is freed from the pancreas to its origin at the celiac axis. The origin of the splenic artery is identified. The left gastric artery is ligated. The celiac and superior mesenteric arteries are isolated at their origins from the aorta. A Feuer maneuver is performed mobilizing the duodenum. Following incision of the suspensory ligaments of the liver and as the thoracic organs are clamped and removed, the aorta and inferior mesenteric vein are infused with synthetic solution. The duodenum is stapled and divided at the pylorus and at the ligament of Treitz. The splenic artery is divided at its origin and the portal vein is transected midway between the pancreas and liver, and the celiac axis at its origin, allowing the liver to be removed. The superior mesenteric artery is divided at its origin allowing the pancreas to be removed. The pancreas is reflushed with synthetic solution on the back table and prepared for preservation or for immediate transplantation.

Description of Procedure (48550)

Procedure includes positioning, prep, and drape of the patient, exploration of the donor through a midline incision from xyphoid to pubis with cruciate incisions as necessary, and manually evaluating the intra-abdominal viscera. The gastrocolic ligament is opened to expose the pancreas, and the vascular anatomy of the liver is assessed to recognize a possible accessory or anomalous right hepatic artery. The porta hepatis is ligated, and the common bile duct is identified and ligated adjacent to the duodenum and divided. Next, the common hepatic artery is identified, and dissected back towards the celiac trunk including dissection and vessel looping of the splenic artery. Dissection of the portal vein is performed, and a generous Kocher maneuver is done to mobilize the head of the pancreas. The nasogastric (NG) tube is positioned through the pylorus into the duodenum and antifungal and antibiotic agents are infused. The NG tube is pulled back into the stomach and a stapler is used to staple the portion of the duodenum just distal to the pylorus as well as the very proximal jejunum distal to the ligament of Treitz. The ligament attachments are taken down between the spleen and the abdominal wall, colon, and kidney, and the tail of the pancreas is mobilized. The mesocolon is then dissected and the middle colonic vessels identified. The superior mesenteric arterial cascade distal to the pancreatic uncinate is also identified. The patient is heparinized and the infrarenal aorta and inferior mesenteric vein are cannulated. Vascular clamps are applied to the suprahepatic aorta and the infrarenal aorta and inferior mesenteric vein are flushed with cold preservation solution. A topical cold solution is applied, and the amount of flushing of the pancreas through the splenic artery and superior mesenteric artery is controlled. The portal vein is divided, as well as the splenic artery and superior mesenteric artery. The middle colonic vessel is also divided, either with the stapler or individual suture ligatures. The small bowel mesenteric vascular arcade is also divided in a similar manner (stapler or individual suture ligatures). The pancreaticoduodenal allograft is removed, leaving the spleen intact, and the donor common iliac, external iliac, and internal iliac arteries and veins are procured. The physician reexamines the pancreaticoduodenal allograft on the "back table," and this allograft is packaged with vessels in preservation solution in ice for transport. Additional lymph nodes from small bowel mesentery are procured as needed for completion of crossmatching, and the physician closes the cadaver donor incision.

Clinical Example (48551)

A cadaver donor pancreas allograft that has been procured with cold preservation and maintained cold is received at the transplant recipient site of service. Standard backbench preparation, including dissection of the allograft from surrounding soft tissues, splenectomy, duodenotomy, ligation of bile duct, ligation of mesenteric vessels, and Y-graft arterial anastomoses from the iliac artery to the superior mesenteric artery and to the splenic artery, is performed.

Description of Procedure (48551)

The pancreas graft is received in a sterile container and is maintained in cold preservation solution. The surgeon requests and confirms that a sterile backbench is set up in the operating room, with appropriate instruments for the backbench dissection. An appropriate recipient has been identified. The correct identification process is carried out to make sure that the pancreas graft is being allocated to the right recipient. The surgeon must make the appropriate arrangements with the operating room and staff to allow for sterile dissection of the organ in coordination with the recipient procedure. The surgeon scrubs and gowns. The pancreas is removed from the sterile container and placed on a sterile table, on ice, while bathing in cold preservation solution. The pancreas graft is inspected to be certain that it is grossly intact and that its appearance is acceptable.

With continuous bathing in cold preservation solution, a splenectomy is performed by meticulously ligating and dividing the splenic vessels at the hilum of

⃠ =Modifier 51 Exempt   ⊙ =Conscious Sedation   ✛ =Add-on Code

the spleen, taking care not to injure the tail of the pancreas. Next, the duodenum is opened longitudinally across from the Sphincter of Oddi and washed clean of sulcus to locate the position of the sphincter. A catheter may be inserted into the common bile duct and passed through the sphincter to confirm sphincter location. Once the sphincter is located, the duodenum is shortened from both the pyloric end and the distal end. The feeding (mesenteric) vessels are carefully ligated and divided individually as the duodenum is dissected away from the pancreas distally. Proximally, the dissection is extended to remove the pylorus. Once the duodenum is trimmed to the desired length (12-14 cm), both ends are stapled and the ends are then oversewn with a non-absorbable suture for reinforcement. The common bile duct is ligated after the catheter is withdrawn. Next, attention is focused on the middle colic vessels, which must be securely ligated at the base of the transverse mesocolon with either suture ligatures or a staple line. This is followed by either individual or mass suture ligation and/or stapling of the superior mesenteric vessels at the root of small bowel mesentery. A Y-graft is then constructed from the junction of the external and internal (hypogastric) iliac arteries of the donor. An arterial anastomosis is constructed first between one of the Y limbs to the superior mesenteric artery (end-to-end), and a second anastomosis between the second limb of the Y and the splenic artery (end-to-end). These anastomoses are completed with fine monofilament suture under loupe magnification.

The pancreas is kept cold in anticipation of transplantation. If necessary, the pancreas is repackaged in a sterile fashion and maintained cold prior to transplantation.

Clinical Example (48552)

The portal vein on the pancreas allograft is short and requires an extension graft prior to transplantation in the patient. Under loupe magnification, an anastomosis between a conduit (either the common or external iliac vein) and the portal vein is performed on the allograft.

Description of Procedure (48552)

On ice, with continuous bathing in cold preservation solution, a segment of donor, iliac vein with matching diameter to the portal vein (either common or external iliac vein) is anastomosed end-to-end to the portal vein. The anastomosis is performed with fine, monofilament suture under loupe magnification.

Urinary System

Kidney

RENAL TRANSPLANTATION

▶Renal *auto* transplantation includes reimplantation of the autograft as the primary procedure, along with secondary extra-corporeal procedure(s) (eg, partial nephrectomy, nephrolithotomy) reported with modifier 51 (see 50380 and applicable secondary procedure(s)).◀

▶Renal allotransplantation involves three distinct components of physician work:◀

▶1) **_Cadaver donor nephrectomy, unilateral or bilateral_**, which includes harvesting the graft(s) and cold preservation of the graft(s) (perfusing with cold preservation solution and cold maintenance) (use 50300). **_Living donor nephrectomy_**, which includes harvesting the graft, cold preservation of the graft (perfusing with cold preservation solution and cold maintenance), and care of the donor (see 50320, 50547).◀

▶2) **_Backbench work_**:◀

▶Standard preparation of a cadaver donor renal allograft prior to transplantation including dissection and removal of perinephric fat, diaphragmatic and retroperitoneal attachments; excision of adrenal gland; and preparation of ureter(s), renal vein(s), and renal artery(s), ligating branches, as necessary (use 50323).◀

▶Standard preparation of a living donor renal allograft (open or laparoscopic) prior to transplantation including dissection and removal of perinephric fat and preparation of ureter(s), renal vein(s), and renal artery(s), ligating branches, as necessary (use 50325).◀

▶Additional reconstruction of a cadaver or living donor renal allograft prior to transplantation may include venous, arterial, and/or ureteral anastomosis(es) necessary for implantation (see 50327-50329).◀

▶3) **_Recipient renal allotransplantation_**, which includes transplantation of the allograft (with or without recipient nephrectomy) and care of the recipient (see 50360, 50365).◀

▲ **50300** Donor nephrectomy (including cold preservation); from cadaver donor, unilateral or bilateral

▲ **50320** open, from living donor

● **50323** Backbench standard preparation of cadaver donor renal allograft prior to transplantation, including dissection and removal of perinephric fat, diaphragmatic and retroperitoneal attachments, excision of adrenal gland, and preparation of ureter(s), renal vein(s), and renal artery(s), ligating branches, as necessary

▶(Do not report 50323 in conjunction with 60540, 60545)◀

● **50325** Backbench standard preparation of living donor renal allograft (open or laparoscopic) prior to transplantation, including dissection and removal of perinephric fat and preparation of ureter(s), renal vein(s), and renal artery(s), ligating branches, as necessary

● **50327** Backbench reconstruction of cadaver or living donor renal allograft prior to transplantation; venous anastomosis, each

● **50328** arterial anastomosis, each

● **50329** ureteral anastomosis, each

▲ **50360** Renal allotransplantation, implantation of graft; without recipient nephrectomy

50380 Renal autotransplantation, reimplantation of kidney

(For ▶renal autotransplantation◀ extra-corporeal ▶(bench)◀ surgery, use autotransplantation as the primary procedure and report secondary procedure▶(s)◀ (eg, partial nephrectomy, nephrolithotomy) ▶with◀ modifier 51)

Ø =Modifier 51 Exempt   ⊙ =Conscious Sedation   ✚ =Add-on Code

Rationale

Five new codes were added to the Renal Transplantation subsection of the Urinary System section to describe backbench preparation of donor renal allograft. Codes 50300, 50320, 50360, and 50547 were revised. Three new parenthetical notes were added, and one was revised. New guidelines were added following the Renal Transplantation heading that indicate the services that are included in renal autotransplantation, as well as the three distinct components of physician work involved in renal allotransplantation.

Code 50323 was added to describe backbench preparation of cadaver donor renal allograft prior to transplantation. Code 50325 was added to describe backbench preparation of living donor renal allograft, either open or laparoscopic, prior to transplantation. Codes 50327, 50328, and 50329 were added to describe backbench reconstruction of cadaver or living donor renal allograft anastomosis prior to transplantation. Code 50327 should be reported for venous anastomosis. Code 50328 should be reported for arterial anastomosis. Code 50329 should be reported for ureteral anastomosis. As indicated by the descriptors of these codes, each anastomosis is separately reported.

Code 50300 was revised to include cold preservation and to exclude preparation and maintenance of the allograft. Code 50321 was revised with the removal of the repetitive donor nephrectomy language, and with the removal of the parenthetical note stating "excluding preparation and maintenance of allograft." Code 50360 was revised to describe renal allotransplantation with implantation of graft without recipient nephrectomy.

A parenthetical note was added following code 50323 instructing users not to report code 50323 in conjunction with codes 60540 and 60545. The parenthetical note following code 50380 was revised to instruct users to report autotransplantation as the primary procedure and then add the second procedure for renal autotransplantation. Two new parenthetical notes were added instructing users to use code 50325 for backbench renal allograft standard preparation prior to transplantation and to see codes 50327 through 50329 for backbench renal allograft reconstruction prior to transplantation.

Clinical Example (50300)

The patient is brain-dead or is on life support.

Description of Procedure (50300)

A long, xiphoid to pubis incision is used to expose the organs to be removed. Careful dissection prepares both kidneys and a long segment of the ureters. The kidneys are removed with all major vessels attached (ie, aortic cuff and vena cava). The renal grafts are then prepared for preservation or for immediate transplantation.

Clinical Example (50320)

The donor is a healthy, related sibling/parent/child of a patient suffering from chronic renal failure.

Description of Procedure (50320)

Through a generous flank/abdominal incision, the kidney is removed and is carefully dissected with particular attention being paid to the renal and ureteral blood supply. A long length of ureter (level of iliac artery) is dissected. The renal artery and vein are dissected to their origins (aorta and vena cava, respectively). After removal, the kidney is perfused and readied for immediate transplantation.

 Clinical Example (50323)

A cadaver whole renal graft that has been procured with cold preservation and maintained cold is received at the transplant recipient site of service and requires preparation prior to transplantation. Standard backbench dissection and removal of perinephric fat, diaphragmatic, and retroperitoneal attachments, excision of adrenal gland, and preparation of renal vein(s), renal artery(ies), and ureter(s), ligating branches, as necessary, is performed.

Description of Procedure (50323)

The renal graft is received in a sterile container and is maintained in cold preservation solution. The surgeon requests and confirms that a sterile backbench is set up in the OR, with appropriate instruments for the backbench dissection. An appropriate recipient has been identified. The correct identification process is carried out to make sure that the renal graft is being allocated to the right recipient. The surgeon must make the appropriate arrangements with the operating room and staff to allow for sterile dissection of the organ in coordination with the recipient procedure. The surgeon scrubs and gowns. The renal graft is removed from the sterile container and placed on a sterile table, on ice, while bathing in cold preservation solution. The renal graft is inspected to be certain that it is grossly intact and that its appearance is acceptable.

With continuous bathing in cold preservation solution, the aortic cuff is first identified in order to determine the presence or absence of aberrant renal arteries. The renal vein(s) is (are) then identified. The adrenal and gonadal veins are identified, ligated and divided. Gerota's fascia and the perinephric adipose tissue is removed carefully avoiding capsular injuries, and identifying and sparing aberrant renal arteries that enter the kidney directly. The renal artery(ies) is(are) dissected clear of surrounding soft tissues. The adrenal gland is identified and gently dissected away from the upper pole of the kidney. The ureter(s) is(are) inspected and trimmed free of retroperitoneal structures and fat avoiding skeletonization of the ureter to ensure adequate blood supply.

The renal graft is then re-perfused with cold preservation solution and kept cold in anticipation of transplantation. If necessary, the renal graft is repackaged in a sterile fashion and maintained cold prior to transplantation.

 Clinical Example (50325)

A living donor renal allograft is received at the transplant recipient site of service in a sterile container, maintained in cold preservation solution. Standard backbench dissection and removal of perinephric fat and preparation of renal vein(s), renal artery(ies), and ureter(s), ligating branches, as necessary, is performed.

⊘ =Modifier 51 Exempt   ⊙ =Conscious Sedation   ✚ =Add-on Code

Description of Procedure (50325)

The renal graft is received in a sterile container and is maintained in cold preservation solution. The surgeon requests and confirms that a sterile backbench is set up in the OR, with appropriate instruments for the backbench dissection. An appropriate recipient has been identified. The correct identification process is carried out to make sure that the renal graft is being allocated to the right recipient. The surgeon must make the appropriate arrangements with the operating room and staff to allow for sterile dissection of the organ in coordination with the recipient procedure. The surgeon scrubs and gowns. The renal graft is removed from the sterile container and placed on a sterile table, on ice, while bathing in cold preservation solution. The renal graft is inspected to be certain that it is grossly intact and that its appearance is acceptable.

With continuous bathing in cold preservation solution, the aortic cuff is first identified in order to determine the presence or absence of aberrant renal arteries. The renal vein(s) is(are) then identified. Gerota's fascia and the perinephric adipose tissue is removed carefully avoiding capsular injuries, and identifying and sparing aberrant renal arteries that enter the kidney directly. The renal vein(s), renal artery(ies), and ureter(s) are prepared for implantation, ligating branches as necessary.

The renal graft is then re-perfused with cold preservation solution and kept cold in anticipation of transplantation. If necessary, the renal graft is repackaged in a sterile fashion and maintained cold prior to transplantation.

Clinical Example (50327)

The renal vein of a right, renal allograft from a deceased donor is short and thin, and requires elongation prior to transplantation in the patient. A backbench, vena cava, extension graft or vein patch (venoplasty) is performed on the allograft.

Description of Procedure (50327)

On ice, with continuous bathing in cold preservation solution, the renal, vein, extension graft is constructed in continuity with the renal vein by using a vascular stapler across the vena cava both above and below the renal vein(s), so that a tube of cava can serve as the extension graft. This requires two applications of the stapler and oversewing of the staple lines for reinforcement, as necessary. If the superior aspect of the cava is short and cannot accommodate a staple line without compromising the lumen of the renal vein(s), a venoplasty is required; a triangulated vein patch is used to cover the deficit by using two suture lines of fine monofilament suture in the superior aspect of the extension.

Clinical Example (50328)

Two renal end arteries are present on a renal allograft. Backbench, arterial anastomosis, either end-to-end or side-to-side, is performed on the allograft to create a single arterial lumen for transplantation.

Description of Procedure (50328)

Work is performed on ice, with continuous bathing in cold preservation solution. The main renal artery is kept attached to the aortic patch of the donor, and if the ostia of the aberrant artery is greater than 1.0 cm apart, the aortic patch is shortened by cutting out a redundant portion of aortic patch and reconstituting continuity with a single layer of fine monofilament suture. Alternatively, the aberrant artery is reimplanted onto the main renal artery either end-to-side or side-to-side forming a single arterial lumen for transplantation in the patient.

 Clinical Example (50329)

Double ureters are present on a renal allograft. Backbench, ureteral anastomosis is performed on the allograft creating a ureteroureterostomy, so that there will be one ureteral orifice for the transplantation ureteroneocystostomy anastomosis (transplantation work is reported separately).

Description of Procedure (50329)

On ice, with continuous bathing in cold preservation solution, the ureters are joined distally by a side-to-side ureteral anastomosis with running absorbable monofilament.

INTRODUCTION

● **50391**   Instillation(s) of therapeutic agent into renal pelvis and/or ureter through established nephrostomy, pyelostomy or ureterostomy tube (eg, anticarcinogenic or antifungal agent)

 Rationale

Code 50391 was added to describe instillation(s) of therapeutic agent into the renal pelvis and/or ureter. This procedure is usually done to treat urothelial tumors in patients where preserved renal function is advantageous to total/partial nephrectomy or multiple endoscopic tumor ablations (eg, those with solitary kidney or compromised renal function who develop ureteral or pelvic carcinoma). Intravesical bacillus Calmette-Guerin (BCG) instillations (known to enhance the body's immune response) are instilled into the upper tract by either antegrade nephrostomy tube or retrograde stent irrigation.

Instillation of anti-fungal agents is also used to treat renal pelvis fungal infections primarily *Candida albicans*, which can form fungal balls that obstruct the ureter and cause urosepsis. Treatment includes placement of a nephrostomy and subsequent irrigation with anti-fungal agents.

 Clinical Example (50391)

A 58-year-old male with a solitary kidney has known 0.5 cm papillary tumor involving the medial aspect of the renal pelvis with associated hydronephrosis. A prior nephrostomy tube had been placed two weeks ago for renal drainage. After a lengthy discussion of options, a decision is made to utilize infusion of BCG into the right, renal pelvis to destroy the cancer and prevent tumor reoccurrence. BCG is instilled into the renal pelvis via the established nephrostomy tube. One amp of BCG is mixed with normal saline.

Description of Procedure (50391)

The patient is positioned in the flank position. The field is sterilized, prepared, and draped. Under fluoroscopic guidance, the position of the previously placed

⊘ =Modifier 51 Exempt   ⊙ =Conscious Sedation   ✛ =Add-on Code nephrostomy tube is confirmed. Then the anti-neoplastic agent (eg, BCG) is prepared per protocol. The irrigant is poured into a syringe connected to the nephrostomy tube. The patient is kept in this position for an appropriate time. Then the fluid is allowed to drain from the kidney and disposed of according to OSHA protocol. Finally, the nephrostomy tube is reconnected to the drainage system.

LAPAROSCOPY

50541   Laparoscopy, surgical; ablation of renal cysts

▲ 50547   donor nephrectomy (including cold preservation), from living donor

(For open procedure, use 50320)

▶(For backbench renal allograft standard preparation prior to transplantation, use 50325)◀

▶(For backbench renal allograft reconstruction prior to transplantation, see 50327-50329)◀

Rationale

Code 50547 in the Laparoscopy subsection was revised to include cold preservation and with the removal of the parenthetical note stating "excluding preparation and maintenance of allograft." Two cross-references were added following 50547 referring to codes 50325 and 50327-50329.

Clinical Example (50547)

A male or female without major medical problems consents to donate a kidney to a relative or close acquaintance with renal failure. Following an extensive medical and psychosocial evaluation confirming the health of the prospective donor, the donor is accepted for the procedure. The laparoscopic procedure is associated with decreased pain, length-of-stay, and morbidity in comparison to those of the traditional open procedure.

Description of Procedure (50547)

The patient is under general anesthesia. The abdomen is insufflated with CO_2. Four ports are placed. The left colon is reflected, the spleen is reflected, the renal vessels are isolated to the aorta, the ureter is divided at the iliac vessel, the kidney is completely freed up. A 6 cm incision for extraction of the kidney is made near the umbilicus, the renal artery and vein are stapled, the kidney is placed in a large retrieval bag and gently pulled out through the extraction incision. The incisions for the four ports and extraction are closed.

ENDOSCOPY

(For supplies and materials, use 99070)

50551   Renal endoscopy through established nephrostomy or pyelostomy, with or without irrigation, instillation, or ureteropyelography, exclusive of radiologic service;

50557   with fulguration and/or incision, with or without biopsy

▶(50559 has been deleted)◀

50570 Renal endoscopy through nephrotomy or pyelotomy, with or without irrigation, instillation, or ureteropyelography, exclusive of radiologic service;

50576   with fulguration and/or incision, with or without biopsy

▶(50578 has been deleted)◀

Ureter

ENDOSCOPY

50951 Ureteral endoscopy through established ureterostomy, with or without irrigation, instillation, or ureteropyelography, exclusive of radiologic service;

50957   with fulguration and/or incision, with or without biopsy

▶(50959 has been deleted)◀

50970 Ureteral endoscopy through ureterotomy, with or without irrigation, instillation, or ureteropyelography, exclusive of radiologic service;

50976   with fulguration and/or incision, with or without biopsy

▶(50978 has been deleted)◀

 Rationale

Codes 50559, 50578, 50959 and 50978 have been deleted and can be reported in the rare instance when these procedures are performed by utilizing the appropriate radiation oncology codes (eg, 77778). Invasive transitional cell cancer of the upper urinary tract which is fairly uncommon is rarely treated through combined endoscopic and radiation therapy. If radiation therapy is given, then it can be reported separately by reporting the appropriate radiation oncology codes (eg, 77778).

Bladder

TRANSURETHRAL SURGERY

Urethra and Bladder

▲ **52234** Cystourethroscopy, with fulguration (including cryosurgery or laser surgery) and/or resection of; SMALL bladder tumor(s) (0.5 up to 2.0 cm)

Ureter and Pelvis
▶(52347 has been deleted)◀

▶(For transurethral resection or incision of ejaculatory ducts, use 52402)◀

Rationale

Code 52234 has been editorially revised to clarify that this code is intended to encompass fulguration or resection of small tumors greater than or equal to 0.5 cm to those measuring less than 2.0 cm.

Code 52347 has been deleted and replaced by code 52402. This replacement represents a relocation of code 52347, since this code is more appropriately placed as a Vesical Neck and Prostate code. The parenthetic note identifying the deletion has been included in this section as well as a cross-reference subsequent to the listing of code 52347, directing users to the correct code to report for this procedure.

VESICAL NECK AND PROSTATE

●**52402** Cystourethroscopy with transurethral resection or incision of ejaculatory ducts

 Rationale

Code 52402 represents a relocation of code 52347, since this code is more appropriately placed as a Vesical Neck and Prostate code. A parenthetic note identifying the deletion and a cross-reference has been included subsequent to the listing of code 52347, directing users to the correct code to report for this procedure.

Male Genital System

Penis

INCISION

▶(For abdominal perineal gangrene debridement, see 11004-11006)◀

54000 Slitting of prepuce, dorsal or lateral (separate procedure); newborn

 Rationale

A cross-reference has been added preceding code 54000 to direct the users to codes 11004-11006 for abdominal perineal gangrene debridement.

Testis

EXCISION

▶(For abdominal perineal gangrene debridement, see 11004-11006)◀

54500 Biopsy of testis, needle (separate procedure)

 Rationale

A cross-reference has been added preceding code 54500 to direct the users to codes 11004-11006 for abdominal perineal gangrene debridement.

Prostate

EXCISION

55859 Transperineal placement of needles or catheters into prostate for interstitial radioelement application, with or without cystoscopy

(For interstitial radioelement application, see 77776-►77784◄)

 Rationale

The cross-reference following code 55859 has been revised to include codes 77781-77784 for high-intensity brachytherapy in the interstitial radioelement application code range 77776-77784.

Female Genital System

Vagina

REPAIR

+●57267 Insertion of mesh or other prosthesis for repair of pelvic floor defect, each site (anterior, posterior compartment), vaginal approach (List separately in addition to code for primary procedure)

►(Use 57267 in addition to 45560, 57240-57265)◄

 Rationale

Code 57267 was established as an add-on code to describe insertion of mesh or other prosthesis for repair of pelvic floor defect via vaginal approach. A parenthetical note following code 57267 was added to indicate that code 57267 should be reported in addition to the primary procedure code(s) 45560, 57240-57265.

Occasionally, with many reconstructive procedures performed for the anterior and posterior compartments of the vagina (eg, procedures described by codes 57240, 57250, 57260, 57265, 45560), the native tissues are determined to be weak and inadequate for repair, especially in patients who have had previous attempts at repair. Consequently, the decision is made to insert an intervening prosthetic material (eg, autograft, allograft, xenograft, synthetic), which involves attachment of the graft to the surrounding tissues in addition to the routine vaginal repair(s). The physician work involved in performing the insertion of prosthetic material, including placing extra separate sutures, preparing the prosthesis for insertion (sizing), and ensuring proper placement for repair of pelvic floor defect(s), is distinct from the physician work involved in performing the primary pelvic floor defect repair(s) which primarily involves re-approximation of pelvic fascial tissues only. Therefore, code 57267 should be reported in addition to the primary vaginal repair procedure.

▲ **57282**   Colpopexy, vaginal; extra-peritoneal approach (sacrospinous, iliococcygeus)

● **57283**   intra-peritoneal approach (uterosacral, levator myorrhaphy)

Corpus Uteri

EXCISION

58260   Vaginal hysterectomy, for uterus 250 grams or less;

58262   with removal of tube(s), and/or ovary(s)

58263   with removal of tube(s), and/or ovary(s), with repair of enterocele

▶(Do not report 58263 in addition to 57283)◀

✍️ Rationale

Code 57282 was revised to describe a vaginal extra-peritoneal colpopexy with sacrospinous or iliococcygeus ligament fixation. Code 57283 was added to describe a vaginal intra-peritoneal colpopexy which involves utilizing the uterosacral ligament or levator musculature for suspension points. Both these procedures are performed to treat vaginal prolapse.

Previously, code 57282 described sacrospinous ligament fixation via an extra-peritoneal approach. Many gynecologic and urologic surgeons also perform similar suspensions with similar work, using primarily iliococcygeus fixation. The iliococcygeus ligament tissue for fixation is located within two centimeters of the sacrospinous ligament fixation point so these procedures require basically the same dissection (extra-peritoneal), same area of suture placement, and same work requirement. Therefore, the description of code 57282 was revised to better describe the range of physician work.

Many gynecologic and urologic surgeons also perform similar vaginal suspensions utilizing an intra-peritoneal approach (often performed in conjunction with hysterectomies) by using the uterosacral ligaments or the levator musculature for the suspension points. Unlike sacrospinous ligament fixation, these approaches require some additional intra-service work (ie, opening and entering the peritoneal cavity through the vagina, packing of bowel, and the identification of the ureter bilaterally required for both uterosacral ligaments or bilateral levator muscle attachments). The physician work involved in performing a uterosacral suspension is distinct from the physician work involved in performing a sacrospinous ligament fixation and therefore code 57283 was added.

In addition, a parenthetical note following code 58263 was added to preclude the reporting of code 57283 with code 58263, as code 58263 is considered to be an inclusive component of 57283.

🩺 Clinical Example (57267)

A 65-year-old, gravida 4 para 4, female patient presents complaining of vaginal pressure, discomfort, and bulging exacerbated by lifting and straining. She has had a previous attempt at repair of rectocele and has no history of urinary incontinence. Her past medical history is negative. Her pertinent physical examination reveals a significant loss of support of the rectum to 2 cm beyond the hymen. Vaginal apical support is adequate but the intervening native, endopelvic, fascial, supportive tissues are very poor. The surgeon considers them inadequate to provide future support alone. He/she performs rectocele repair. Because of the lack of reasonable tissue strength, the surgeon inserts a prosthetic graft over the native tissues to buttress the weak endopelvic fascia between the vagina and rectum.

Description of Procedure (57267)

The physician examines the vaginal defect. He/she prepares the surgical graft material and cuts the graft material to the correct size. Next, dissection deep in the pelvis is done to identify ischial spines and surrounding ligamentous tissues for attachment. The sutures are placed deep into the pelvis beyond the vaginal apex for initial attachment. The graft is attached to the stay sutures and tied to suspend deep in the pelvis. Several subsequent sutures are placed in the graft in the levator muscles and the lateral vagina and attached to the graft along the full length of the vagina bilaterally. Additional sutures are placed through the distal, perineal muscles and the graft to attach to the distal vagina. The excess vaginal epithelium is resected and irrigated copiously. The remaining vaginal epithelium is closed with running suture. Finally, the vagina is packed with gauze.

 ### Clinical Example (57282)

A 62-year-old, gravida 3, para 3, female patient presents complaining of vaginal pressure, discomfort, and heaviness, as well as vaginal bulging exacerbated by lifting and prolonged standing. There is no history of incontinence, but she has some bladder pressure and urinary frequency. Her past medical history is negative. Her pertinent physical examination reveals significant prolapse of the vaginal apex to 3 cm beyond the hymen. There is also moderate loss of support of the bladder (cystocele), rectum (rectocele), and an enterocele is present. The physician is trained in pelvic reconstructive surgery and performs suspension of the vaginal apex to the sacrospinous or iliococcygeus ligaments. Colpopexy, vaginal; extra-peritoneal approach (sacrospinous, iliococcygeus), as well as repair of cystocele, rectocele and enterocele.

Description of Procedure (57282)

Pre-service activities consist of hospital admission, history and physical examination, record review, chart preparation, review of laboratory tests, pre-operative discussion and evaluation, waiting time, scrub time, positioning of the patient, checking equipment, and waiting time during anesthesia induction.

A vaginal colpopexy is a procedure developed to correct the defect in the support of the vaginal apex. This can occur in association with uterine prolapse or after hysterectomy. Available ligamentous structures in the pelvis which are accessible via the extra-peritoneal approach through the vagina include the sacrospinous ligament(s) and the iliococcygeus ligament(s). Access to these structures is via dissection into the para-rectal space posteriorly or the para-vesical space anteriorly; both of these are via an extra-peritoneal route. To complete the vaginal colpopexy, permanent sutures are placed through these pelvic ligaments

Ⓝ=Modifier 51 Exempt   ⊙=Conscious Sedation   ✚=Add-on Code

and then through the apex of the vagina inclusive of the anterior and/or posterior endopelvic fascia and tied to suspend the vagina deep into the pelvis to a more normal position and reduce and repair the apical prolapse. The operator must be completely knowledgeable of the anatomy of the entire pelvic region to avoid hemorrhage and potential damage to vital structures, blood vessels and nerves within the operative field.

The physician writes orders for post-operative care, accompanies the patient to the recovery room, and speaks with the patient's family members. The patient is visited in the hospital until discharged. She returns for office visits during the global period.

Clinical Example (57283)

A 71-year-old, gravida 3, para 3, female patient presents complaining of vaginal pressure, discomfort, and heaviness as well as vaginal bulging exacerbated by lifting and prolonged standing. There is no history of incontinence but she has some bladder pressure and urinary frequency. Her past medical history is negative. Her pertinent physical examination reveals significant inversion of the vaginal apex 2 cm beyond the level of the hymen. In addition, an enterocele is demonstrated at the vault of the apex. The physician is trained in pelvic, reconstructive surgery and performs transvaginal colpopexy with entrance into the peritoneal cavity through the enterocele sac and bilateral attachment of the vaginal apex (anterior and posterior, endopelvic fascia) to the uterosacral ligaments or levator musculature with enterocele repair.

Description of Procedure (57283)

The physician first examines the vaginal defect. He/she then opens the vaginal mucosa at the apex of the vagina. Next the anterior and posterior endopelvic fascia is dissected away from the mucosa exposing the enterocele. The peritoneum is identified and entered sharply under direct visualization. The bowel is retracted away and packed with a laparotomy towel. Then the ureters are identified and palpated bilaterally. The uterosacral ligaments are identified on each side. The uterosacral ligaments high in the pelvis are grasped with clamps and placed on traction. Next, a series of interrupted sutures is placed through the uterosacral ligaments on both sides. A culdeplasty is performed to obliterate the culdesac. The physician brings the sutures through the exposed anterior (pubocervical) and posterior (rectovaginal) endopelvic fascia. Then the sutures are tied to suspend the vagina deep in the pelvis. The vaginal vault is closed with interrupted sutures. A catheter is placed and left in for bladder drainage. Finally, the vagina is packed with gauze.

INTRODUCTION

●58356   Endometrial cryoablation with ultrasonic guidance, including endometrial curettage, when performed

▶(Do not report 58356 in conjunction with 58100, 58120, 58340, 76700, 76856)◀

Rationale

CPT code 58356 was established to report uterine cryoablation therapy previously reported with Category III code 0009T. This procedure utilizes extreme cold and ultrasound as opposed to thermal ablation, which utilizes heat and hysteroscopy. Uterine cyroablation does not require general anesthesia and thus may be performed in the physicians's office or in an outpatient hospital setting. This procedure is designed to diagnose/treat excessive, frequent or irregular menstruation, metrorrhagia and premenopausal menorrhagia. Suction curettage is recommended to thin the endometrial lining prior to cryotherapy. If curettage is performed, it is included in code 58356, and should not be reported separately.

Widespread market acceptance and clinical efficacy of uterine cryoablation therapy has been confirmed since the establishment of Category III code 0009T (endometrial cryoablation with ultrasonic guidance) in CPT 2002, which has resulted in the fulfillment of the requirements for conversion of the Category III code to Category I.

A parenthetical note was added after code 58356 to indicate that the procedures described by codes 58100, 58120, 58340, 76700, 76856 are inclusive components and should not be reported separately when performed in conjunction with the endometrial cryoablation procedure (58356).

Clinical Example (58356)

The typical patient is a premenopausal woman who presents with menorrhagia due to benign causes and for whom childbearing is complete. Appropriately selected patients include women with heavy menstrual bleeding where conservative therapy (hormonal therapy and/or dilation and curretage) has failed and hysterectomy is the next treatment option considered by her physician.

Uterine cryoablation therapy is contraindicated in patients with known or suspected endometrial carcinoma or premalignant changes in the endometrium, or any anatomic or pathologic condition in which weakness of the myometrium could exist. Active genital infection, active pelvic inflammatory disease, active urinary tract infection (UTI), or intrauterine device (IUD) currently in place is ruled out.

Before scheduling a patient for uterine cryoablation therapy, the physician first attempts to determine the cause of the woman's abnormal uterine bleeding. The patient's diagnostic work-up includes blood tests to rule out any bleeding disorders, thyroid disease, and pregnancy. In addition, the physician obtains visualization of the endometrium by vaginal ultrasound, sonohysterogram or diagnostic hysteroscopy. An endometrial biopsy is performed, as well as a Pap smear.

Description of Procedure (58356)

It is recommended that the lining of the uterine cavity be thinned prior to the cryoablation procedure by administering a gonadotropin releasing hormone (GnRH) agonist (Lupron) 21 to 28 days prior to the procedure. If a GnRH agonist is not used, cryoablation may be performed any time during the menstrual cycle, but a suction curettage may be performed immediately prior to cryoablation to thin the lining.

The site of service is decided by the physician in consultation with the patient, and can include a hospital outpatient, ambulatory surgery center, or physician's office.

In the hospital, the patient is placed into dorsal lithotomy position. In the office, the patient reclines, with her legs placed in stirrups. The patient is prepped and draped in a sterile manner.

When the procedure is performed in a hospital setting, the patient is typically given intravenous (IV) sedation or general anesthesia. In addition, some physicians will perform a paracervical block on the patient. When the procedure is performed in an office setting, physicians typically recommend their patients take oral medications (eg, non-steroidal anti-inflammatory drugs, diazepam, etc) one hour before the treatment. A topical anesthetic spray is sometimes applied to the cervix and cervical canal. A paracervical block is administered.

The sterile, disposable cryoablation control unit is locked onto the cryoablation console and the sterile drape is deployed. The cryoablation console needs to be pre-cooled before starting the procedure. Particularly in the office setting, it is important to allow the paracervical block to set in for five to ten minutes before starting the procedure.

A full bladder is required to provide a good backdrop to enhance the ultrasound image of the uterus. For patients treated in the hospital, a Foley catheter is typically placed and the bladder is filled. For patients in the office setting, many physicians will encourage the patient not to void prior to the procedure to ensure an appropriately filled bladder.

If necessary, a single tooth tenaculum is placed on the anterior cervical lip and the physician applies gentle traction to straighten out the uterus. The uterus is sounded; first in the center and then in both cornu to determine the symmetrical nature of the cavity. The physician also checks the cervical canal diameter to determine passage of the 5.5 mm cryoprobe. At this point, the physician will dilate the cervix to 6.0 mm, if dilation is necessary.

When performed in the hospital, hysteroscopy may be performed. Suction curettage is recommended to thin the endometrial lining if pre-treatment with a GnRH agonist was not utilized.

Probe Placement with Ultrasound Guidance
The ultrasound probe is placed on the lower abdomen to locate the uterus. The ultrasound is lined up so that the longitudinal axis of the uterus is displayed. The physician then applies gentle traction on the tenaculum and carefully inserts the cryoprobe into the uterus, through the cervix, observing its path on the ultrasound. With the probe gently touching the fundus, the physician notes the appearance of the cryoprobe on the ultrasound, ensuring that the probe has not created a false passage or perforated the uterus. The physician compares the depth of the cryoprobe to the depth noted when the uterus was sounded, in order to confirm that a uterine perforation has not occurred. The procedure is terminated if the uterus is perforated.

The physician then redirects the tip of the cryoprobe towards one cornu. The ultrasound is repositioned so the uterus is viewed in a horizontal axis. The cryoprobe is slowly moved in and out for a distance of about a centimeter and its position in the cornu confirmed with the ultrasound.

The probe placement under ultrasound guidance has similarities to the probe placement that is performed with prostate cryoablation procedures. The primary difference is that with prostate cancer, the probe placement is performed with multiple probes each placed once, while with cryoablation of the uterus, placement is performed multiple times with a single probe.

First Freeze Monitored with Ultrasound Guidance
Approximately 5 cc of sterile saline is injected through the bottom injection port of the cryoprobe. The injection of saline removes air from the uterus and provides better visualization of the uterine cavity and probe placement.

In order to begin the initial freeze, the physician depresses the "minus" button on the cryoprobe handle. The physician maintains the cryoprobe and tenaculum pressure until the cryoprobe tip temperature reaches minus 60°C. The tension on the cryoprobe and tenaculum are relaxed and gradual expansion of the cryozone is observed on the ultrasound. The cryoprobe tip temperature is monitored and shown on the cryoablation console. The tip temperature should reach negative 80°C within three minutes of starting the procedure.

A black area corresponding to the formation of ice along and extending out from the cryoprobe appears. The first treatment session lasts for four minutes, or the physician stops the procedure if the cryozone gets within 2 mm of the serosa of the uterus. Clinical safety and effectiveness data in the Federal Drug Administration (FDA) premarket approval was derived from a four-minute freeze followed by a six-minute freeze; however, some physicians may choose to freeze longer, using ultrasound guidance, in order to get more complete coverage of the uterus. It is important that the cryozone not extend beyond the serosa of the surface as this could cause serious complications associated with freezing adjacent organs and structures.

Once adequate freezing is achieved, the physician depresses the plus button to stop freezing and to start heating the probe. The skills associated with monitoring the extent of the cryozone and deciding on the appropriate time to stop treatment are similar to the skills required during a cryoablation of the prostate.

Remove Cryoprobe and Reposition to Contralateral Cornu
Once the tip temperature of the cryoprobe reaches positive 20°C, the probe can be removed from the cryozone. The physician gently rotates the cryoprobe back and forth and slowly withdraws the cryoprobe from the first cryozone. It is not necessary to remove the cryoprobe from the uterus, but it must be withdrawn out to or near the internal cervical os.

The cryoprobe is then repositioned into the contralateral cornu. The cryoprobe is swung 90° (toward the patient's opposite leg) to be sure that the cryoprobe is being placed into the contralateral cornu. The physician applies gentle traction on the tenaculum and gently slides the cryoprobe next to the initial cryozone into the untreated cornu. In repositioning the cryoprobe tip, the initial cryozone is often encountered. If resistance is encountered, the cryoprobe is placed on the cryozone, angled toward the targeted cornu, and the heater on the cryoprobe is used to melt a pathway for the cryoprobe to be placed into the second cornu. The injection of warm saline may also be used to facilitate the passage of the cryoprobe.

Probe Placement Confirmation
The physician confirms by ultrasound that the cryoprobe is at the fundus and in the untreated cornu. The physician will also use ultrasound to confirm that a perforation has not occurred. The temperature on the console should register greater than positive 10°C. If the tip reading is below 10°C, the physician rechecks the probe placement to be sure that the cryoprobe has not been placed in the original cryozone.

Second Freeze Monitored with Ultrasound Guidance
Approximately 5 cc of sterile saline is injected through the bottom injection port of the cryoprobe. The physician maintains counter traction on the tenaculum and depresses the minus button to start the second freeze cycle. Once the cryoprobe tip reaches minus 60°C, tension may be relaxed. The physician monitors the developing cryozone as previously outlined. Observation of cryozone growth is best viewed through the horizontal plane. The physician continues freezing for six minutes or stops if the advancing edge of the cryozone reaches within 2 mm of the serosa. Again, it is important that the physician monitor the cryozone to ensure it does not extend beyond the uterus. The second cryozone should completely merge with the first cryozone, creating one single large ice ball.

Once adequate freezing is achieved, the physician depresses the "plus" button to stop freezing and to start heating the probe. At 20°C, the physician rotates the cryoprobe and removes it.

Alternate Freeze Pattern Third Freeze
Some physicians may choose to perform a third freeze in the lower uterine segment, particularly for patients with a uterus that sounds to larger than 9 cm.

Procedure Completion and Recovery
Once all freezes are complete, the cryoprobe is removed. The tenaculum is then removed from the cervix. Hemostasis of the cervix is achieved, as necessary. If a Foley catheter has been used, the patient's bladder is emptied and the catheter removed. The speculum is removed. The patient is typically sent to a recovery room or an appropriate waiting area for observation and recovery from the anesthesia.

LAPAROSCOPY/HYSTEROSCOPY

58558 Hysteroscopy, surgical; with sampling (biopsy) of endometrium and/or polypectomy, with or without D & C

●**58565**   with bilateral fallopian tube cannulation to induce occlusion by placement of permanent implants

    ▶(Do not report 58565 in conjunction with 58555 or 57800)◀

    ▶(For unilateral procedure, use modifier 52)◀

 Rationale

Code 58565 was established for reporting hysteroscopic fallopian tube cannulation and placement of permanent tiny implants for elective female sterilization. Since this procedure avoids abdominal incisions, it is considered less invasive than more traditional methods of sterilization.

A cross-reference has been included after code 58565 to indicate that diagnostic hysteroscopy (58555) and cervical dilation (57800) are inclusive components and should not be reported separately when performed in conjunction with the hysteroscopic sterilization (58565). A second reference was added to indicate that modifier 52 should be used when this procedure is performed unilaterally.

 Clinical Example (58565)

A 37-year-old, multiparous female desires permanent sterilization. She is a poor candidate for laparoscopy in that she is obese and has had several, previous, abdominal, surgical procedures. She has been counseled regarding the various options available to her and her partner including vasectomy, minilaparotomy, open laparoscopy as well as hysterscopic techniques and has opted for the hysterscopic approach.

Description of Procedure (58565)

Following induction of appropriate anesthesia, a pelvic exam is performed. A perineal/vaginal prep is performed. Sterile drapes are placed. A speculum is inserted into the vagina and a single-toothed tenaculum is placed on the anterior lip of the cervix. A paracervical block is performed. The cervix is serially dilated. The operative hysterscope is introduced through the dilated cervix. A complete diagnostic survey of the uterine cavity is performed. Access to both fallopian tube ostia is assessed for adequacy. Each tube is cannulated, then microinserts are placed bilaterally. The hysteroscope is removed from the uterus. The tenaculum is removed and bleeding from the site controlled, if necessary. The patient is transferred to a stretcher and escorted to the recovery room.

                    ⊘=Modifier 51 Exempt   ⊙=Conscious Sedation   ✚=Add-on Code

Ovary

EXCISION

● **58956** Bilateral salpingo-oophorectomy with total omentectomy, total abdominal hysterectomy for malignancy

▶(Do not report 58956 in conjunction with 49255, 58150, 58180, 58262, 58263, 58550, 58661, 58700, 58720, 58900, 58925, 58940)◄

 Rationale

Code 58956 was established for reporting bilateral salpingo-oophorectomy with total omentectomy and total abdominal hysterectomy for malignancy. A parenthetical note with a list of exclusionary codes was also added following code 58956.

This procedure is performed in women with gynecological malignancies (eg, endometrial, ovarian, tubal and primary peritoneal) with omental metastasis. Many times, the appropriate treatment will be to perform a total abdominal hysterectomy and bilateral salpingoophorectomy (TAH BSO) with omentectomy, but not remove the pelvic or paraaortic lymph nodes. For example, women with metastatic endometrial cancer to the omentum should be treated with a TAH BSO omentectomy, but do not need to have a pelvic and paraaortic lymph node dissection for staging because the disease has already spread intra-abdominally. It also may be clinically appropriate to perform a TAH BSO and omentectomy without a nodal dissection in situations where ovarian, tubal and primary peritoneal cancer exists.

 Clinical Example (58956)

A 67-year-old female presents with postmenopausal bleeding for 18 months duration. A biopsy reveals a FIGO, grade 3, endometrial carcinoma. The patient is taken for exploratory laparotomy. At the time of surgery, there are several 2 cm implants found in the omentum. There is no adenopathy and no peritoneal implants. The patient undergoes TAH BSO and a complete omentectomy to remove all gross disease. The patient receives the usual follow-up care in the hospital and office during the 90-day global period.

Description of Procedure (58956)

The patient is positioned on the table and an exam under anesthesia is performed. The patient is prepared and draped and an abdominal incision is made. A thorough exam of the abdomen and pelvis is done which reveals multiple omental metastases that involve the greater and lesser omentum. There does not appear to be other intraperitoneal disease and there is no retroperitoneal lymphadenopathy. A retractor is placed and a complete TAH BSO is performed. The lymph nodes and retroperitoneal spaces are carefully inspected. After completion of the TAH BSO a complete omentectomy is perfomed. The omentum is freed from the transverse colon and the omentum is taken off the greater curvature of the stomach up to the splenic hilum. All of the metastatic disease is resected with the omentectomy. Hemostasis is ensured and the abdomen is irrigated, and closed.

Parathyroid, Thymus, Adrenal Glands, Pancreas, and Carotid Body

EXCISION

60540 Adrenalectomy, partial or complete, or exploration of adrenal gland with or without biopsy, transabdominal, lumbar or dorsal (separate procedure);

60545 with excision of adjacent retroperitoneal tumor

▶(Do not report 60540, 60545 in conjunction with 50323)◀

✎ Rationale

An exclusionary cross-reference has been added following code 60545 to preclude the use of the renal transplantation code 50323 with codes 60540 and 60545.

Nervous System

Skull, Meninges, and Brain

TWIST DRILL, BURR HOLE(S), OR TREPHINE

61105 Twist drill hole for subdural or ventricular puncture;

⊘**61107** for implanting ventricular catheter or pressure recording device

(For intracranial neuroendoscopic ventricular catheter placement, use 62160)

▶(For twist drill or burr hole performed to place thermal perfusion probe, use Category III code 0077T)◀

✎ Rationale

A cross-reference has been added following code 61107 to direct the users to Category III code 0077T for twist drill or burr hole performed to place a thermal perfusion probe.

NEUROSTIMULATORS (INTRACRANIAL)

▲**61885** Insertion or replacement of cranial neurostimulator pulse generator or receiver, direct or inductive coupling; with connection to a single electrode array

61888 Revision or removal of cranial neurostimulator pulse generator or receiver

▶(Do not report 61888 in conjunction with 61885 or 61886 for the same pulse generator)◀

✍ Rationale

Code 61885 was revised to maintain consistency with other similar codes for implantation of stimulation or drug delivery devices with the addition of replacement and to clarify the intent of the use of code 61885 for the equivalent work of replacement of a neurostimulator device. A cross-reference was added to code 61888 to indicate that as revision and replacement procedures are distinct, code 61888 would not be reported in addition to 61885 or 61886 for the same pulse generator.

🩺 Clinical Example (61885)

A 45-year-old male presents with essential tremor that has become quite severe and is disabling. He has had the disease for 8 years and has failed to obtain tremor relief using various oral medications and physical therapy. He is not a candidate for direct brain resection or an ablative brain procedure because of the severity of his tremor and the length of symptoms. His history also includes implantation of a deep brain stimulator electrode array, which upon stimulation, eliminated 80% of the patient's tremor. He undergoes internalization of the tail of the electrode array and placement and connection of a subcutaneous stimulator generator for long-term brain stimulation.

Description of Procedure (61885)

Under general anesthesia, the cranial lead is recovered from the subgaleal space. A linear incision is made just below the clavicle over a distance of approximately 3 cm. A subcutaneous pocket is created under this incision. The cephalic wound is re-opened where the electrode array had been placed. A small incision is made at approximately the level of the mastoid and the electrode extension passer is passed from the cephalic wound down a subgaleal tract and out the mastoid wound. Using this passer, the lead is pulled through the subcutaneous tract. The same passer is passed from the mastoid wound down another subcutaneous tract and out the clavicular wound, pulling the electrode tail and extension wire through this subcutaneous tract. A sleeve is placed on the distal tail of the electrode array. The array tail is inserted into the proximal end of the extension wire and tightened. The sleeve is placed over the connection and tied in place with 0-silk suture. The boot and connector are placed in the subgaleal space while the proximal end of the extension wire is secured to the skull. The distal end of the extension wire is inserted into the generator and tightened. Excess extension wire is coiled behind the stimulator generator. The stimulator generator is sutured into place in the subcutaneous tissue. The stimulator is tested, under sterile technique, to determine the impedance of the connections and to rule out an electrical short. The skin and subcutaneous tissues of all wounds are closed with deep sutures and skin staples.

Spine and Spinal Cord

POSTERIOR EXTRADURAL LAMINOTOMY OR LAMINECTOMY FOR EXPLORATION/DECOMPRESSION OF NEURAL ELEMENTS OR EXCISION OF HERNIATED INTERVERTEBRAL DISKS

●**63050** Laminoplasty, cervical, with decompression of the spinal cord, two or more vertebral segments;

●**63051** with reconstruction of the posterior bony elements (including the application of bridging bone graft and non-segmental fixation devices (eg, wire, suture, mini-plates), when performed)

▶(Do not report 63050 or 63051 in conjunction with 22600, 22614, 22840-22842, 63001, 63015, 63045, 63048, 63295 for the same vertebral segment(s))◀

Rationale

Two new laminoplasty codes (63050, 63051) have been added for decompression of the cervical spine in the treatment of cervical spondylosis with myelopathy, ossification of the posterior longitudinal ligament, and cervical stenosis. Unlike the existing posterior cervical decompression codes included in CPT that involve complete removal of the posterior elements of the spine (63015, 63001), the new codes involve procedures which leave portions of the posterior elements intact. Laminoplasty is an alternative approach for posterior decompression of the cervical spinal cord. A unilateral osteotomy is made between the facet joint and the lamina, and a partial osteotomy is made on the contralateral side creating a "swinging door" to allow expansion of a stenotic spinal canal. Bone graft and or non-segmental fixation may be used to secure the lamina in the 'open' position. A list of the codes which are inherently included in 63050 and 63051 that should not be reported separately are listed in the exclusionary note following 63051 and include 22600, 22614, 22840-22842, 63001, 63015, 63045, 63048.

Clinical Example (63050)

A 46-year-old male has a six-month history of progressive hand weakness, paresthesias, and gait difficulty. He has hand intrinsic weakness and upper extremity sensory loss with lower extremity hyperreflexia and positive Babinski signs. He undergoes a cervical laminoplasty from C3 to C7 for decompression of the spinal cord. Post operative hospital care and office visits are conducted as necessary through the 90-day global period.

Description of Procedure (63050)

A midline, posterior, cervical incision is made and the paraspinous muscles are reflected out to the facet joints, exposing the laminae, spinous processes and facet joints from C3 to C7. A high-speed drill is used to create a multisegment osteotomy through the junction of the lamina and facet joints on the right side from C7 up through and including C3. The underlying ligamentum flavum is sectioned with micro Kerrison rongeurs. On the left side, the junction of the facet and lamina at each level is scored with the drill from C7 to C3 to create a stress riser in the bone. A small Key elevator is then placed into the right side osteotomy, between the lamina and facet joint, and the laminae are sequentially

∅=Modifier 51 Exempt ☉=Conscious Sedation ✚=Add-on Code

cracked back to expand the spinal canal. Hemostasis is achieved and the incision is closed in layers.

 Clinical Example (63051)

A 32-year-old female has episodic paresthesias radiating into all limbs with cervical extension. She has upper limb weakness and sensory loss with lower extremity hyperreflexia and positive Babinski signs. She undergoes a cervical laminoplasty from C3 to C7 for decompression of the spinal cord and reconstruction of the posterior spinal structures using an iliac crest allograft and non-segmental fixation.

Description of Procedure (63051)

A midline posterior cervical incision is made and the paraspinous muscles are reflected out to the facet joints, exposing the laminae, spinous processes and facet joints from C3 to C7. A high-speed drill is used to create a multisegment osteotomy through the junction of the lamina and facet joints on the right side from C7 up through and including C3. The underlying ligamentum flavum is sectioned with micro rongeurs. On the left side, the junction of the facet and lamina at each level is scored with the drill from C7 to C3 to create a stress riser in the bone. An elevating device is then placed into the right side osteotomy, between the lamina and facet joint, and the laminae are sequentially cracked back to expand the spinal canal. An iliac crest allograft is shaped, fashioned (reported separately), and then fit into the right side osteotomy to keep the space open, posteriorly. Absorbable miniplates are then applied to each segment of the posterior cervical spine, with the plate spanning the osteotomy and iliac bone allograft. Then 3 mm absorbable screws are placed through the plate at each level into the facet and the lamina, securing the plate and maintaining the canal expansion. Hemostasis is achieved and the incision is closed in layers.

EXCISION BY LAMINECTOMY OF LESION OTHER THAN HERNIATED DISK

+●63295   Osteoplastic reconstruction of dorsal spinal elements, following primary intraspinal procedure (List separately in addition to code for primary procedure)

▶(Use 63295 in conjunction with 63172, 63173, 63185, 63190, 63200-63290)◀

▶(Do not report 63295 in conjunction with 22590-22614, 22840-22844, 63050, 63051 for the same vertebral segment(s))◀

 Rationale

Code 63295 was added as an add-on code for osteoplastic reconstruction commonly performed in pediatric patients following primary intraspinal procedures (eg, removal of spinal cord tumors, arteriovenous malformations, or dorsal rhizotomies). The standard laminectomy procedures (eg, 63001) include the removal of the dorsal elements of the spine which are considered part of the pathologic process. However, in the pediatric population, laminectomy without reconstruction has been shown to have a high incidence of post-operative kyphotic spinal deformity. To limit post-surgical spinal deformity, the dorsal elements of the spinal segment, including the the laminae, spinous processes, and ligamentous structures, are replaced into the spine to recreate normal anatomic architecture and biomechanical properties. A list of the codes which are inherently included in 63295 are listed in the exclusionary note and include 22590-22614, 22840-22844.

 Clinical Example (63295)

A 12-year-old boy, undergoing a laminectomy for a cervical spinal cord tumor, is at significant risk for developing a postoperative kyphotic deformity. An osteoplastic reconstruction of the dorsal spinal elements is performed as an add-on procedure, following the primary laminectomy procedure.

Description of Procedure (63295)

Following the closure of the dura, the previously removed dorsal spinal elements (ie, laminae, spinous process and supporting ligaments) are returned to an anatomic position for reconstruction. Using a fine drill bit, holes are drilled into the lateral aspect of each lamina and heavy sutures, wires, or miniplates are used to secure the dorsal elements, fixing the bone in position.

NEUROSTIMULATORS (SPINAL)

▲ **63685**   Insertion or replacement of spinal neurostimulator pulse generator or receiver, direct or inductive coupling

▶(Do not report 63685 in conjunction with 63688 for the same pulse generator or receiver)◀

 Rationale

Code 63685 was revised to maintain consistency with other similar codes for implantation of stimulation or drug delivery devices with the addition of replacement and to clarify the intent of the use of code 63685 for the equivalent work of replacement of a neurostimulator device. A cross-reference was added following code 63685 to indicate that as revision and replacement procedures are distinct, code 63688 would not be reported in addition to 63685 for the same pulse generator.

Extracranial Nerves, Peripheral Nerves, and Autonomic Nervous System

NEUROSTIMULATORS (PERIPHERAL NERVE)

▲ **64590**   Insertion or replacement of peripheral neurostimulator pulse generator or receiver, direct or inductive coupling

▶(Do not report 64590 in conjunction with 64595)◀

 Rationale

Code 64590 was revised to maintain consistency with other similar codes for implantation of stimulation or drug delivery devices with the addition of

---

⊘=Modifier 51 Exempt   ⊙=Conscious Sedation   ✚=Add-on Code

"replacement" and to clarify the intent of the use of code 64590 for the equivalent work of replacement of a neurostimulator device. A cross-reference was added following code 64590 to indicate that as revision and replacement procedures are distinct, code 64595 would not be reported in addition to 64590 for the same pulse generator.

Eye and Ocular Adnexa

Anterior Segment

IRIS, CILIARY BODY

Destruction

66700   Ciliary body destruction; diathermy

▲**66710**   cyclophotocoagulation, transscleral

●**66711**   cyclophotocoagulation, endoscopic

►(Do not report 66711 in conjunction with 66990)◄

 Rationale

Code 66711 was added to describe endoscopic photocoagulation of the ciliary body for the treatment of glaucoma. This technique requires a surgical incision for insertion of the endoscope through the anterior segment to provide direct visualization of the tissue to be coagulated. The existing photocoagulation code 66710 has been revised to indicate that this procedure is performed externally (or transscleral) without an incision (which was the only surgical approach in use at the time it was added to the CPT code set in 1992). Although the endoscopic approach has been in use since 1995, the endoscopic procedure was not captured in the CPT code set. The add-on code 66990 for ophthalmic endoscopy is intended to be used when this technique is combined with other more extensive intraocular primary procedures (ie, 65820, 65875, 65920, 66985, 66986, 67038, 67039, 67040). The new code, 66711, which includes the endoscopic approach, differentiates the intraocular cyclophotocoagulation from the extra-ocular procedure described in code 66710, which carries lesser surgical risk. Likewise, code 66711 is not reported in addition to 66990 as the endoscopic approach, which makes this procedure much safer, has been included in the procedure.

Clinical Example (66711)

A 66-year-old patient with a history of chronic glaucoma has progressive optic nerve damage and elevated intraocular pressure that has not been controlled by medical therapy and a previous filtering operation. The patient is pseudophakic with a miotic pupil.

Description of Procedure (66711)

Anesthesia is begun with periocular local anesthetic. A cleansing prep is performed of the conjunctiva, followed by placement of a drape. A lid speculum is inserted to allow adequate visualization. A clear corneal incision is made with the diamond blade approximately 3.4 mm in width, usually temporally. Viscoelastic material is injected into the anterior chamber over the pupil and lens to increase and maintain anterior chamber depth. Viscoelastic is then injected under the iris for 180° to visualize the ciliary body processes with the endoscope. The endoscope is inserted through the temporal incision viewing the nasal ciliary processes. The ciliary processes are coagulated through the endoscope with the endpoint of shrinkage and whitening. The endoscope is moved in an arc allowing treatment of the processes over an arc of 180°. A second corneal incision is made 90° away and 180° of ciliary processes are treated. At the end of the procedure, the surgeon has completed coagulation of 270° of angle. After completion of laser therapy, the viscoelastic material is removed from the anterior segment of the eye with an irrigation and aspiration device to prevent intraocular pressure spikes. The eye is reformed with balanced salt solution. The wounds are checked for leakage and if necessary sutures are placed to seal the wound.

Radiology

The guideline additions to the Radiology section of the CPT book for this year are to provide greater clarity in coding. Guidelines have been added to clarify appropriate reporting for diagnostic angiographies in the Aorta and Arteries, Veins and Lymphatics, and Transcatheter Procedures subsections of Radiology. In addition, new guidelines define and clarify ultrasound imaging services in the Abdomen and Peritoneum and Non-Obstetrical subsections of Radiology. New codes include services for fetal ultrasound, and substantial revisions in the Therapeutic Nuclear Medicine subsection. Also for 2005, attenuation correction services are now included due to revisions of the myocardial perfusion imaging codes.

Radiology

Diagnostic Radiology (Diagnostic Imaging)

Spine and Pelvis

72192   Computed tomography, pelvis; without contrast material

72193   with contrast material(s)

72194   without contrast material, followed by contrast material(s) and further sections

▶(For computed tomographic colonography, see Category III codes 0066T, 0067T. Do not report 72192-72194 in conjunction with 0066T, 0067T)◀

(For coronal, sagittal, and/or oblique sections, use 76375.)

 Rationale

Parenthetical notes have been included following codes 72192, 72193, and 72194 to direct the user to report computed tomographic colonography or virtual colonography codes 0066T, 0067T. Use of codes for computed tomography of the pelvis are exclusive of the computed tomographic colonography codes.

Abdomen

74150   Computed tomography, abdomen; without contrast material

74160   with contrast material(s)

74170   without contrast material, followed by contrast material(s) and further sections

(For coronal, sagittal, and/or oblique sections, use 76375)

▶(For computed tomographic colonography, see Category III codes 0066T, 0067T. Do not report 74150-74170 in conjunction with 0066T, 0067T)◀

 Rationale

Parenthetical notes have been included following code 74150 to direct the user to report computed tomographic colonography or virtual colonography codes 0066T, 0067T. Use of codes for computed tomography of the abdomen are exclusive of the computed tomographic colonography codes.

▶Vascular Procedures◀

AORTA AND ARTERIES

Selective vascular catheterizations should be coded ...

Additional second and/or third order arterial ...

▶For angiography performed in conjunction with therapeutic transcatheter radiological supervision and interpretation services, see the Radiology Transcatheter Procedures guidelines.◀

▶Diagnostic angiography (radiological supervision and interpretation) codes should NOT be used with interventional procedures for:◀

▶1) Contrast injections, angiography, roadmapping, and/or fluoroscopic guidance for the intervention,◀

▶2) Vessel measurement, and◀

▶3) Post-angioplasty/stent angiography◀

▶as this work is captured in the interventional procedure code(s).◀

▶Diagnostic angiography performed at the time of an interventional procedure is separately reportable if:◀

▶1) No prior catheter-based angiographic study is available and a full diagnostic study is performed, and the decision to intervene is based on the diagnostic study, OR◀

▶2) A prior study is available, but as documented in the medical record:◀

▶a) The patient's condition with respect to the clinical indication has changed since the prior study, OR◀

▶b) There is inadequate visualization of the anatomy and/or pathology, OR◀

▶c) There is a clinical change during the procedure that requires new evaluation outside the target area of intervention◀

▶Diagnostic angiography performed at a separate setting from an interventional procedure is separately reported.◀

▶Diagnostic angiography performed at the time of an interventional procedure is NOT separately reportable if it is specifically included in the interventional code descriptor.◀

(For intravenous procedure, see 36000-36013, 36400-36425 and 36100-36248 for intra-arterial procedure)

✐ Rationale

The introductory guidelines to instruct appropriate reporting for the CPT subsections related to selective vascular catheterization imaging have been revised to clarify the circumstances under which a provider should report both a diagnostic angiogram/venogram radiological supervision and interpretation service and an interventional therapeutic vascular radiological supervision and interpretation service.

The guideline revisions and additions clarify the conditions under which it is appropriate for a provider to report both a diagnostic angiogram/venogram radiological supervision and interpretation service and an interventional therapeutic vascular radiological supervision and interpretation service.

VEINS AND LYMPHATICS

▶For venography performed in conjunction with therapeutic transcatheter radiological supervision and interpretation services, see the Radiology Transcatheter Procedures guidelines.◀

⊘=Modifier 51 Exempt   ⊙=Conscious Sedation   ✚=Add-on Code

►Diagnostic venography (radiological supervision and interpretation) codes should NOT be used with interventional procedures for:◄

►1) Contrast injections, venography, roadmapping, and/or fluoroscopic guidance for the intervention,◄

►2) Vessel measurement, and◄

►3) Post-angioplasty/stent venography◄

►as this work is captured in the interventional procedure code(s).◄

►Diagnostic venography performed at the time of an interventional procedure is separately reportable if:◄

►1) No prior catheter-based venographic study is available and a full diagnostic study is performed, and decision to intervene is based on the diagnostic study, OR◄

►2) A prior study is available, but as documented in the medical record:◄

►a) The patient's condition with respect to the clinical indication has changed since the prior study, OR◄

►b) There is inadequate visualization of the anatomy and/or pathology, OR◄

►c) There is a clinical change during the procedure that requires new evaluation outside the target area of intervention◄

►Diagnostic venography performed at a separate setting from an interventional procedure is separately reported.◄

►Diagnostic venography performed at the time of an interventional procedure is NOT separately reportable if it is specifically included in the interventional code descriptor.◄

✎ Rationale

The introductory guidelines to instruct appropriate reporting for the CPT subsections related to selective vascular catheterization imaging have been revised to clarify the circumstances under which a provider should report both a diagnostic angiogram/venogram radiological supervision and interpretation service and an interventional therapeutic vascular radiological supervision and interpretation service.

The guideline revisions and additions clarify the conditions under which it is appropriate for a provider to report both a diagnostic angiogram/venogram radiological supervision and interpretation service and an interventional therapeutic vascular radiological supervision and interpretation service.

TRANSCATHETER PROCEDURES

►Therapeutic transcatheter radiological supervision and interpretation code(s) include the following services associated with that intervention:◄

►1) Contrast injections, angiography/venography, roadmapping, and fluoroscopic guidance for the intervention,◄

▶2) Vessel measurement, and◀

▶3) Completion angiography/venography (except for those uses permitted by 75898).◀

▶Unless specifically included in the code descriptor, diagnostic angiography/venography performed at the time of transcatheter therapeutic radiological and interpretation service(s) is separately reportable (eg, no prior catheter-based diagnostic angiography/venography study of the target vessel is available, prior diagnostic study is inadequate, patient's condition with respect to the clinical indication has changed since the prior study or during the intervention). See 75600-75893.◀

🖎 Rationale

The introductory guidelines to instruct appropriate reporting for the CPT subsections related to selective vascular catheterization imaging have been revised to clarify the circumstances under which a provider should report both a diagnostic angiogram/venogram radiological supervision and interpretation service and an interventional therapeutic vascular radiological supervision and interpretation service.

The guideline revisions and additions clarify the conditions under which it is appropriate for a provider to report both a diagnostic angiogram/venogram radiological supervision and interpretation service and an interventional therapeutic vascular radiological supervision and interpretation service.

75952 Endovascular repair of infrarenal abdominal aortic aneurysm or dissection, radiological supervision and interpretation

▶(For radiologic supervision and interpretation of endovascular repair of abdominal aortic aneurysm involving visceral vessels, see Category III codes 0078T-0081T)◀

🖎 Rationale

A cross-reference has been added following code 75952 referring to codes 0078T-0079T for endovascular repair of abdominal aortic aneurysm or dissection involving visceral vessels using fenestrated modular bifurcated prostheses.

▲**75960** Transcatheter introduction of intravascular stent(s), (except coronary, carotid, and vertebral vessel), percutaneous and/or open, radiological supervision and interpretation, each vessel

(For radiologic supervision and interpretation for transcatheter placement of extracranial ▶vertebral or intrathoracic carotid◀ artery stent(s), ▶see◀ Category III codes ▶0075T, 0076T◀)

(For procedure, see 37205-37208)

🖎 Rationale

Concurrent with the conversion of the carotid stent introduction services from a service formerly reported by Category III codes 0005T and 0006T to Category I codes 37215 and 37216, and revision and renumbering of Category III codes 0005T, 0006T and 0007T to Category III codes 37215 and 37216, the cross-reference following code 75960 has been revised to indicate that radiologic supervision and interpretation for transcatheter placement of extracranial vertebral or intrathoracic carotid artery stents is now reported and included within

Category III codes 0075T and 0076T. This is a departure from the structure of the original Category III codes 0005T, 0006T and 0007T, as radiologic supervision and interpretation was previously reported separately with code 0007T.

Other Procedures

▲76075 Dual energy x-ray absorptiometry (DXA), bone density study, one or more sites; axial skeleton (eg, hips, pelvis, spine)

76076 appendicular skeleton (peripheral) (eg, radius, wrist, heel)

●76077 vertebral fracture assessment

(To report dual energy x-ray absorptiometry (▶DXA◀) body composition study, one or more sites, use Category III code 0028T)

✍ Rationale

Code 76075 and its corresponding cross-reference were revised to indicate that the nomenclature for this technology has been revised to be referred to as DXA (Dual energy X-ray Absorptiometry), as the recognized acronym for this technology. In addition, code 76077 was added to identify vertebral fracture assessment (VFA) using DXA technology.

Clinical Example (76075)

A 55-year-old menopausal female presents with a family history of osteoporosis, and is considering estrogen therapy.

Description of Procedure (76075)
Calibration and quality control (eg, measurement of phantom) of the device is performed. Anatomic markings are appropriately displayed and are in proper position.

Clinical Example (76077)

A 65-year-old female, 15 years post-menopause, undergoes a bone mineral density exam (DXA scan) to determine her bone density diagnosis (World Health Organization definition of normal, osteopenia, osteoporosis) and assessment of her relative and absolute risk for a future osteoporotic fracture. The DXA scan results disclose a T-score of –1.9 at the lumbar spine and total hip (the T-score is a comparison to a young adult mean in standard deviations). The patient's diagnosis is osteopenia by World Health Organization criteria. This patient has a 5- and 6-fold increased risk of future fracture at the lumbar spine and total hip respectively (site specific), and a 2-fold increased risk of future fracture anywhere in the body (global risk) as compared to an age-matched female with a T-score of 0.0. The National Osteoporosis Foundation suggests that postmenopausal women with a bone density T-score of less than –2 should be treated. Thus the value of this patient's T-score of –1.9 (osteopenia) would not necessarily be an indication for medical therapy. A vertebral fracture assessment using DXA equipment was used to obtain an image of the patient's thoracic and lumbar spine to determine if a previous thoracic and lumbar spine vertebral fracture had occurred. Although the patient had no history of spinal pain, 2 compression fractures were found by vertebral fracture assessment. The presence of 2 prevalent vertebral fractures using Vertebral Fracture Assessment (VFA) by DXA imaging indicates a 7-fold increased risk for future vertebral fractures independent of the patient's bone mineral density. Pharmacological intervention is indicated due to the presence of prevalent, vertebral fractures.

Description of Procedure (76077)

The physician reviews the VFA images obtained and the post-processed measurements to assure that the measurements were accurately done and that scanning technique was satisfactory. The physician interprets the VFA thoracic and lumbar images (anterior/posterior (AP) and lateral views) using accepted fracture assessment methodology, the Semiquantitative Analysis of Genant and Quantitative Morphometry, to determine the number and severity of fractures present. The physician compares the results of the VFA interpretation to previous radiographic or VFA images to determine if a significant change in vertebral anatomy has occurred in the interim. The physician dictates the report for the medical record.

76375   Coronal, sagittal, multiplanar, oblique, 3-dimensional and/or holographic reconstruction of computed tomography, magnetic resonance imaging, or other tomographic modality

(Use 76375 in addition to code for imaging procedure)

▶(For computed tomographic colonography, see Category III codes 0066T, 0067T. Do not report 76375 in conjunction with 0066T, 0067T)◀

 Rationale

Parenthetic notes have been included following code 76375 to notify users that these codes should be used for computed tomographic colonography (CT colonography, or virtual colonography codes 0066T, 0067T). All components of the CT colonography procedure are included as part of the 0066T and 0067T codes. Therefore, since specific codes exist that identify all elements of CT colonography, image reconstruction is inherently included as part of the CT colonography procedure and not separately reported. Code 76375 should not be reported with 0066T or 0067T.

76394   Magnetic resonance guidance for, and monitoring of, visceral tissue ablation

(For percutaneous radiofrequency ablation, use 47382)

▶(For focused ultrasound ablation treatment of uterine leiomyomata, see Category III codes 0071T, 0072T)◀

 Rationale

A cross-reference has been added directing users to Category III codes 0071T and 0072T for focused ultrasound ablation treatment of uterine leiomyomata.

⊘ =Modifier 51 Exempt   ⊙ =Conscious Sedation   ✚=Add-on Code

Diagnostic Ultrasound

▶All diagnostic ultrasound examinations require permanently recorded images with measurements, when such measurements are clinically indicated. For those codes whose sole diagnostic goal is a biometric measure (ie, 76514, 76516, and 76519), permanently recorded images are not required. A final, written report should be issued for inclusion in the patient's medical record. The prescription form for the intraocular lens satisfies the written report requirement for 76519. For those anatomic regions that have "complete" and "limited" ultrasound codes, note the elements that comprise a "complete" exam. The report should contain a description of these elements or the reason that an element could not be visualized (eg, obscured by bowel gas, surgically absent, etc).◀

▶If less than the required elements for a "complete" exam are reported (eg, limited number of organs or limited portion of region evaluated), the "limited" code for that anatomic region should be used once per patient exam session. A "limited" exam of an anatomic region should not be reported for the same exam session as a "complete" exam of that same region.◀

▶Doppler evaluation of vascular structures (other than color flow used only for anatomic structure identification) is separately reportable. To report, see Non-Invasive Vascular Diagnostic Studies (93875-93990).◀

▶Ultrasound guidance procedures also require permanently recorded images of the site to be localized, as well as a documented description of the localization process, either separately or within the report of the procedure for which the guidance is utilized.◀

▶Use of ultrasound, without thorough evaluation of organ(s) or anatomic region, image documentation, and final, written report, is not separately reportable.◀

Definitions

> ***A-mode*** implies a one-dimensional ultrasonic measurement ...

> ***M-mode*** implies a one-dimensional ultrasonic measurement ...

> ***B-scan*** implies a two-dimensional ultrasonic scanning ...

> ***Real-time scan*** implies a two-dimensional ultrasonic scanning procedure with display of both two-dimensional structure and motion with time.

(To report diagnostic vascular ultrasound studies, see 93875-93990)

▶(For focused ultrasound ablation treatment of uterine leiomyomata, see Category III codes 0071T, 0072T)◀

 Rationale

Guidelines were added at the beginning of the Diagnostic Ultrasound subsection of the Radiology section to assist users in determining the appropriate criteria for reporting ultrasound examinations. A cross-reference has been added directing users to Category III codes 0071T and 0072T for focused ultrasound ablation treatment of uterine leiomyomata.

Head and Neck

●**76510**   Ophthalmic ultrasound, diagnostic; B-scan and quantitative A-scan performed during the same patient encounter

▲**76511**   quantitative A-scan only

▲**76512**   B-scan (with or without superimposed non-quantitative A-scan)

 Rationale

The ophthalmic ultrasound codes have been revised to distinguish unique services by separating out B-scan probe (76512) from diagnostic quantitative A-scan (76511), to reflect the differences in difficulty and time required to perform this procedure. The quantitative diagnostic A-scan described by code 76511 is done at a few centers for the management of intraocular tumors. The non-quantitative A-scan described by code 76512 is built into some of the B-scan instrumentation, and is not related to the diagnostic A-scan which measures the height, internal reflectivity, and dimensions of the lesion. Code 76510 has been added to describe performance of both a B-scan and quantitative A-scan performed during the same patient-physician encounter.

 Clinical Example (76510)

A 67-year-old, white male is found to have a mass in the temporal retina and is referred for diagnostic ultrasound evaluation.

Description of Procedure (76510)

The B-scan probe is then placed on the cornea and the lesion localized. Multiple views are taken in all quadrants. Any shadowing and reflected patterns are documented. The nature of the mass is evaluated and possible extension is documented. The presence and nature of vitreous cells and overlying retinal detachment is evaluated and documented. Multiple images are taken and clinical correlation is done. The B-scan probe is removed and the physician places an A-scan probe on the globe with the beam passing perpendicularly through the lesion. Multiple images in all quadrants are examined to determine diameter, elevation, and nature of internal reflectivity. Possible breach of Bruch's membrane and choroidal extension is determined. Appropriate views are documented during the scan. Integration of ultrasound findings with clinical presentation is evaluated. The physician formulates the clinical diagnosis.

Clinical Example (76511)

A 68-year-old white male is found to have a mass in the temporal retina and is referred for a diagnostic A-scan to include measurement of the height, internal reflectivity, and dimensions of the lesion.

Description of Procedure (76511)

The lesion is inspected and the cornea is anesthetized. The physician places an A-scan probe on the lids or globe with the beam passing perpendicularly through the lesion. Multiple images in all quadrants are examined to determine diameter, elevation, and nature of internal reflectivity. Possible breach of Bruch's membrane and choroidal extension is determined. Appropriate views are documented during

⊘=Modifier 51 Exempt   ⊙=Conscious Sedation   ✚=Add-on Code

the scan. Integration of ultrasound findings with clinical presentation is evaluated. The physician formulates a clinical diagnosis.

 Clinical Example (76512)

A 68-year-old white male is found to have elevated retina in the temporal posterior segment and is referred for a diagnostic contact B-scan.

Description of Procedure (76512)

The lesion is inspected and the cornea is anesthetized. The physician places an A-scan probe on the lids or globe with the beam passing perpendicularly through the lesion. Multiple images in all quadrants are examined to determine diameter, elevation, and nature of internal reflectivity. Possible breach of Bruch's membrane and choroidal extension is determined. Appropriate views are documented during the scan. Integration of ultrasound findings with clinical presentation is evaluated. The physician formulates a clinical diagnosis.

Abdomen and Retroperitoneum

▶A complete ultrasound examination of the abdomen (76700) consists of B mode scans of: liver, gall bladder, common bile duct, pancreas, spleen, kidneys, and the upper abdominal aorta and inferior vena cava including any demonstrated abdominal abnormality.◀

▶A complete ultrasound examination of the retroperitoneum (76770) consists of B mode scans of: kidneys, abdominal aorta, common iliac artery origins, and inferior vena cava, including any demonstrated retroperitoneal abnormality. Alternatively, if clinical history suggests urinary tract pathology, complete evaluation of the kidneys and urinary bladder also comprises a complete retroperitoneal ultrasound.◀

▶Use of ultrasound, without thorough evaluation of organ(s) or anatomic region, image documentation and final, written report, is not separately reportable.◀

76700 Ultrasound, abdominal, B-scan and/or real time with image documentation; complete

 Rationale

Guidelines have been added to the Abdomen and Retroperitoneum Ultrasound subsection of the Radiology section to assist users in determining the appropriate criteria for reporting ultrasound services. The guidelines define a complete abdominal ultrasound and a complete retroperitoneal ultrasound, and define the services included (eg, written report) in the codes in this section.

Pelvis

OBSTETRICAL

●**76820** Doppler velocimetry, fetal; umbilical artery

●**76821**   middle cerebral artery

▲ **76827**   Doppler echocardiography, fetal, pulsed wave and/or continuous wave with spectral display; complete

76828   follow-up or repeat study

(To report the use of color mapping, use 93325)

 Rationale

Two codes have been added to assess blood flow of umbilical artery (76820) and the fetal middle cerebral artery (76821) to evaluate fetal anemia and fetal growth restriction caused by placental vascular resistance. Umbilical artery Doppler velocimetry is useful in assessing and timing delivery of the growth restricted fetus. Middle cerebral artery peak velocity is useful in evaluating fetuses at risk of anemia and eliminates the risk of fetal loss associated with invasive techniques (eg, amniocentesis and direct sampling of fetal blood). The existing Doppler fetal echocardiography codes 76827 and 76828 have been revised to exclude the general term "cardiovascular system" since this term is redundant, as by definition echocardiography is an evaluation of the cardiovascular system.

 Clinical Example (76820)

A 23-year-old female is referred for evaluation of uterine size less than dates. Her current gestational age is 32 weeks. Review of her history demonstrates a certain last menstrual period confirmed by a 10 week ultrasound performed at the time of her first prenatal visit. Uterine size had been consistent with menstrual dates up until approximately 20 weeks. Since that time there has been a progressive lag in uterine size as compared to her known menstrual age. An obstetrical ultrasound examination is performed. That study demonstrates composite fetal measurements consistent with 29 weeks and significant head/abdomen circumference discrepancy suggesting asymmetric fetal growth retardation. The amniotic fluid volume is normal. Doppler velocimetry of the umbilical artery is performed to further evaluate fetal well-being and determine the need for further intervention.

Description of Procedure (76820)

The physician reviews the prenatal records and reviews previous ultrasound reports and/or films. Next, a visualization is obtained of a segment of the umbilical cord, and a duplex Doppler sampling gate is placed over a portion of an umbilical artery most perpendicular to the axis of the gate. Gain and filters are adjusted to ensure adequate recording of diastolic flow. Two to four waveforms are recorded during period when fetus is inactive and fetal breathing is absent. Electronic calipers are used to measure peak systolic and end diastolic frequency shift. One of several commonly used indices is then calculated.

An average of the results of two to four waveforms is obtained, and comparison of specific normal values to gestational age is made.

 Clinical Example (76821)

The patient is a 25-year-old gravida 3, para 1, ab 1 female who became Rh-D sensitized when she did not receive Rhesus immune globulin at the time of a spontaneous miscarriage in her first pregnancy. In her second pregnancy she had minimal elevation of anti-D titers. In the current (third) pregnancy, the patient's

⊘ =Modifier 51 Exempt   ⊙ =Conscious Sedation   ✚ =Add-on Code

initial antibody screen at 20 weeks' gestation revealed an anti-D titer of 1:128. Middle cerebral artery Doppler studies are performed at 22 weeks gestation in order to assess the risk of ongoing anemia and need for further intervention.

Description of Procedure (76821)
A review of the prenatal records, laboratory data, and/or previous ultrasound reports and/or films is provided.

A real time ultrasound is performed to locate the fetal head. In addition, the anterior wing of the sphenoid bone is identified. Color flow Doppler is used to image the Circle of Willis. A pulsed Doppler gate is placed over the middle cerebral artery near its origin from the Circle of Willis, and transducer probe orientation or gate orientation is adjusted to ensure angle of insonance is close to zero degrees. Two to four measurements are then obtained and the highest velocity is recorded. A comparison of peak systolic velocity is performed to published gestational age-specific norms. The patient is informed of the results. The results are then communicated, and recommendations made to the referring physician. The written report is then prepared and signed.

NON-OBSTETRICAL

▶Code 76856 includes the complete evaluation of the female pelvic anatomy. Elements of this examination include a description and measurements of the uterus and adnexal structures, measurement of the endometrium, measurement of the bladder (when applicable), and a description of any pelvic pathology (eg, ovarian cysts, uterine leiomyomata, free pelvic fluid).◀

▶Code 76856 is also applicable to a complete evaluation of the male pelvis. Elements of the examination include evaluation and measurement (when applicable) of the urinary bladder, evaluation of the prostate and seminal vesicles to the extent that they are visualized transabdominally, and any pelvic pathology (eg, bladder tumor, enlarged prostate, free pelvic fluid, pelvic abscess).◀

▶Code 76857 represents a focused examination limited to the assessment of one or more elements listed in code 76856 and/or the reevaluation of one or more pelvic abnormalities previously demonstrated on ultrasound. Code 76857, rather than 76770, should be utilized if the urinary bladder alone (ie, not including the kidneys) is imaged, whereas code 51798 should be utilized if a bladder volume or post-void residual measurement is obtained without imaging the bladder.◀

▶Use of ultrasound, without thorough evaluation of organ(s) or anatomic region, image documentation, and final, written report, is not separately reportable.◀

76830   Ultrasound, transvaginal

 Rationale
The Non-Obstetrical subheading has been relocated to the Pelvis subsection of the Radiology section, and introductory language added following the Non-Obstetrical heading to assist users in determining if the required criteria are met when reporting non-obstetrical pelvic ultrasound services. The language defines the elements included in the non-obstetrical pelvic ultrasound examination. The language clarifies that code 76856 should be used to report a complete male pelvic ultrasound. Limited ultrasound is also defined in the new introductory language.

Radiation Treatment Delivery

(Radiation treatment delivery (77401-77416) recognizes the technical component and the various energy levels.)

(77400 has been deleted)

▶(For stereotactic body radiation therapy treatment delivery, use Category III code 0082T)◀

 Rationale

A cross-reference has been included to identify the intended use of Category III code 0082T for stereotactic body radiation therapy treatment delivery.

▲77418 Intensity modulated treatment delivery, single or multiple fields/arcs, via narrow spatially and temporally modulated beams, binary, dynamic MLC, per treatment session

(For intensity modulated treatment planning, use 77301)

▶(For compensator-based beam modulation treatment delivery, use Category III code 0073T)◀

 Rationale

Code 77418 was revised by removing the "eg" parenthetical. In addition, a cross-reference has been added to direct the user to the appropriate code for reporting compensator-based modulation treatment delivery, Category III code 0073T. See code 0073T for more information.

Radiation Treatment Management

77432 Stereotactic radiation treatment management of cerebral lesion(s) (complete course of treatment consisting of one session)

▶(For stereotactic body radiation therapy treatment management, use Category III code 0083T)◀

 Rationale

A cross-reference has been added to direct the use of Category III code 0083T to report stereotactic radiation treatment management.

Clinical Brachytherapy

▲77750 Infusion or instillation of radioelement solution (includes three months follow-up care)

(For administration of radiolabeled monoclonal antibodies, ▶use◀ 79403)

▶(For non-antibody radiopharmaceutical therapy by intravenous administration only, not including three month follow-up care, use 79101)◀

 Rationale

Code 77750 was revised to include a parenthetical to clarify the timeframe for follow-up care. In addition, a cross-reference was added to direct users to report

79101 for non-antibody radiopharmaceutical therapy by intravenous administration only, not including three month follow-up care.

Nuclear Medicine

Listed procedures may be performed independently …

Radioimmunoassay tests are found …

The services listed do not include the provision of radium or other radioelements. ▶Diagnostic and therapeutic radiopharmaceuticals supplied by the physician should be reported separately.◀

 Rationale

The Nuclear Medicine guidelines were editorially revised to be consistent with the deletion of code 78990 and 79900, and to indicate that diagnostic and therapeutic radiopharmaceuticals supplied by the physician should be reported separately.

Diagnostic

GASTROINTESTINAL SYSTEM

▲ **78267**   Urea breath test, C-14 (isotopic); acquisition for analysis

78268   analysis

 Rationale

Code 78267 was revised to clarify that this code describes urea breath test studies using C-14 isotope, a radioactive substance. This revision is consistent with concurrent revisions to codes 83013, 83014, and 91065 and the addition of code 83009.

 Clinical Example (78267)

A 39-year-old female has had epigastric pain for 3 weeks, and had reached a level of severity which led her to seek consultation with her primary care physician. Her doctor referred her for evidence of *H. pylori* infection, and ordered a urea breath test. The first part of the procedure, the acquisition of the breath sample, is normally administered by a technologist under the guidance of a physician; the second part of the procedure is the analysis, which involves measurement of the level of radioactivity in the sample using a liquid scintillation counter; the physician supervises the quality of the measurement, reviews the results and reports on the significance of the results to the attending physician.

Description of Procedure (78267)

The physicain supervises data acquisition and processing of data. Next, the data is analyzed and reprocessed as necessary. The study is monitored and an interpretation of the results is provided. The physician then compares the results in relation to current diagnosis and past treatment or examination, if appropriate.

CARDIOVASCULAR SYSTEM

78460   Myocardial perfusion imaging; (planar) single study, at rest or stress (exercise and/or pharmacologic), with or without quantification

▲**78464**   tomographic (SPECT), single study (including attenuation correction when performed), at rest or stress (exercise and/or pharmacologic), with or without quantification

▲**78465**   tomographic (SPECT), multiple studies (including attenuation correction when performed), at rest and/or stress (exercise and/or pharmacologic) and redistribution and/or rest injection, with or without quantification

✍ Rationale

Codes 78464 and 78465 have been revised to include attenuation correction when performed, in order to report myocardial perfusion single photon emission computed tomography (SPECT) imaging with attenuation correction requiring professional interpretation of data generated by the system. These code revisions incorporate into the existing codes the additional professional, technical, and acquisition time as well as additional hardware and software resources associated with the attenuation correction techniques. Attenuation correction imaging corrects distortions in SPECT images caused by overlying tissue and scattered photons. The procedure requires professional interpretation of data generated by an attenuation correction system, differentiates attenuation artifact from coronary artery disease when performing myocardial perfusion SPECT imaging, and consists of both the device and software. Scatter correction is important for more accurate measures of myocardial uptake values and to assist in minimizing artifacts that can result from subdiaphragmatic activity in proximity to the heart.

OTHER PROCEDURES

▶(78810 has been deleted. To report, see 78811-78813)◀

▶(For PET of brain, see 78608, 78609)◀

▶(For PET myocardial imaging, see 78491, 78492)◀

●**78811**   Tumor imaging, positron emission tomography (PET); limited area (eg, chest, head/neck)

●**78812**   skull base to mid-thigh

●**78813**   whole body

●**78814**   Tumor imaging, positron emission tomography (PET) with concurrently acquired computed tomography (CT) for attenuation correction and anatomical localization; limited area (eg, chest, head/neck)

●**78815**   skull base to mid-thigh

●**78816**   whole body

▶(Report 78811-78816 only once per imaging session)◀

▶(Computed tomography (CT) performed for other than attenuation correction and anatomical localization is reported using the appropriate site specific CT code with modifier 59)◀

⊘=Modifier 51 Exempt   ⊙=Conscious Sedation   ✚=Add-on Code

Rationale

Six new codes for reporting tumor imaging by positron emission tomography (PET) and computed tomography (CT) procedures have been added to the Nuclear Medicine Diagnostic subsection of CPT. Code 78810 has been deleted and a cross-reference has been added to direct users to the appropriate PET procedures.

Codes 78811-78816 differentiate the three different levels of work associated with PET and PET/CT imaging.

Code 78811 is intended to report a PET study for a limited area (eg, chest, head/neck), while code 78812 is intended to describe a PET study of the skull base to mid-thigh. Code 78813 is intended to describe a PET study of the whole body.

Code 78814 describes the reporting of a PET procedure with concurrently acquired CT for attenuation correction and anatomical localization of a limited area (eg, chest, head/neck). Code 78815 similarly describes a study using PET with concurrently acquired CT for attenuation correction and anatomical localization of the skull base to mid-thigh. Finally, code 78816 is intended to report a whole body study using PET with concurrently acquired CT for attenuation correction and anatomical localization. A cross-reference following this series of codes was added to instruct the user to report 78811-78816 only once per imaging session.

In addition to the establishment of codes 78811-78816, a series of cross-references have been added to direct the user to the appropriate PET codes for brain studies (78680, 78609); direct the user to the appropriate PET codes for myocardial studies (78491, 78492); instruct the user that these procedures should be reported one time per imaging session; and inform the user that the site-specific CT codes with modifier 59 should be used if CT is performed for other than attenuation correction and anatomical localization.

Clinical Example (78811)

The patient is a 42-year-old female with a history of invasive, ductal carcinoma of the left breast. The initial tumor was 4.5 cm in largest diameter by mammography. She has now completed neoadjuvant chemotherapy and assessment of treatment response is requested prior to surgical resection. A limited PET scan of the chest is performed.

Description of Procedure (78811)

An appropriate dose of radiopharmaceutical is prescribed by the physician. The physician supervises a certified technologist who assays the dose of the radiopharmaceutical, instructs the patient on the procedure, and injects the radiopharmaceutical in a designated injection room where the patient remains during the uptake period. The physician supervises the technologist in the acquisition and reconstruction of the data in multiple planes including transmission scans, and for the non-attenuation corrected and attenuation corrected emission scans. The physician reviews the study for adequacy and need for additional acquisitions. All images are interpreted by the physician including correlation with prior imaging studies. Quantification of an abnormality is made by the calculation of the standardized uptake value (SUV) when clinically indicated. The physician dictates the report for the medical record.

Clinical Example (78812)

A 59-year-old male with a long history of smoking presents with a new 2.0 cm nodule on chest x-ray. A computed tomography (CT) scan of the chest is performed and demonstrates an indeterminate solitary pulmonary nodule. A transthoracic needle aspiration biopsy demonstrates a non-small, cell, lung cancer. A position emission tomography (PET) scan is performed from skull base to mid thigh for initial staging of the lung cancer.

Description of Procedure (78812)

An appropriate dose of radiopharmaceutical is prescribed by the physician. The physician supervises a certified technologist who assesses the dose of the radiopharmaceutical, instructs the patient on the procedure, and injects the radiopharmaceutical in a designated injection room where the patient remains during the uptake period. The physician supervises the technologist in the acquisition and reconstruction of the data in multiple planes including transmission scans, and for the non-attenuation corrected and attenuation corrected emission scans. The physician reviews the study for adequacy and need for additional acquisitions. All images are interpreted by the physician including correlation with prior imaging studies. Quantification of an abnormality is made by the calculation of the standardized uptake value (SUV) when clinically indicated. The physician dictates the report for the medical record.

Clinical Example (78813)

The patient is a 33-year-old male with a history of a malignant melanoma resected from his back, inferior to the right scapula, eight months previously. A small, non-painful, left axillary lymph node has developed in the previous month. All recent laboratory and imaging studies have been unremarkable. He is referred for staging prior to left, axillary resection. A whole-body PET scan is performed.

Description of Procedure (78813)

An appropriate dose of radiopharmaceutical is prescribed by the physician. The physician supervises a certified technologist who assays the dose of the radiopharmaceutical, instructs the patient on the procedure, and injects the radiopharmaceutical in a designated injection room where the patient remains during the uptake period. The physician supervises the technologist in the acquisition and reconstruction of the data in multiple planes including transmission scans, and for the non-attenuation corrected and attenuation corrected emission scans. The physician reviews the study for adequacy and need for additional acquisitions. All images are interpreted by the physician including correlation with prior imaging studies. Quantification of an abnormality is made by the calculation of the standardized uptake value (SUV) when clinically indicated. The physician dictates the report for the medical record.

⊘=Modifier 51 Exempt   ⊙=Conscious Sedation   ✚=Add-on Code

Clinical Example (78814)

The patient is a 52-year-old male with a remote history of adenoid, cystic carcinoma of the left, parotid gland. The patient recently re-presents with facial weakness and paresthesia. Magnetic resonance imaging (MRI) shows abnormal tissue in the parotid bed, but it is unclear whether this is recurrent tumor or post-operative scar. A PET-CT scan of the head/neck and chest is performed to evaluate the extent of recurrent tumor and document precise anatomic distribution prior to consideration for surgery and/or radiation therapy.

Description of Procedure (78814)

An appropriate dose of radiopharmaceutical is prescribed by the physician. The physician supervises a certified technologist who assays the dose of the radiopharmaceutical, instructs the patient on the procedure, and injects the radiopharmaceutical in a designated injection room where the patient remains during the uptake period. The physician supervises the acquisition of CT data in the areas of interest. The physician supervises the technologist in the acquisition and reconstruction of the PET data in multiple planes including transmission scans, and for the non-attenuation corrected and attenuation corrected emission scans. The interpreting physician, using a computer workstation, creates or directly supervises the creation of composite images for anatomic correlation by precisely overlying PET and CT images. The physician reviews 3 sets of images: emission PET scans, the CT anatomical localization data, and a fusion of the two images which contains the PET and CT data anatomically superimposed over each other. PET images are interpreted by the physician and correlated with the CT localization data obtained as well as with relevant prior imaging studies. Quantification of an abnormality is made by the calculation of the standardized uptake value (SUV) when clinically indicated. The physician dictates the report for the medical record.

Clinical Example (78815)

A 67-year-old female with colon carcinoma has had a right hemicolectomy, radiation, and chemotherapy, and is asymptomatic but now has rising carcinoembryonic antigen (CEA) tumor markers. A positron emission tomography-computed tomography (PET-CT) scan from skull base to mid thigh is performed to assess tumor recurrence and document precise anatomic distribution.

Description of Procedure (78815)

An appropriate dose of radiopharmaceutical is prescribed by the physician. The physician supervises a certified technologist who assays the dose of the radiopharmaceutical, instructs the patient on the procedure, and injects the radiopharmaceutical in a designated injection room where the patient remains during the uptake period. The physician supervises the acquisition of CT data in the areas of interest. The physician supervises the technologist in the acquisition and reconstruction of the PET data in multiple planes including transmission scans, and for the non-attenuation corrected and attenuation corrected emission scans. The interpreting physician, using a computer workstation, creates or directly supervises the creation of composite images for anatomic correlation by precisely overlying PET and CT images. The physician reviews 3 sets of images: emission PET scans, the CT anatomical localization data, and a fusion of the two images which contains the PET and CT data anatomically superimposed over each other. PET images are interpreted by the physician and correlated with the CT localization data obtained as well as with relevant prior imaging studies. Quantification of an abnormality is made by the calculation of the standardized uptake value (SUV) when clinically indicated. The physician dictates the report for the medical record.

 ### Clinical Example (78816)

A 47-year-old female had a malignant melanoma resected from her scalp 14 months previously, followed by right, supraclavicular, nodal recurrence eight months later. Imaging studies, including a positron emission tomography (PET) scan, were abnormal only in that known, recurrence site. She has undergone further resection and is now referred for evaluation of her response to chemotherapy and for whole body restaging. A whole body positron emission tomography-computed tomography (PET-CT) scan is performed.

Description of Procedure (78816)

An appropriate dose of radiopharmaceutical is prescribed by the physician. The physician supervises a certified technologist who assays the dose of the radiopharmaceutical, instructs the patient on the procedure, and injects the radiopharmaceutical in a designated injection room where the patient remains during the uptake period. The physician supervises the acquisition of CT data in the areas of interest. The physician supervises the technologist in the acquisition and reconstruction of the PET data in multiple planes including transmission scans, and for the non-attenuation corrected and attenuation corrected emission scans. The interpreting physician, using a computer workstation, creates or directly supervises the creation of composite images for anatomic correlation by precisely overlying PET and CT images. The physician reviews 3 sets of images: emission PET scans, the CT anatomical localization data, and a fusion of the two images which contain the PET and CT data anatomically superimposed over each other. PET images are interpreted by the physician and correlated with the CT localization data obtained as well as with relevant prior imaging studies. Quantification of an abnormality is made by the calculation of the standardized uptake value (SUV) when clinically indicated. The physician dictates the report for the medical record.

78890   Generation of automated data: interactive process involving nuclear physician and/or allied health professional personnel; simple manipulations and interpretation, not to exceed 30 minutes

78891   complex manipulations and interpretation, exceeding 30 minutes

►(78990 has been deleted)◄

 ### Rationale

Code 78990 has been deleted. HCPCS Level II codes may be used to report the diagnostic radiopharmaceuticals used.

Ø=Modifier 51 Exempt   ⊙=Conscious Sedation   ✚=Add-on Code

Therapeutic

▶The oral and intravenous administration codes in this section are inclusive of the mode of administration. For intra-arterial, intra-cavitary, and intra-articular administration, also use the appropriate injection and/or procedure codes, as well as imaging guidance and radiological supervision and interpretation codes, when appropriate.◀

▶(79000, 79001 have been deleted. To report, use 79005)◀

● **79005** Radiopharmaceutical therapy, by oral administration

▶(79020, 79030, 79035 have been deleted. To report, use 79005)◀

▶ (79100 has been deleted. To report, use 79101)◀

● **79101** Radiopharmaceutical therapy, by intravenous administration

▶(Do not report 79101 in conjunction with 36400, 36410, 79403, 90780, 90784, 96408)◀

▶(For radiolabeled monoclonal antibody by intravenous infusion, use 79403)◀

▶(For infusion or instillation of non-antibody radioelement solution that includes three months follow-up care, use 77750)◀

▲ **79200** Radiopharmaceutical therapy, by intracavitary administration

▲ **79300** Radiopharmaceutical therapy, by interstitial radioactive colloid administration

▶(79400 has been deleted. To report, use 79101)◀

79403 Radiopharmaceutical therapy, radiolabeled monoclonal antibody by intravenous infusion

(For pre-treatment imaging, see 78802, 78804)

(Do not report 79403 in conjunction with ▶79101◀)

▶(79420 has been deleted. To report use 79445)◀

▲ **79440** Radiopharmaceutical therapy, by intra-articular administration

● **79445** Radiopharmaceutical therapy, by intra-arterial particulate administration

▶(Do not report 79445 in conjunction with 90783, 96420)◀

▶(Use appropriate procedural and radiological supervision and interpretation codes for the angiographic and interventional procedures provided pre-requisite to intra-arterial radiopharmaceutical therapy)◀

▶(79900 has been deleted)◀

▲ **79999** Radiopharmaceutical therapy, unlisted procedure

✍ Rationale

Comprehensive revisions to the Therapeutic Radiology subsection include new introductory guidelines to explain the appropriate use of the injection codes and redefinition of the 79000 series codes. The revised descriptors are differentiated by route of administration (ie, intravascular, intra-articular, intracavitary, etc)

Codes 79000, 79001, 79020, 79030 and 79035 have been deleted and code 79005 has been established for reporting radiopharmaceutical therapy by oral administration. A related cross-reference has been added to direct users to the appropriate code to report for radiopharmaceutical therapy by oral administration.

Codes 79100 and 79400 have also been deleted and code 79101 has been established for reporting radiopharmaceutical therapy by intravenous administration. In conjunction with these revisions, a series of parenthetical notes has been added to:

1) Direct users to the appropriate code to report for radiopharmaceutical therapy, by intravenous administration (79101), oral administration (79005), or by intra-arterial particulate administration (79445).

2) Exclude the use of code 79101 in conjunction with codes 36400, 36410, 79403, 90780, 90784, 96408.

3) Direct users to code 79403 for reporting radiolabeled monoclonal antibody by intravenous infusion.

4) Direct users to code 77750 for reporting for infusion of instillation of non-antibody radioelements solution that includes three months follow-up care.

Code 79420 was deleted and code 79445 was added for reporting radiopharmaceutical therapy by intra-arterial administration. Two cross-references have been added following code 79445. The first parenthetical excludes the use of 79445 in conjunction with 90783 and 96420. The second cross-reference instructs users to the appropriate procedure and radiological supervision and interpretation codes for the angiographic and interventional procedures provided pre-requisite to intra-arterial radiopharmaceutical therapy.

Codes 79200, 79300, and 79440 were revised to indicate route of administration (eg, intracavitary, interstitial, intra-articular). Code 79999 was revised for consistency with other new unlisted Radiology codes.

Code 79900 has been deleted. HCPCS Level II codes may be used to report the use of therapeutic radiopharmaceuticals.

The descriptor for the unlisted procedure code 79999 has been revised to conform with the other radiopharmaceutical therapy codes.

 ### Clinical Example (79005)

A 56-year-old female presents with symptoms of hyperthyroidism. On physical examination, she had an enlarged, nodular, thyroid gland. The 24-hour thyroid uptake was 43% and a thyroid scan indicated a diffusely enlarged gland with multiple areas of both increased and decreased activity bilaterally. She was referred for I131 therapy for toxic multinodular goiter.

Description of Procedure (79005)

An appropriate dose of radiopharmaceutical is prescribed. The qualified physician supervises a certified technologist who assays the dose of the radiopharmaceutical, instructs the patient on the procedure, and in a designated therapy room assists

⊘=Modifier 51 Exempt   ☉=Conscious Sedation   ✚=Add-on Code

the patient in drinking the radiolabeled drug, mixed in water. The physician reviews post therapy, exposure measurements. The physician discharges the patient with instructions.

 Clinical Example (79101)

A 67-year-old male presents with known prostate carcinoma and has extensive skeletal metastases. He complains of increasing pain in the chest, mid-thoracic and lumbar spine, and legs. He has had spot external beam radiation but now has more diffuse and generalized bone pain and requires narcotics throughout the day to obtain some relief. He also requires narcotics to sleep through the night. He is referred for Strontium 89 therapy as palliation for painful, bony metastases.

Description of Procedure (79101)

An appropriate dose of radiopharmaceutical is prescribed. The qualified physician supervises a certified technologist who assays the dose of the radiopharmaceutical and obtains intravenous (IV) access. The radiopharmaceutical is administered slowly by the physician. (It typically takes up to 10 minutes.) The physician reviews post therapy, exposure measurements. The physician discharges the patient with instructions.

Clinical Example (79445)

A 56-year-old male with colorectal cancer developed multiple, liver metastases. Because of the number of liver metastases, local therapy (eg, surgical resection, radiofrequency ablation) was not an option, and he had failed systemic chemotherapy. The patient had no evidence of metastasis elsewhere. He was referred for possible intra-arterial radiotherapy.

Description of Procedure (79445)

An appropriate dose of radiopharmaceutical is prescribed. The qualified physician supervises a certified technologist who assays the dose of the radiopharmaceutical. Coordination with physicians obtaining appropriate intra-arterial access is obtained, the prerequisite arterial access, selective vascular selection(s), angiogram(s), and intervention(s) are performed and are separately coded by the relevant providing physician(s). In coordination with the operating interventionalist, the physician supervises the administration of the radiopharmaceutical. Post injection scintigraphic images are acquired and interpreted to assess the final distribution of the intra-arterial injection. The physician reviews post therapy, exposure measurements and imaging data. The physician discharges the patient with instructions.

Pathology and Laboratory

For 2005, codes and cross-references have been added to report *Helicobacter pylori* testing, a series of procedures has been added to report flow cytometry testing and interpretation, and extensive additions and revisions have been made to the morphometric analysis codes in the Surgical Pathology subsection of Pathology and Laboratory.

In conjunction with the addition of Appendix I for Molecular Genetics Testing, guidelines have been added to the Molecular Diagnostics and Cytogenetics subsections of Pathology and Laboratory.

Pathology and Laboratory

82040	Albumin; serum
82042	urine or other source, quantitative, each specimen
82043	urine, microalbumin, quantitative
82044	urine, microalbumin, semiquantitative (eg, reagent strip assay)
	(For prealbumin, use 84134)
●82045	ischemia modified

 Rationale

Code 82045 was established to report the different methodologies of albumin testing for cardiovascular events preceded by ischemia.

Clinical Example (82045)

A patient presents at the emergency room or outpatient setting with chest pain and other symptoms of possible cardiovascular ischemia.

A routine venipuncture is performed to obtain a venous blood specimen. The specimen is tested in the hospital laboratory using the Albumin Cobalt Binding test to assess if biochemical features of ischemia are present.

Positive results are indicative of a true cardiovascular event and result in further workup and probable admission. Negative results suggest that symptoms are non-ischemic in nature.

●82656	Elastase, pancreatic (EL-1), fecal, qualitative or semi-quantitative

Rationale

Code 82656 has been added to report a non-invasive stool test for the determination of exocrine pancreatic function. Code 82656 describes a new analyte utilizing an existing methodology, enzyme-linked immunosorbent assay (ELISA). The fecal pancreatic elastase-1 (PE1) test uses a monoclonal antibody specific to human PE1. In the assay, an aliquot of fecal specimen is emulsified in the extraction buffer and the diluted specimen is transferred to the microtiter well. The test kit contains immobilized monoclonal antibody against PE1. If detectable levels of PE1 are present in the specimen, the PE1 binds to the immobilized antibody. A second monoclonal antibody that is biotinylated binds to PE1 during a second incubation. This is then detected by a peroxidase oxidation reaction yielding a color change when PE1 is present.

Although the measurement of PE1 utilizes an existing methodology, there were no codes that apply specifically to PE1, a new analyte, nor are there any codes that address the specimen preparation that is required before the actual analysis can take place.

Clinical Example (82656)

A 58-year-old white male presented to his primary care physician with a history of chronic diarrhea for the past 2 and one half months. His symptoms include nocturnal diarrhea and recent weight loss (4 pounds). His clinical signs included some steatorrhea and very malodorous and pale stools.

Results from initial investigations, including CBC, ESR, CRP, routine electrolytes, nitrogen, creatinine, LFTs, serum calcium, B12 levels, folate, Fe status, thyroid function, and celiac serology, were all negative. Results from stool culture and microscopy for parasites and yeast were also normal. Because the patient's symptoms indicated possible malabsorption, he was referred to a gastroenterologist. Colonoscopy was done to assess the stool quality and biopsies of the colon were done to rule out other causes of bowel pathology. These investigations yielded negative findings.

The gastroenterologist then needed to assess malabsorption and pancreatic function. The following tests were initially considered: secretin-pancreozymin test; 72-hour fecal fat; acid steatocrit; or chymotrypsin assays. Of these, only the secretin-pancreozymin test demonstrates diagnostic specificity for pancreatic insufficiency; however, it is quite expensive and inconvenient to perform. The human-specific test for pancreatic dysfunction was chosen—fecal pancreatic elastase-1 (PE1). PE1 is currently the preferred noninvasive test for exocrine pancreatic dysfunction. The patient took home the specimen collection kit, collected the stool specimen, and sent the sample to the laboratory for analysis. The sample was sent overnight in a neat vial specimen container at room temperature for processing. The patient was discovered to have PE1 levels below the established reference range (<200 mcg/gm) indicating pancreatic exocrine insufficiency. The patient was subsequently given a trial of pancreatic enzymes and his symptoms rapidly improved.

● 83009   Helicobacter pylori, blood test analysis for urease activity, non-radioactive isotope (eg, C-13)

▶(For H. pylori, breath test analysis for urease activity, see 83013, 83014)◀

▲ 83013   Helicobacter pylori; breath test analysis for urease activity, non-radioactive isotope (eg, C-13)

▲ 83014   drug administration

(For H. pylori, stool, use 87338. For H. pylori, liquid scintillation counter, see 78267, 78268. For H. pylori, enzyme immunoassay, use 87339)

▶(For H. pylori, blood test analysis for urease activity, use 83009)◀

Rationale

The Radiology, Pathology and Laboratory, and Medicine sections of the CPT code set have been updated to include codes and instructional cross-references for reporting *Helicobacter pylori* breath test and blood test analyses.

In the Radiology section, code 78267 was revised to clarify its use of the radioactive (C14) isotope. In the Pathology and Laboratory section codes 83013 and 83014 were revised to clarify that the intent of these procedures is to report

⊘ =Modifier 51 Exempt   ⊙ =Conscious Sedation   ✚ =Add-on Code

breath test analysis for urease activity. In addition, code 83009 was added to describe a blood test analysis for urease activity. Finally, for consistency, the Medicine section has been updated to include a cross-reference following revised code 91065 to direct users to 83013 for non-radioactive (C13) isotope analysis; to 78267 for radioactive (C14) isotope analysis.

Clinical Example (83009)

A serum specimen is collected and analyzed for the presence of urease activity. The patient results are received and the patient is treated accordingly.

Clinical Example (83013)

The typical patient presents with symptoms consisting of burning pain between the breast bone and belly button, pain when their stomach is empty, pain between meals and in the early morning hours, pain relief when eating or taking antacids, nausea, vomiting, and loss of appetite.

●**83630**   Lactoferrin, fecal, qualitative

Rationale

Code 83630 was established to report qualitative determination of lactoferrin in feces. Previously, no code in the CPT code set specifically identified the specific analyte being measured.

Code 83630 is intended to describe a test to determine the presence of intestinal inflammation, differentiate inflammatory from non-inflammatory gastrointestinal disease, monitor patient response to therapy, and predict inflammatory bowel disease recurrence.

Clinical Example (83630)

A 56-year-old male patient presented with diarrhea (of two weeks duration) containing a significant amount of blood and mucus. A test for *Clostridium difficile* was ordered and a sigmoidoscopy performed. The sigmoidoscopy revealed little or no ulceration extending beyond the rectal area. Due to the acute onset of the diarrhea and age of the patient, there was no strong indication of inflammatory bowel disease. Fecal lactoferrin levels were elevated (2500 mcg/mL), indicating significant intestinal inflammation. Test results for Clostridium difficile toxin were negative.

Patient was placed on oral prednisone and enemas containing non-steroidal anti-inflammatory medications. The patient did not respond to treatment and returned to the physician after one week complaining of continued diarrhea with blood loss and subsequent weakness. The patient was immediately admitted to a hospital where a colonoscopy was performed. This showed ulceration far into the colon beyond the small section initially observed during sigmoidoscopy. The fecal lactoferrin level was now 9000 mcg/mL.

The patient was placed on an antiinflamatory agent, an antibiotic, and other medication.

After five days symptoms resolved and lactoferrin levels had dropped significantly to 400 mcg/mL. Patient was discharged and told to continue taking Asacol.

One week later lactoferrin levels, which were being monitored on a daily basis, began to rise (7000 mcg/mL). Medication was changed to a slow release capsule before any diarrhea symptoms reappeared. After one week fecal lactoferrin levels had dropped to less than 7 mcg/mL

Codes 83890-83912 are intended for use ...

Codes 83890-83912 are coded by procedure ...

Code separately for each procedure used ...

▶When molecular diagnostic procedures are performed to test for infectious disease, oncology, hematology, neurology or inherited disorder, use the appropriate modifier to specify probe type or condition tested. (See Appendix I).◀

(For microbial identification, see 87797, 87798)

83890   Molecular diagnostics; molecular isolation or extraction

 Rationale

In an effort to address advances in technology, capture specific data for tracking utilization and provide diagnostic granularity and specific information to allow payors to adjudicate claims for such analyses, a list of Genetic Testing Modifiers has been added, with the inclusion of the new Appendix I. This numeric-alpha modifier coding system is arranged in a hierarchial system with the first (numeric) digit indicating the disease type and the second (alpha) digit indicating the disease/gene. This system allows complete capture of the human genome and presents a viable solution to the expected growth of molecular genetics testing in clinical practice over the next decade, while the technology and nomenclature systems mature.

In addition to the list of Genetic Testing Modifiers in Appendix I, and for consistency purposes, reporting guidelines have been added to the molecular diagnostic and cytogenetic subsections of Pathology and Laboratory to direct users to see Appendix I for a list of appropriate modifiers to report with molecular diagnostic and cytogenetic procedures.

Appendix I is listed in the Appendices section of this book.

● **84163**   Pregnancy-associated plasma protein-A (PAPP-A)

 Rationale

Code 84163 was established to describe testing for pregnancy associated plasma protein-A (PAPP-A). PAPP-A is a screening test to identify women at highest risk of carrying a fetus with Down syndrome, trisomy 18, or other chromosomal abnormality. An increased risk result does not mean the pregnancy is affected with the condition but rather indicates that further testing such as chorionic villus sampling (CVS) or amniocentesis to determine the fetal karyotype is warranted.

⊘=Modifier 51 Exempt   ⊙=Conscious Sedation   ✚=Add-on Code

Clinical Example (84163)

A 28-year-old gravida 2, para 1, female at 12 weeks gestation with no prior history of Down syndrome was offered a first trimester Down syndrome screening test to assess her specific risk of carrying a fetus with Down syndrome. An ultrasound examination was performed in which crown-rump length (CRL) was measured to accurately date the pregnancy and fetal nuchal translucency (NT) was measured according to an internationally recognized standard. CRL measured 55 mm, confirming her gestational age as 12.0 weeks, and the nuchal translucency measured 1.8 mm. At the time of the ultrasound exam, a dried maternal blood sample was obtained via finger stick and forwarded to the laboratory. Free-beta hCG and pregnancy associates plasma protein-A (PAPP-A) were found to be 1.12 and 0.88 multiples of the median (MoM) respectively.

The patient's risk for Down syndrome and trisomy 18 were calculated based on maternal age and the nuchal translucency, free-Beta hCG and PAPP-A values. The patient's risk before this screening test was 1 in 755 based on maternal age alone and after this screening test was 1 in 7541. This risk is much less than the screen cut-off of 1 in 250 therefore no further testing is indicated and the patient is reassured.

▲**84165** Protein; electrophoretic fractionation and quantitation, serum

●**84166**   electrophoretic fractionation and quantitation, other fluids with concentration (eg, urine, CSF)

(For Western Blot tissue analysis, use 88371)

 Rationale

Code 84165 was revised and 84166 was added in the Chemistry subsection to provide a more specific and accurate description of electrophoresis methods and specimen sources for protein and immunofixation electrophoresis procedures. Code 84165 was revised to specify analysis of serum. Code 84166 was established to describe a protein electrophoresis procedure for fluids other than serum with concentration.

 Clinical Example (84165)

Evaluation and report of protein electrophoresis and related laboratory data from a 59-year-old male with elevated total serum protein and bony defects of the skull.

Description of Procedure (84165)
The test result is interpreted. The results are compared to previous study reports. Relevant statistical variations are considered. Clinically meaningful findings are identified. Literature and other results are reviewed during examination of the test result. The provider performs any dictation or report preparation during examination of the test result.

 Clinical Example (84166)

A patient presents with a fifth lumbar vertebra break with bone pain and anemia. Serum electrophoresis indicated a large protein of restricted mobility, which suggested the possibility a monoclonal gammopathy. Subsequent use of immunofixation electrophoresis characterized the protein as an IgG kappa immunoglobulin.

85004 Blood count; automated differential WBC count

▲ **85046** reticulocytes, automated, including one or more cellular parameters (eg, reticulocyte hemoglobin content (CHr), immature reticulocyte fraction (IRF), reticulocyte volume (MRV), RNA content), direct measurement

85049 platelet, automated

Rationale

Indented code 85046 was revised to describe multiple different, yet clinically similar automated cellular parameters and to clarify that this code describes a direct measurement.

Clinical Example 1 (85046)

A neonate developed jaundice shortly after birth and was found to have a hemoglobin of 9.5 g/dL and hematocrit of 29% with otherwise normal red cell indices. Consideration is given to the need for red cell transfusion, but there is the desire to avoid exposure to allogenic blood products. A reticulocyte analysis by automated methods allowing the measurement of an immature reticulocyte fraction (IRF) is ordered, which shows a normal reticulocyte count, but an elevated IRF at 0.41 (normal range 0.1–0.3). Evaluation for active hemolysis (blood smear review, haptoglobin, DAT) were all negative. The elevated IRF is indicative of active erythropoiesis, hence the decision for transfusion was postponed due to the evidence of bone marrow activity and the lack of evidence of a hemolytic process. During the next few days, the hemoglobin and hematocrit begin to rise and a follow-up reticulocyte count showed elevated reticulocyte levels and a persistent elevation of the IRF. The need for transfusion was then judged to be nil.

Clinical Example 2 (85046)

A 64-year-old male with mild osteoarthritis and non-insulin dependent diabetes was found to have a single guiac positive stool. During further evaluation he was found to have a mildly microcytic anemia. The differential diagnosis included blood loss, iron deficiency, and anemia of chronic disease. Reticulocyte analysis by automated methods was performed and revealed a normal reticulocyte count, normal IRF, normal reticulocyte cell volume (MRV) and normal reticulocyte hemoglobin content (CHr). These laboratory values indicated the cause of the anemia to be chronic disease, which was further confirmed by normal iron studies.

Clinical Example 3 (85046)

A 73-year-old female presented with intermittent dyspnea upon exertion without other known medical problems was found upon a routine medical examination to have a borderline normochromic anemia. Reticulocyte analysis indicated a high normal reticulocyte count, but an elevated IRF with normal CHr and MRV. A subsequent cardiac evaluation indicated aortic stenosis. A nearly compensated hemolytic anemia on a mechanical basis was then considered as the cause for the borderline anemia, which was subsequently confirmed by decreased haptoglobin levels.

Immunology

●**86064**   B cells, total count

▶(For flow cytometric immunophenotyping for the assessment of potential hematolymphoid neoplasia, see 88182, 88184-88189)◀

 Rationale

The number of clinical flow cytometric applications has grown significantly in the past few years as has the number of antibodies used to evaluate hematologic conditions. To address the changing medical environment, three new procedure codes have been established in the Immunology section to describe total B cell (86064), Natural Killer (NK) cells (86379), and stem cells (86587). Cross-references also have been added following codes 86064, 86379 and 86587 to report flow cytometric immunophenotyping for the assessment of potential hematolymphoid neoplasia. Additionally, unlisted antigen code 86586 has been added and is intended to be reported for each antigen tested.

Code 86064 is intended to report total count of B cells. Code 86379 is intended to report Natural Killer (NK) cells, total count. Code 86587 describes total count of stem cells (ie, CD34). These codes are to be used only for quantitative analyses such as those used to assess for immunodeficiency and do not include an interpretive report. When one is assessing for hematolymphoid neoplasia, codes 88182 and 88184-88189 should be used.

 Clinical Example (86064)

Peripheral blood immunophenotyping is performed on a 6-year-old patient with recurrent atypical infections to assess for potential immunodeficiency.

▲**86334**   Immunofixation electrophoresis; serum

●**86335**   other fluids with concentration (eg, urine, CSF)

(Lymphocytes immunophenotyping, ▶see 88182, 88189◀ for cytometry; see 88342, 88346 for microscopic techniques)

 Rationale

Code 86334 was revised and 86335 was added to provided a more accurate description of electrophoresis methods. Code 86334 was revised to specify analysis of serum and 86335 was established for reporting immunofixation electrophoresis procedures for fluids other than serum with concentration.

A cross-reference has been included following code 88353 referring to codes 88182, 88189 for cytometry for lymphocyte immunophenotyping and to codes 88342, 88346 for microscopic techniques.

Clinical Example (86334)

Evaluation and report of the immunofixation electrophoresis study in an 84-year-old male with abnormal electrophoretic peak and equivocal immunoelectrophoretic study of serum protein.

Clinical Example (86335)

A patient presents with a fifth lumbar vertebra break with bone pain and anemia. Serum electrophoresis indicated a large protein of restricted mobility, which suggested the possibility of monoclonal gammopathy. Subsequent use of capillary immunosubtraction electrophoresis identified the protein as an IgG kappa monoclonal gammopathy.

● **86379**   Natural killer (NK) cells, total count

▶(For flow cytometric immunophenotyping for the assessment of potential hematolymphoid neoplasia, see 88182, 88184-88189)◀

Rationale

The rationale for code 86379 is included under code 86064.

● **86587**   Stem cells (ie, CD34), total count

▶(For flow cytometric immunophenotyping for the assessment of potential hematolymphoid neoplasia, see 88182, 88189)◀

Rationale

The rationale for code 86587 is included under code 86064.

Microbiology

87040   Culture, bacterial; blood, aerobic, with isolation and presumptive identification of isolates (includes anaerobic culture, if appropriate)

▲ **87046**   stool, aerobic, additional pathogens, isolation and presumptive identification of isolates, each plate

87301   Infectious agent antigen detection by enzyme immunoassay technique, qualitative or semiquantitative, multiple step method; adenovirus enteric types 40/41

87335   Escherichia coli O157

(For giardia antigen, use ▶87329◀)

Rationale

Code 87046 was revised to provide a mechanism to report each plate. Additionally, the cross-reference for giardia antigen was revised to direct users to the correct code.

87802   Infectious agent antigen detection by immunoassay with direct optical observation; Streptococcus, group B

87803   Clostridium difficile toxin A

⊘=Modifier 51 Exempt   ⊙=Conscious Sedation   ✚=Add-on Code

87804	Influenza
●87807	respiratory syncytial virus

 Rationale

Code 87807 was established to report detection of respiratory synctial viral antigen by immunoassay with direct optical observation. Currently codes do exist for respiratory syncytial virus antigen by immunofluorescent technique (87280) and by enzyme immunoassay technique (multiple step method) (87420); however, there is no code for respiratory syncytial virus (RSV) for tests using antigen detection by immunoassay with direct optical observation.

 Clinical Example (87807)

A 2-year-old infant presents to the pediatric clinic with symptoms of fever (102°), cough and malaise, all occurring within the last 24 hours. It is late autumn and both influenza and respiratory syncytial virus have been reported locally. A clinical decision must be made whether this child has a viral or bacterial infection, and if antibiotics should be prescribed. In addition, if the infection is determined to be respiratory syncytial virus, a decision must be made as to whether the infant should be hospitalized and isolated. Also, the clinic is part of the sentinel physicians surveillance network, reporting respiratory syncytial virus to both the Centers for Disease Control and Prevention (CDC) and state public health offices in order to track viral activity from October though May. A nasal wash is performed and the specimen is tested for respiratory syncytial virus. Results are positive for respiratory syncytial virus. Because the infant does not have a bacterial co-infection, antibiotics are not prescribed. The symptoms are sufficiently severe that the infant is admitted to the hospital for oxygen therapy and isolation. A confirmed case of respiratory syncytial virus is reported to the CDC and state public health influenza surveillance programs.

Description of Procedure (87807)

The service includes physician performance or supervision of a nasal wash to collect a suitable specimen. Alternatively, a nasal swab can be used to collect a nasal specimen and then dipping the swab containing the specimen into a solution provided with the test kit. A measured sample of the prepared solution or nasal wash (100 uL) is pipetted onto the rapid test and in 15 minutes the test results are read and interpreted as positive or negative. Built-in procedural controls are reviewed to determine if the test is performed properly. If the test comes from a new kit, external positive and negative controls will be run on two tests to confirm quality assurance.

Cytopathology

▶(88180 has been deleted. To report, see 88182, 88189)◀

88182	Flow cytometry; cell cycle or DNA analysis
●88184	Flow cytometry, cell surface, cytoplasmic, or nuclear marker, technical component only; first marker

---

+●88185   each additional marker (List separately in addition to code for first marker)

▶(Report 88185 in conjunction with 88184)◀

●88187   Flow cytometry, interpretation; 2 to 8 markers

●88188   9 to 15 markers

●88189   16 or more markers

Rationale

The number of clinical flow cytometric applications has grown significantly in the past few years as has the number of antibodies used to evaluate hematologic conditions. In response to the changing medical environment, two codes have been established to report the technical component of flow cytometry and three codes to report flow cytometric interpretations. Code 88184 and add-on code 88185 describe the technical component of flow cytometry procedures. Codes 88187, 88188, and 88189 are intended to describe flow cytometry interpretation. Codes 88180 and 88182 continue to describe flow cytometry procedures for each cell surface, cell cycle or DNA analysis. A cross-reference was added following code 88185 to direct users to report code 88185 in conjunction with code 88184.

In conjunction with these changes to the Cytopathology subsection, three additional cross-references were added in the Immunology subsection following codes 86064, 86379, and 86587 to direct the user to report 88180 and 88182 for flow cytometric immunophenotyping for the assessment of potential hematolymphoid neoplasia. For consistency purposes, code 88180 has been deleted and an instructional cross-reference has been added to direct users to the appropriate codes to report.

Cytogenetic Studies

▶When molecular diagnostic procedures are performed to test for oncologic or inherited disorders, use the appropriate modifier to specify probe type or condition tested. (See Appendix I).◀

(For acetylcholinesterase, use 82013)

(For alpha-fetoprotein, serum or amniotic fluid, see 82105, 82106)

(For laser microdissection of cells from tissue sample, see 88380)

88230   Tissue culture for non-neoplastic disorders; lymphocyte

Rationale

As mentioned before, in addition to the inclusion of Appendix I, general guidelines have been added to the molecular diagnostic and cytogenetic subsections of the Pathology and Laboratory section to direct users to see Appendix I for a list of appropriate modifiers to report with molecular diagnostic and cytogenetic procedures.

88342 Immunohistochemistry (including tissue immunoperoxidase), each antibody

▶(Do not report 88342 in conjunction with 88360 or 88361 for the same antibody)◀

(For quantitative or semiquantitative immunohistochemistry, ▶see 88360,◀ 88361)

88355 Morphometric analysis; skeletal muscle

88356 nerve

88358 tumor (eg, DNA ploidy)

(Do not report 88358 with 88313 unless each procedure is for a different special stain)

●**88360** Morphometric analysis, tumor immunohistochemistry (eg, Her-2/neu, estrogen receptor/progesterone receptor), quantitative or semiquantitative, each antibody; manual

▲**88361** using computer-assisted technology

(Do not report ▶88360,◀ 88361 with 88342 unless each procedure is for a different antibody)

▶(For morphometric analysis, in situ hybridization, see 88367, 88368)◀

(When semi-thin plastic-embedded sections are performed in conjunction with morphometric analysis, only the morphometric analysis should be reported; if performed as an independent procedure, see codes 88300-88309 for surgical pathology.)

▲**88365** In situ hybridization (eg, FISH), each probe

▶(Do not report 88365 in conjunction with 88367, 88368 for the same probe)◀

●**88367** Morphometric analysis, in situ hybridization, (quantitative or semi-quantitative) each probe; using computer-assisted technology

●**88368** manual

✐ Rationale

In situ hybridization (ISH) has rapidly gained acceptance in the pathology and oncology communities as a definitive diagnostic marker for certain cancers. In response to the changing clinical practice, the following changes have been added for 2005:

1) code 88360 established to describe manual morphometric analysis and codes 88361 and 88365 revised for number sequencing purposes;

2) codes 88367 and 88368 established to describe morphometric analysis in situ hybridization differentiated as manual and computer-assisted;

3) a parenthetical note added following code 88342 to preclude the reporting of 88360 or 88361 in conjunction with 88342 for the same antibody;

4) an existing cross-reference revised following code 88342 to reflect the addition of code 88360;

5) a cross-reference added following code 88361 to preclude reporting of code 88360 or 88361 with 88342 for the same antibody;

6) a cross-reference added following code 88361 to direct the user to see codes 88367, 88368 for morphometric analysis;

7) a cross-reference added following code 88365 to preclude reporting 88365 in conjunction with codes 88367 or 88368 for the same probe.

Fluorescent in situ hybridization (FISH) involves comparing double-stranded DNA from a patient sample with that of a labeled control sample using fluorescence for signal detection. Both samples are treated to render them single-stranded. Pairing (hybridization) of the single strands then occurs. The amount of pairing is measured and is indicative of the genomic relationship between the two. The nucleic acid probe result may be confirmatory or exclude the possibility of a specific condition. Similar studies are also performed with chromogenic labels (CISH), differing only by the type of signal that is visualized.

There are, however, other situations where relative gene copy number carries significant prognostic and therapeutic implications. The most common example of this is ISH for HER-2/neu amplification in which individual cells are examined by fluorescent microscopy and each probe signal is counted per cell, and a ratio is calculated in comparison to a centromere marker. HER-2/neu gene amplification is defined as a ratio over 2.0. The additional quantitative steps reflect distinctly more work in comparison to the qualitative analysis. Quantitative ISH studies are currently coded as 88358 for morphometric analysis and 88365 for the ISH preparation. Utilization of quantification performed as an adjunct procedure to the hybridization has increased and this has led payors payment policy for these services.

Clinical Example (88360)

A 54-year-old female has previously been diagnosed with invasive ductal carcinoma of the breast with axillary nodal metastasis identified by sentinel lymph node biopsy. Stained slides are analyzed by immunohistochemistry, along with reference positive and negative controls, first determining the appropriate areas of the tumor to evaluate and then interpreting the analysis as amplification of the HER2 gene.

Clinical Example (88361)

A 54-year-old female has previously been diagnosed with ductal carcinoma of the breast with axillary nodal metastasis identified on sentinel lymph node biopsy. The stained slides are analyzed by the pathologist, along with reference positive and negative samples, to determine if the staining process is interpretable and therefore warrants a semiquantitative or quantitative interpretation. The immunoassay is positive for estrogen receptors and evaluation is performed. A semiquantitative or quantitative interpretation is provided using a computer assisted methodology.

⊘ =Modifier 51 Exempt   ⊙ =Conscious Sedation   ✚ =Add-on Code

Description of Procedure (88361)

Tumor tissue is submitted for immunohistchemical staining using a monoclonal antibody that is complementary to the human estrogen receptor. Interpretation of the stained slides is performed to determine if a semiquantitative/quantitative procedure is needed. Interpretation of the preparation is performed visually using manual microscopy. Comparison to previous study reports is performed. Relevant statistical variations are considered. Clinically meaningful findings are identified. Review of research literature, if any, during examination of the test results is performed. Dictation or report preparation during examination of the test results is performed.

Clinical Example (88365)

A 47-year-old male who had received a heart transplant two years previously and has been on maintenance immunosuppression developed bowel obstruction and was found to have a post transplant lymphoproliferative disorder of monomorphic large cell type. Stained slides of the tumor are analyzed by chromogenic in situ hybridization (CISH) for RNA associated with the Epstein Barr virus (EBV) by the pathologist, along with reference positive and negative controls. The pathologist first identifies the areas of the slide containing appropriate neoplasm for evaluation, and then interprets the CISH preparations as demonstrating the presence of EBV in the tumor cells.

Clinical Example (88367)

A 54-year-old female has previously been diagnosed with invasive ductal carcinoma of the breast with axillary nodal metastasis identified by sentinel lymph node biopsy. Stained slides are analyzed by fluorescence in situ hybridization (FISH) by the pathologist at a FISH workstation, along with reference positive and negative controls, first determining the appropriate areas of the tumor to evaluate, followed by interpretation of the FISH, quantifying amplification of the *HER2* gene.

Clinical Example (88368)

A 54-year-old female has previously been diagnosed with invasive ductal carcinoma of the breast with axillary nodal metastasis identified by sentinel lymph node biopsy. Stained slides are analyzed by fluorescence in situ hybridization (FISH) by the pathologist at a FISH workstation, along with reference positive and negative controls, first determining the appropriate areas of the tumor to evaluate and then interpreting the FISH quantifying amplification of the *HER2* gene.

Reproductive Medicine Procedures

89250   Culture of oocyte(s)/embryo(s), less than 4 days;

▶(To report Hyaluronan binding assay (HBA), use Category III code 0087T)◀

89342   Storage, (per year); embryo(s)

89343   sperm/semen

89344   reproductive tissue, testicular/ovarian

▲ **89346**   oocyte(s)

 Rationale

Code 89346 was editorially revised to replace the word "oocyte" with "oocyte(s)."
Reproductive procedures were added to the CPT book in 2004. For more detailed
information see *CPT Changes: An Insider's View 2004.*

⊘=Modifier 51 Exempt   ⊙=Conscious Sedation   ✚=Add-on Code

Medicine

Among the changes in the Medicine section for 2005, substantial revisions have been made to the vaccine administration procedure codes, the gastric testing codes and the acupuncture codes. Revisions have also been made to the neurostimulator codes to clarify reporting for initial and subsequent programming services and to the echocardiography guidelines for clarification of the requirements for reporting these services.

Medicine

Immunization Administration for Vaccines/Toxoids

Codes ▶90465◀-90474 must be reported in addition to the vaccine and toxoid code(s) 90476-90749.

▶Report codes 90465-90468 only when the physician provides face-to-face counseling of the patient and family during the administration of a vaccine. For immunization administration of any vaccine that is not accompanied by face-to-face physician counseling to the patient/family, report codes 90471-90474.◀

● **90465** Immunization administration under 8 years of age (includes percutaneous, intradermal, subcutaneous, or intramuscular injections) when the physician counsels the patient/family; first injection (single or combination vaccine/toxoid), per day

▶(Do not report 90465 in conjunction with 90467)◀

+● **90466** each additional injection (single or combination vaccine/toxoid), per day (List separately in addition to code for primary procedure)

▶(Use 90466 in conjunction with 90465 or 90467)◀

● **90467** Immunization administration under age 8 years (includes intranasal or oral routes of administration) when the physician counsels the patient/family; first administration (single or combination vaccine/toxoid), per day

▶(Do not report 90467 in conjunction with 90465)◀

+● **90468** each additional administration (single or combination vaccine/toxoid), per day (List separately in addition to code for primary procedure)

▶(Use 90468 in conjunction with 90465 or 90467)◀

 Rationale

A new series of codes (90465-90468) for immunization administration which incorporates the work of physician immunization counseling for young children (under 8 years of age) has been added. The majority of vaccines are mandated for early childhood when reactions can be both more frequent and more severe. Children react differently to vaccines due to the physiologic differences inherent in developing brains, with associated neurological events such as seizures and sequelae of an encephalopathic nature. The increased attention to claims of associated developmental problems and risks related to vaccines has increased families' concerns and the need for physician counseling prior to administration. Lastly, since many vaccines are mandated, physicians often spend additional time counseling those families who choose not to immunize their children.

 Clinical Example (90465)

An 18-month-old girl is seen for a well-child visit. In accordance with national recommendation for childhood immunizations, the pediatrician determines that the child should receive a diphtheria, tetanus, and pertussis (DTaP) vaccination.

Description of Procedure (90465)

The physician first reviews the patient's previous experience with the vaccine and determines if there are any contraindications prior to proceeding. A vaccine information sheet (VIS) is given to the parent/guardian for the DTaP vaccine, and in keeping with state and federal laws, the information including risks and benefits of DTaP vaccine is discussed with the parent/guardian in detail, and a discussion occurs about the vaccine and the diseases it protects against. Appropriate documentation is entered into the patient record. The documentation for the vaccine includes: which VIS was given; the date of the publication of the VIS; the date the VIS was given; the name, address, and title of the person who administered the vaccine; the date of administration; the vaccine manufacturer; and the vaccine lot number. Additionally, the appropriate types and doses of medications to alleviate fever and pain at the injection site are discussed. Since the physician participates in the Vaccines for Children (VFC) program, the nurse obtains the vaccine from the appropriate inventory, making sure to document which supply of vaccines was used for this particular patient. Although federal law does not mandate separate vaccine inventories, the Centers for Disease Control and Prevention (CDC) strongly recommend them for reasons of accountability. Informed consent is obtained by the physician who then orders the nurse to prepare the vaccine. The nurse prepares the DTaP vaccine using a safe, sharp syringe and administers the vaccine. The patient is observed in the office for an immediate allergic reaction and then is discharged home by the nurse. The immunization tracking number is entered into a computerized statewide registry.

▲ 90471   Immunization administration (includes percutaneous, intradermal, subcutaneous, or intramuscular injections); one vaccine (single or combination vaccine/toxoid)

▶(Do not report 90471 in conjunction with 90473)◄

✚ 90472   each additional vaccine (single or combination vaccine/toxoid) (List separately in addition to code for primary procedure)

(Use 90472 in conjunction with 90471 ▶or 90473◄)

90473   Immunization administration by intranasal or oral route; one vaccine (single or combination vaccine/toxoid)

▶(Do not report 90473 in conjunction with 90471)◄

✚ 90474   each additional vaccine (single or combination vaccine/toxoid) (List separately in addition to code for primary procedure)

(Use 90474 in conjunction with ▶90471 or◄ 90473)

✍ Rationale

Code 90471 has been revised to eliminate the phrase "jet injection," as this route of administration is not commonly performed. Two parenthetical notes were added following codes 90471 and 90473 to preclude the reporting of both codes 90471 and 90473 together. In addition, the parenthetical notes following codes 90472 and 90474 have been revised for consistency.

⊘=Modifier 51 Exempt   ⊙=Conscious Sedation   ✚=Add-on Code

Vaccines, Toxoids

Codes 90476-90748 identify the vaccine product only. To report the administration of a vaccine/toxoid, the vaccine/toxoid product codes 90476-90749 must be used in addition to an immunization administration code(s) ▶90465-90474◀. Do not append modifier 51 to the vaccine/toxoid product codes 90476-90749.

If a significantly separately identifiable …

To meet the reporting requirements of immunization registries …

Separate codes are available for combination vaccines …

(For immune globulins, see codes 90281–90399, and 90780–90784 for administration of immune globulins)

90476   Adenovirus vaccine, type 4, live, for oral use

⊘●**90656**   Influenza virus vaccine, split virus, preservative free, for use in individuals 3 years and above, for intramuscular use

⊘▲**90700**   Diphtheria, tetanus toxoids, and acellular pertussis vaccine (DTaP), for use in individuals younger than 7 years, for intramuscular use

✍ Rationale

The descriptor language of code 90700 was revised to reflect the age group (younger than 7 years) for which this toxoid/vaccine was intended.

Code 90656 has been established to report injection of thimerosal-free influenza injections for individuals 3 years and above. In addition, the code range for the immunization administration codes (90465-90474) was added to the introductory language. In addition, the guidelines have been revised to reflect the new range of codes for immunization administration (90465–90474).

Therapeutic, Prophylactic or Diagnostic Injections

90782   Therapeutic, prophylactic or diagnostic injection (specify material injected); subcutaneous or intramuscular

(For administration of vaccines/toxoids, see ▶90465◀-90472)

✍ Rationale

The parenthetical note included subsequent to the heading for this section was revised to include the new codes for pediatric immunization administration (90465-90468).

Biofeedback

90911   Biofeedback training, perineal muscles, anorectal or urethral sphincter, including EMG and/or manometry

(For incontinence treatment by pulsed magnetic neuromodulation, use Category III code 0029T)

▶(For testing of rectal sensation, tone and compliance, use 91120)◀

 Rationale

A parenthetical note has been added following code 90911 directing users to code 91120 for reporting testing of rectal sensation, tone and compliance.

Gastroenterology

▶(91032 and 91033 have been deleted. To report, see 91034, 91035)◀

● **91034**   Esophagus, gastroesophageal reflux test; with nasal catheter pH electrode(s) placement, recording, analysis and interpretation

● **91035**   with mucosal attached telemetry pH electrode placement, recording, analysis and interpretation

● **91037**   Esophageal function test, gastroesophageal reflux test with nasal catheter intraluminal impedance electrode(s) placement, recording, analysis and interpretation;

● **91038**   prolonged (greater than 1 hour, up to 24 hours)

● **91040**   Esophageal balloon distension provocation study

▶(For balloon dilatation with endoscopy, see 43220, 43249, 43456, or 43458)◀

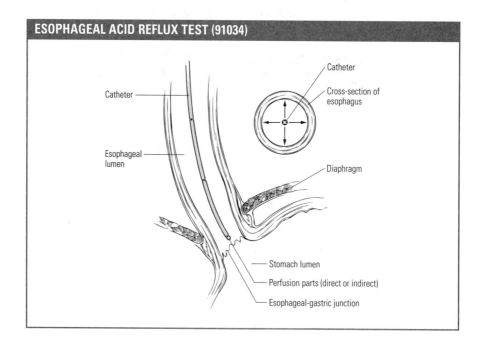

ESOPHAGEAL ACID REFLUX TEST (91034)

Ø=Modifier 51 Exempt   ⊙=Conscious Sedation   ✚=Add-on Code

✍️ Rationale

Codes 91032 and 91033 were deleted and replaced by codes 91034 and 91035. These codes have been added to CPT to specifically identify nasal insertion of pH catheters (91034) or mucosal attachment of telemetry pH electrodes (91035) for detection of gastroesophageal reflux disease (GERD). In addition, the language was revised to allow for testing of both acid and non-acidic reflux, replacing acid with reflux.

These codes describe important tests for the diagnosis of GERD. GERD results from the abnormal reflux of stomach contents into the esophagus. This can result in heartburn and other serious problems such as dysphagia, dysphonia, asthma and Barrett's esophagus. Measuring the level of acid in the esophagus is an important step in the diagnosis of patients with symptomatic GERD and establishing treatment plans. Further, pH monitoring can be used to determine the effectiveness of treatment and the potential need for additional medical, pharmacologic, endoscopic, and/or surgical intervention.

Traditionally, ambulatory pH monitoring was accomplished by use of a catheter that was passed through the patient's nose and connected to a recording device (previously 91032 and 91033, now represented by code 91034). Ideally, the recording was performed for a 24-hour period. Because of the discomfort associated with the intranasal catheter, patients frequently changed their daily activity during the day of the test. For example, patients often self-reported that they stayed home from work and ate different foods. This leads to test results that were not representative of a "normal" day. A number of patients refused to have the test performed.

A newer method of monitoring intra-esophageal pH levels has become available in recent years. This is a telemetry-based system for measuring acid reflux (91035). The system involves the placement of a monitoring capsule that is temporarily inserted and attached to the patient's esophagus. The capsule monitors the presence of acid and transmits pH levels via radiofrequency telemetry to an external receiver that the patient wears for up to 72 hours. After a period of several days, the capsule is sloughed by the body and passes through the patient's digestive tract. Use of this method generally results in greater patient compliance with normal daily routines and greater acceptance to have the test performed than catheter-based systems.

Codes 91037 and 91038 are used to describe gastroesophageal impedance monitoring. Prolonged gastroesophageal reflux impedance testing monitors all reflux, both acid and non-acid, over a prolonged period. Code 91038 includes a specific time range in its descriptor to clearly define what constitutes a prolonged period for monitoring intraluminal impedance testing. Impedance is utilized for this procedure since use of this modality provides a comprehensive definition of all reflux regardless of acidity. Nonacid reflux is associated with symptoms such as chest pain, regurgitation, cough, asthma, laryngitis, wheezing, and recurrent pneumonia in patients.

To perform this procedure, a pressure sensing catheter is inserted trans-nasally down to the esophagus to measure sphincter function and esophageal muscular

---

function. The manometry test quantifies sphincter location, length and closure pressure, function, and peristaltic muscular activity of the esophagus during swallow challenges of liquid material. During esophageal function testing, a bolus transit impedance catheter that includes incremental impedance sensors is inserted trans-nasally. The impedance test quantifies bolus transit dynamics and bolus transit effectiveness of the esophagus. Both liquid and viscous swallow challenges are used to optimally test the peristaltic process. Therefore, the new procedure code differs since assessment of both muscular activity and bolus transit dynamics are determined in a single procedure.

The proposed modification gives clarification to where and how the test is done to account for dynamic readings and clarifies the meaning of prolonged as greater than 1 hour and less than 24 hours.

Code 91040 is used to report an esophageal balloon distension provocation study. For this procedure, serial insufflations of air or water are used to determine the threshold which reproduces symptomatic response in the patient. These insufflations are performed with the patient blind to the volume of substance infused to allow accurate results. The results are used by the physician to evaluate recurrent unexplained chest pain and dysphagia. Esophageal balloon provocation has been shown to be sensitive and specific in pointing to an esophageal source for chest pain in patients with or without GERD.

Non-cardiac chest pain remains a common and vexing clinical problem. Provocative esophageal testing can help to identify an esophageal cause for the pain. Current gastrointestinal (GI) procedures used to evaluate non-cardiac chest pain are insufficient for identifying this type of problem as these procedures either lack the sensitivity and specificity, are only able to detect gastroesophageal reflux, or focus on acid causes for chest pain.

 Clinical Example (91034)

A 54-year-old female presents with a three-year history of heartburn, regurgitation and throat soreness. She has no dysphagia, weight loss, or gastrointestinal (GI) bleeding. She has not improved with over the counter medications. Her diagnostic testing, including an upper GI and esophagogastroduodenoscopy (EGD), was normal. She is suspected to have gastroesophageal reflux disease (GERD) and was placed on pharmacological agents with initial improvement, but continues to have breakthrough regurgitation symptoms despite adjusting pharmacological management.

Description of Procedure (91034)

Following nasal spray administration of anesthetic, a thin, plastic catheter is passed through one nostril, down the back of the throat, and into the esophagus as the patient swallows. The tip of the catheter contains a sensor that is positioned in the esophagus so that it is just above the lower esophageal sphincter. In this position, the sensor records each reflux of acid. The catheter protruding from the nose is connected to a recorder that registers each reflux of acid. The patient is counseled again to go about his or her usual activities, for example, eating, sleeping, and working. Meals, periods of sleep, and symptoms are recorded by the patient in a diary and/or by pushing buttons on the recorder. The patient is discharged with the catheter and recorder in place. The patient returns to the site of service, typically the next day, and the catheter is removed.

 Clinical Example (91035)

A 40-year-old male presents with severe chest pain. A thorough cardiac evaluation suggested no cardiac abnormality. The patient was placed on pharmacological agents, but symptoms have persisted. An esophagogastroduodenoscopy (EGD) revealed mild, distal, esophageal erythema, otherwise unremarkable.

Description of Procedure (91035)

Following administration of anesthetic, a capsule that contains an acid sensing probe, a battery, and a transmitter is introduced into the esophagus on a catheter through the nose or mouth and is attached to the lining of the esophagus with a clip. The catheter is detached from the capsule and removed. The patient is counseled again to go about his or her usual activities, for example, eating, sleeping, and working. Meals, periods of sleep, and symptoms are recorded by the patient in a diary and/or by pushing buttons on the recorder. The patient is discharged with a recorder in place. The patient returns to the site of service, typically the next day, to return the recorder. Note: The capsule can transmit for two days, and then the battery dies. Five to seven days later, the capsule falls off and is passed in the stool.

 Clinical Example (91037)

A 56-year-old female is referred for evaluation of difficulty in swallowing and heartburn. The patient has tried a variety of pharmacologic agents without relief of symptoms.

Description of Procedure (91037)

Following nasal spray administration of anesthetic, a multi-channel catheter with impedance sensors is inserted via the nose to a depth of 60 cm. The patient was allowed some time to accommodate the catheter. The catheter's distal impedance sensor is then positioned 5 centimeters above the lower esophageal sphincter (LES). The patient is instructed to perform 10 swallows of 5 mL saline material at 20-30 second intervals. Time and impedance measurements are taken as the bolus material moves through the esophagus into the stomach. The patient is then instructed to perform 10 swallows of 5 mL viscous material at 20-30 second intervals. Time and impedance measurements are recorded as the bolus material moves through the esophagus into the stomach. At the conclusion of the procedure, the catheter is withdrawn and the patient is discharged to home.

 Clinical Example (91038)

The patient is a 44-year-old male with a complaint of frequent heartburn. The patient has tried a variety of pharmacologic agents without relief of symptoms. An esophagogastroduodenoscopy (EGD) was unremarkable. An esophageal pH test failed to elucidate the etiology of the patient's symptoms.

Description of Procedure (91038)

Following nasal spray administration of anesthetic, a multi-channel catheter with impedance sensors is inserted via the nose to a depth of 60 centimeters. After the catheter is positioned, it is taped securely at the nares to prevent movement over the prolonged monitoring period. The patient is then instructed in the usage of a recording device to monitor symptom occurrences, body position and meal periods. After completing the patient instructions, the recording is started and the patient is discharged from the laboratory. The patient is instructed to keep a log book of symptoms. Upon completion of the monitoring period, the patient returns to the lab, the catheter is withdrawn, and the patient is discharged.

 ### Clinical Example (91040)

A 45-year-old male is referred for evaluation of recurrent, unexplained, chest pain and dysphagia. Cardiac workup and EGD have been unremarkable.

Description of Procedure (91040)

After informed consent is obtained, the patient is brought to the gastroenterology laboratory. Following topical anesthesia of a naris, a 4.5-millimeter catheter with a 45-millimeter, latex balloon attached to a single, air-perfusion port is inserted into the middle esophagus. Serial insufflations using air or water are performed in 2 cc increments from 0 to 30 cc, with the patient blinded to the volume infused. With each insufflation, the patient is asked if he/she experienced reproduction of symptoms. Once a positive response was obtained, several insufflations at similar volumes and sham insufflations are performed to confirm the positive response. A record of the insufflation volume and symptoms generated is kept. At the completion of the test, the catheter is withdrawn, and the patient is discharged.

▲91065   Breath hydrogen test (eg, for detection of lactase deficiency, fructose intolerance, bacterial overgrowth, or oro-cecal gastrointestinal transit)

▶(For H. pylori breath test analysis, use 83013 for non-radioactive (C-13) isotope or 78268 for radioactive (C-14) isotope)◀

 ### Rationale

Code 91065 is used to identify hydrogen breath testing, utilizing the ability to determine malabsorption of dietary saccharides through use of a breath sample as opposed to an aspirate of gastric contents (sample of the contents of the stomach). Hydrogen breath testing for bacterial overgrowth requires different substrates and a different testing protocol than that used for lactose intolerance. The test is noninvasive and is, therefore, more readily tolerated by patients than alternative testing that requires jejunal intubation and aspiration of contents for detection of bacteria.

A parenthetic note has been included following code 91065 to direct users to the correct coding for H. pylori breath testing.

Hydrogen breath testing has been an established test for measuring gastrointestinal function for more than 20 years. It has been used to determine malabsorption of dietary saccharides such as lactose, the presence of bacterial overgrowth, and intestinal transit. Prior to this revision, the hydrogen breath test procedure, used to determine lactose malabsorption, was only available to test for intolerance using a direct absorption testing through duodenal and jejunal

○=Modifier 51 Exempt   ⊙=Conscious Sedation   ✦=Add-on Code intubation. Due to the type of sample used for this procedure, this code may now be used to report breath hydrogen testing for other disorders as well.

Fructose intolerance is a common and treatable condition in patients with unexplained chronic diarrhea, bloating due to gaseousness, and abdominal pain. It affects patients of all ages from infants as well as the elderly. The problem has become much more common since the food industry began to use high fructose corn syrup as a sweetener in place of sucrose.

Bacterial overgrowth is particularly common and treatable in patients with unexplained chronic diarrhea and malabsorption, in diabetics with chronic diarrhea, in selected patients with refractory irritable bowel syndrome, as well as elderly patients with malabsorption. Since measurement of oro-cecal transit is useful in detecting motor disorders involving the stomach and small bowel such as diabetic gastroparesis, pseudo-obstruction secondary to scleroderma, diabetes or dumping syndromes, it is of use in patients with symptoms of unexplained bloating and distension, diarrhea or constipation, nausea and vomiting and abdominal pain. The test is useful in all age groups from infancy to the elderly. Differentiation from small bowel bacterial overgrowth is important and can be difficult because overgrowth and delayed transit can co-exist.

Clinical Example 1 (91065)

A 60-year-old female is referred for evaluation of recurrent diarrhea, abdominal bloating and weight loss. Radiologic and endoscopic studies have been unremarkable.

Description of Procedure (91065 Example 1):
Following an eight-hour fast, and after informed consent is obtained, the patient is brought to the gastroenterology diagnostic laboratory, where a baseline breath hydrogen measurement is taken. The patient swallows 75 grams of glucose dissolved in 250 cc of water. Measurements of end-expiratory breath hydrogen are collected every 30 minutes for three hours and analyzed using a gas chromatograph. The patient is asked to keep a diary of any gastrointestinal symptoms experienced during the test. The patient is monitored for any adverse effects. Post-procedure vital signs are assessed, and the patient is discharged. The measurements are plotted graphically and analyzed. The results are interpreted by the physician, and a report is generated.

Clinical Example 2 (91065)

A 45-year-old male is referred for evaluation of recurrent abdominal pain, gaseousness and diarrhea. He had been seen by multiple physicians and told that he had irritable bowel syndrome. Upper and lower endoscopic studies, stool studies and a breath test for lactose intolerance are all within normal limits.

Description of Procedure (91065 Example 2):
Following instructions for a low fiber, low residue diet and an overnight fast, the patient reported to the gastroenterology diagnostic laboratory. Once informed consent is obtained, a baseline breath hydrogen specimen is collected. The patient

is given 25 grams of fructose in 250 cc of water to ingest. Measurements of end-expiratory breath specimens are collected every 30 minutes for three hours, and are analyzed using a gas chromotograph. The patient is asked to keep a diary of any gastrointestinal symptoms experienced during the test. The patient is monitored for any adverse effects. Post-procedure vital signs are assessed, and the patient is discharged. The measurements are plotted graphically and analyzed. The results are interpreted by the physician, and a report is generated.

Clinical Example 3 (91065)

A 50-year-old male with longstanding diabetes mellitus is referred for evaluation of persistent unexplained chronic diarrhea. Colonoscopy and small bowel radiologic studies are normal.

Description of Procedure (91065 Example 3):
Following an 8-hour fast, the patient reports to the Gastroenterology Diagnostic Laboratory. Once informed consent is obtained, a fasting baseline breath hydrogen measurement is taken. The patient is then given 10 grams of lactulose syrup to ingest. Measurements of end-expiratory breath hydrogen are collected every 30 minutes for two hours and analyzed using a gas chromatograph. The patient is asked to keep a diary of any gastrointestinal symptoms experienced during the test. The patient is monitored for any adverse effects. Post-procedure vital signs are assessed, and the patient is discharged. The measurements are then plotted graphically and analyzed. Oro-cecal transit is defined as the time from ingestion of lactulose until the substrate reaches the colon resulting in a greater than 20 parts per million rise in hydrogen breath concentration. The results are interpreted by the physician, and a report is generated.

●**91120**   Rectal sensation, tone, and compliance test (ie, response to graded balloon distention)

▶(For biofeedback training, use 90911)◀

▶(For anorectal manometry, use 91122)◀

✍ Rationale

Code 91120 was added to identify measurement of rectal sensation, rectal tone and compliance of the rectal wall as well as assessment of sensory properties of the rectal wall in response to controlled balloon distention of the rectum. Specifically, code 91120 describes a comprehensive assessment of sensory, motor and biomechanical function of the rectum in patients with irritable bowel syndrome, constipation and/or fecal incontinence. Testing is performed at rest and after provocative stimuli. The provocation stimuli include responses of the rectum to a graded balloon distention. The response provides data that the physician is able to analyze to determine information regarding rectal motility and function.

To assist the user in selection of the correct code to identify this procedure, parenthetic notes have been included following code 91120. In addition, other parenthetic notes have been included in other sections to identify non-rectal sensation testing procedures (eg, 90911).

Clinical Example (91120)

A 35-year-old female presents with a three-year history of constipation. She has no desire to defacate and manually disimpacts her bowel once every 2-3 weeks. On examination, the abdomen is distended. Rectal exam shows impaired rectal sensation and hard stools, of which the patient was completely unaware.

Description of Procedure (91120)

Informed consent was obtained and rectal cleansing completed. The patient is placed in the left lateral position. A 5 mm diameter probe, with a 10 cm long, highly compliant balloon was placed into the rectum and taped in position. The balloon was connected to a computerized distending device. Stepwise, graded, balloon distentions were performed to assess the intra-operating pressure (IOP). Baseline rectal tone is assessed over a 30-minute period. Intermittent balloon distensions are then performed at 4 mm Hg increments until the patient reports sensation, desire to defecate, and urgency to defecate. Pain on maximum tolerable volume is recorded. While monitored, the patient is asked to defecate the balloon. After a 15-minute rest, the balloon is re-inserted into the rectum, and then inflated to IOP. The patient is then fed a standardized 1000 calorie meal. Rectal tone and sensory changes are then recorded for a subsequent 60-minute period. The balloon is deflated, and the balloon and probe are removed.

Special Otorhinolaryngologic Services

Audiologic Function Tests With Medical Diagnostic Evaluation

▶(92589 has been deleted)◀

▶(For central auditory function evaluation, see 92620, 92621)◀

Evaluative and Therapeutic Services

● **92620**   Evaluation of central auditory function, with report; initial 60 minutes

● **92621**   each additional 15 minutes

▶(Do not report 92620, 92621 in conjunction with 92506)◀

● **92625**   Assessment of tinnitus (includes pitch, loudness matching, and masking)

Rationale

Code 92589 has been deleted and renumbered to the Evaluative and Therapeutic Services subsection of the CPT book. Two codes have been established to more accurately describe central auditory function testing services as they are currently performed and to allow reporting multiple individual tests performed during a clinic visit. The new codes allow reporting the initial 60 minutes of tests performed and additional reporting for each additional 15 minutes of a central auditory function evaluation in which a single test might be performed repeatedly or a battery of multiple tests performed during a single session. A cross-reference has been added to indicate that codes 92620 and 92621 would not be reported separately in addition to 92506.

As central auditory function has become more understood, testing protocols for evaluation of auditory processing abilities using both speech and non-speech stimuli have become more refined and a variety of more effective test procedures has been developed. Examples of the tests available for evaluating auditory processing include auditory figure-ground tests, a variety of filtered speech tests, accelerated (or compressed) speech, tonal pattern recognition, a variety of competing words and competing sentences tests designed separately for adults and children, speech in noise procedures, and psychoacoustic procedures for detection of acoustic gaps in tones in addition to tonal duration discrimination. While a battery of tests should be used to examine the various components of auditory processing (eg, frequency, temporal, or dichotic/diotic discrimination), the specific number of test procedures varies from one patient to the next dependent upon the patient's age, communication abilities, degree of wellness, and primary language spoken.

 Clinical Example (92620)

A seven-year-old male was referred for a comprehensive evaluation of auditory processing abilities due to academic difficulties and a discrepancy between IQ potential and classroom performance. A prior hearing screening indicated that hearing sensitivity was normal for all test frequencies. Prior psychological and language evaluations revealed IQ scores in the high average range and no difficulties with receptive or expressive language. Although his teacher reported behaviors that resembled attention deficit disorder, psychological testing using a constant vigilance task did not reveal impulsiveness or a breakdown in performance for the duration of the test. The medical history was not significant for serious illnesses, head trauma, or otitis media. A family history of similar difficulties was noted in that his mother reported that she has always had difficulties understanding speech when there was significant noise in the environment.

Description of Procedure (92620)

After greeting the family and bringing them to the audiometric booth, a history was obtained with regard to developmental, familial, and medical factors that may have bearing on the development of auditory processing skills.

The child was then seated in the sound treated room and instructed that he will be listening to words that may be hard to understand. His task is to repeat each word to the best of his abilities and take a guess at individual responses if he is not sure of what the target word is. The audiologist leaves the child in the patient side of the audiometric booth and takes a seat behind the diagnostic audiometer, positioning himself where he can maintain eye contact with the child. Each test is played via CD, routed through the diagnostic audiometer, and presented at an intensity of 50 dB. The audiologist records the child's responses on respective scoring forms for each test. After administration of each test the audiologist determines the raw and standard scores and plots the standard scores for a visual representation of the child's performance. Before the administration of each new test, the child receives instructions through the audiometer and the earphones with regard to the nature of the task and the child's required responses. The audiologist must record the child's responses and monitor the child's performance to ensure that the child remains suitable for testing with regard to attentiveness and fatigue.

After administering all necessary tests, the audiologist compiles the respective scores to derive an interpretation of the age-equivalent performance level and types of stimuli and environments that will cause difficulties for the child's listening abilities. The results, interpretation, and recommendations are then conveyed to the family. For interdisciplinary evaluations, representatives of the other professional disciplines are notified of the test results and interpretation in the event that these findings influence the conclusions and recommendations generated by their respective test results. A report is prepared and forwarded to the referring physician and to the other members of the interdisciplinary team.

● **92625** Assessment of tinnitus (includes pitch, loudness matching, and masking)

▶(Do not report 92625 in conjunction with 92562)◀

▶(For unilateral assessment, use modifier 52)◀

 Rationale
Code 92625 has been established to report tinnitus assessment to include pitch, loudness matching, and masking. A parenthetical note has been added to preclude reporting code 92625 separately in addition to code 92562 for loudness balance testing. As this service is intended for bilateral testing, a second parenthetical has been added to instruct the use of modifier 52 when tinnitus assessment is performed unilaterally.

Tinnitus pitch testing measures the perceptual characteristics of self-perceived sounds. The quantification and documentation of self-perceived pitch are used to document the presence of self-perceived sounds (eg, tinnitus) and to provide baseline information prior to treatment and to monitor the effectiveness of treatment.

Tinnitus loudness testing of perceived sounds is used as a diagnostic aid in documenting the presence and characteristics of tinnitus and as a means of assessing the magnitude of the perceived loudness of tinnitus prior to and following clinical treatment regimen(s) and in judgment of the severity of perceived tinnitus.

Tinnitus masking for establishment of minimum masking levels and tinnitus suppression is used in the treatment of self-perceived sounds (tinnitus). Also, data obtained from the measurement of minimum masking levels and tinnitus suppression provides documentation of the effectiveness of treatment protocols.

 Clinical Example 1 (92625)
A 69-year-old female is reporting the onset of constant, irritating, high pitched sounds in both ears. The sound sensations appeared suddenly after chemotherapy treatments four months ago. The patient reports that the ongoing perception of

these sounds was initially tolerable; however, they have been increasing in perceived loudness over the past six weeks. She now finds that she has considerable difficulty in going to sleep because the perceived loudness appears to increase and is most bothersome during the quiet evening hours. She has tried to keep the television on during the evening in an effort to cover over the tinnitus, but this has proven unsuccessful. Of particular concern is the interference of sleep resulting from these self-perceived sounds.

An audiometric examination performed four weeks prior to the loudness (intensity) measurement revealed the patient to have a sloping mild to moderate high frequency sensori-neural hearing impairment bilaterally, consistent with ototoxicity. Otoacoustic emissions testing showed that the patient has a cochlear end organ impairment that affected outer hair cell function in the high frequencies bilaterally. Tympanometry demonstrated normal mobility of the tympanic membrane and middle ear pressures in both ears. Stapedial reflexes were present at expected stimulus levels bilaterally, consistent with cochlear involvement. The otolaryngologic examination was normal, with the exception of the audiologic studies.

Description of Procedure (92625 Example 1)
The audiologist greets the patient and accompanies her to the testing suite. The audiologist prepares the patient by inserting earphones into each ear canal after otoscopic inspection. The audiologist then sits in the control booth facing the patient in the test booth. All instructions are given to the patient via the talk-over system of the diagnostic audiometer. The patient is instructed regarding the general nature of the procedure and the required responses. The audiologist then performs loudness matching testing by presenting a series of pure tones to the patient. The patient is asked to report if each presented tone is louder, softer or equal in loudness to the self-perceived sound. The frequency selection and intensity values of each tone are under the control of the audiologist. Typically, octave and mid-octave frequencies from 500 Hz to 8000 Hz are presented to the patient's earphone. These nine frequencies (500, 750, 1000, 1500, 2000, 3000, 4000, 6000, and 8000 Hz) are presented at intensity levels slightly above the patient's auditory sensitivity threshold in the test ear at each frequency. The intensity level of the stimulus is increased or decreased in 1 dB steps by the audiologist until a perceived loudness match between the audiometric stimulus and the patient's tinnitus is obtained. When the patient reports the external stimulus as being equal in loudness to the tinnitus, this level is recorded as the tinnitus loudness match (in dB) for that frequency. Equal loudness estimates are calculated in dB SL (SL=Sensation Level, eg, tinnitus loudness match in dB HL minus the auditory threshold in dB HL at that frequency). This loudness matching procedure is performed in each ear separately, thus resulting in eighteen (nine matches per ear) loudness matches between the stimulus (presented tone) and the patient's self-perceived sound. The results of this assessment are presented to the patient. The referring physician is notified by telephone and by report concerning the outcome of the loudness evaluation and resulting recommendations.

Clinical Example 2 (92625)

A 70-year-old male is complaining of the onset of hearing loss with a piercing ringing sound in his right ear six months ago. The onset of the hearing loss and perceived ringing was sudden and noted upon awakening. While the hearing in the right ear has subsequently improved to near-normal levels, the piercing ringing sound has remained constant and unrelenting. The patient expresses considerable irritation with the tinnitus as it causes him sleep disturbance and annoyance throughout each day.

A complete hearing evaluation performed six months ago revealed a moderate sensori-neural hearing loss in the right ear and normal hearing in the left ear. At that time, the patient had a complete otologic evaluation and was subsequently treated with a 10-day tapering course of steroids. A magnetic resonance image (MRI) was ordered and was normal, ruling out an acoustic neuroma. Post-treatment hearing tests demonstrated hearing improvement in the right ear with the most recent evaluation two weeks ago showing symmetrical pure tone auditory sensitivity, with the exception of an isolated high frequency hearing loss in the right ear. Otoacoustic emissions testing showed that the patient has an end organ impairment that affected cochlear outer hair cell function in the high frequencies in the right ear. Immittance audiometry demonstrated normal tympanic membrane mobility and middle ear pressures. Stapedius reflexes were present at expected stimulus levels bilaterally.

Description of Procedure (92625 Example 2)

The audiologist greets the patient and accompanies him into the audiometric testing suite. The patient is seated and prepared for the procedure through the insertion of earphones following otoscopic inspection. All instructions are given to the patient through the talk-over system of the diagnostic audiometer. The patient is instructed regarding the general description of the test procedures and the required responses. The concept of low versus high pitch is initially demonstrated by allowing the patient to listen to low frequency and high frequency tones generated by the clinical audiometer. Pitch (frequency) matching of the tinnitus is accomplished by presenting various audiometric stimuli to the patient through the test earphone. Nine frequencies (500, 750, 1000, 1500, 2000, 3000, 4000, 6000, and 8000 Hz) are individually presented using a two-alternative forced-choice procedure (2AFC) whereby the patient must choose which tone is closest in pitch to his self-perceived tone(s). The audiometric tones are presented at intensity levels slightly above the patient's auditory threshold at each frequency. Interrupted tones are used to avoid confusion between the audiometric stimuli and the patient's tinnitus. The procedure begins with wide frequency spacing with both ascending and descending frequency steps used to avoid order preferences (that is, the tendency to choose the first tone of the two). The patient indicates which tone, the first or the second, sounds closest in pitch to his own tinnitus. This pitch bracketing process continues until the patient reports that the audiometric stimulus is the same as the perceived tinnitus or the tinnitus is fully bracketed between two adjacent half-octave frequencies. The frequency selected the greatest percentage of time is reported as the pitch match. Frequencies at octave intervals relative to the pitch match are then presented to check for octave confusion. (For those patients with bilateral tinnitus, the entire pitch matching procedure would then be performed on the other ear.) The patient is then informed of the outcome of the pitch (frequency) matching evaluation and the potential for effective intervention. The referring physician is notified by telephone and by report regarding the outcome of the evaluation and the recommendations derived from the results.

Description of Procedure (92625 Example 2)
The audiologist greets the patient and accompanies her to the testing suite. The audiologist prepares the patient by inserting earphones into each ear canal after otoscopic inspection. The audiologist then sits at the diagnostic audiometer in the control booth facing the patient in the test booth. Pitch (frequency) matching is accomplished by individually presenting nine frequencies (500, 750, 1000, 1500, 2000, 3000, 4000, 6000 and 8000 Hz) using a two-alternative forced-choice procedure (2AFC) whereby the patient must choose which tone is closest in pitch to her self-perceived tone. The audiometric tones are presented at intensity levels slightly above the patient's auditory threshold at each frequency. The patient describes the pitch of the stimulus as higher, lower, or similar to her perceived sound. This pitch bracketing process continues until the patient states that the stimulus is the same as or very similar to her perceived sound or is fully bracketed between adjacent half-octave frequencies. This procedure is then performed on the patient's other ear. Loudness matching testing is then performed by presenting a series of pure tones and the patient is asked to report if each presented tone is louder, softer or equal in loudness to the self-perceived sound. Typically, octave and mid-octave frequencies from 500 Hz to 8000 Hz are presented at intensity levels slightly above the patient's auditory threshold at each frequency. The intensity level of the stimulus is increased or decreased in 1 dB steps by the audiologist. When the patient reports the external stimulus as being equal in loudness to her self-perceived sound, this level is recorded as the loudness match (in dB) for that frequency. Equal loudness estimates are calculated in dB SL (loudness match in dB HL minus the auditory threshold in dB HL at that frequency). This loudness matching procedure is performed for each ear separately, resulting in eighteen (nine matches per ear) loudness matches between the stimulus and the patient's self-perceived sound. Instructions regarding the masking procedure are then given to the patient and masking stimuli are presented to the same earphone as the perceived tone. Ten individual masking stimuli (nine frequencies of narrow band noise at octave and mid-octave frequencies from 500-8000 Hz as well as wide band noise) are individually increased in intensity from threshold in 1-2 dB steps until masking of the tinnitus is accomplished. The Minimum Masking Level (MML) is recorded in dB SL (SL=Sensation Level, eg, the effective tinnitus masking level in dB HL minus the auditory threshold for the masking stimulus) for each masking stimulus. Comparative measurements between the various forms of maskers are needed to select the masker with the greatest efficiency in providing the most effective masking stimulus. This procedure is performed for each ear independently and for binaural stimulation for those patients with bilateral tinnitus. The audiologist then presents the most effective masking stimulus at +10 to +15 dB SL (above the MML)

continuously for 60 seconds. The patient is asked to report if her perceived tinnitus increased, decreased or was unchanged after cessation of the masking stimulus. The length of time the patient is without perception of the tinnitus is determined and the duration of tinnitus suppression ("residual inhibition") is calculated.

The patient is informed of the outcome of the evaluation and the potential for remediation. The referring physician is notified by telephone and by report concerning the outcome of the evaluation and recommendations for masking therapy.

Cardiovascular

Therapeutic Services

⊙ **92980**   Transcatheter placement of an intracoronary stent(s), percutaneous, with or without other therapeutic intervention, any method; single vessel

✚ ⊙ **92981**   each additional vessel (List separately in addition to code for primary procedure)

(Use 92981 in conjunction with 92980)

▶(Codes 92980, 92981 are used to report coronary artery stenting. Coronary angioplasty (92982, 92984) or atherectomy (92995, 92996), in the same artery, is considered part of the stenting procedure and is not reported separately. Codes 92973 (percutaneous transluminal coronary thombectomy), 92974 (coronary brachytherapy) and 92978, 92979 (intravascular ultrasound) are add-on codes for reporting procedures performed in addition to coronary stenting, atherectomy, and angioplasty and are not included in the "therapeutic interventions" in 92980)◀

(To report additional vessels treated by angioplasty or atherectomy only during the same session, see 92984, 92996)

(To report transcatheter placement of radiation delivery device for coronary intravascular brachytherapy, use 92974)

(For intravascular radioelement application, see 77781- 77784)

 Rationale

An instructional parenthetical has been added following codes 92980 and 92981 to provide instruction for reporting additional CPT codes in conjunction with codes that have with or without other therapeutic intervention in their CPT descriptor, when applicable. The addition of this cross-reference is intended to clarify that codes 92973 (for percutaneous transluminal coronary thombectomy), 92974 (for coronary brachytherapy) and 92978, 92979 (for intravascular ultrasound) are not the "therapeutic interventions" procedures described in code 92980. These codes are, however, considered to be add-on codes which are appropriately reported in addition to codes 92980, 92981, 92982, 92984, 92995 and 92996 for coronary stenting, atherectomy, and angioplasty.

Echocardiography

Echocardiography includes obtaining ultrasonic signals from the heart and great arteries, with two-dimensional image and/or Doppler ultrasonic signal documentation, and interpretation and report. When interpretation is performed separately use modifier 26.

▶Echocardiography is an ultrasound examination of the cardiac chambers and valves, the adjacent great vessels, and the pericardium. A complete transthoracic echocardiogram (93307) is a comprehensive procedure that includes 2-dimensional and selected M-mode examination of the left and right atria, left and right ventricles, the aortic, mitral, and tricuspid valves, the pericardium, and adjacent portions of the aorta. These structures are assessed using multiple views as required to obtain a complete functional and anatomic evaluation, and appropriate measurements are obtained and recorded. Despite significant effort, identification and measurement of some structures may not always be possible. In such instances, the reason that an element could not be visualized must be documented. Additional structures that may be visualized (eg, pulmonary veins, pulmonary artery, pulmonic valve, inferior vena cava) would be included as part of the service.◀

▶A follow-up or limited echocardiographic study (93308) is an examination that does not evaluate or document the attempt to evaluate all the structures that comprise the complete echocardiographic exam. This is typically performed in follow-up of a complete echocardiographic examination when a repeat complete exam is unnecessary due to the more focused clinical concern. In some emergent clinical situations, a limited echocardiographic study may be performed primarily.◀

▶Report of an echocardiographic study, whether complete or limited, includes an interpretation of all obtained information, documentation of all clinically relevant findings including quantitative measurements obtained, plus a description of any recognized abnormalities. Pertinent images, videotape, and/or digital data are archived for permanent storage and are available for subsequent review. Use of echocardiography not meeting these criteria is not separately reportable.◀

▶Use of ultrasound, without thorough evaluation of organ(s) or anatomic region, image documentation and final, written report, is not separately reportable.◀

(For fetal echocardiography, see 76825-76828)

Rationale

New introductory language was added at the beginning of the Echocardiography subsection to define the services that are included in echocardiography. This language will assist users in determining if the required criteria are met when reporting echocardiography.

Other Vascular Studies

▲93741   Electronic analysis of pacing cardioverter-defibrillator (includes interrogation, evaluation of pulse generator status, evaluation of programmable parameters at rest and during activity where applicable, using electrocardiographic recording and interpretation of recordings at rest and during exercise, analysis of event markers and device response); single chamber or wearable cardioverter-defibrillator system, without reprogramming

▶(Do not report 93741 in conjunction with 93745)◀

▲93742   single chamber or wearable cardioverter-defibrillator system, with reprogramming

⊘=Modifier 51 Exempt   ⊙=Conscious Sedation   ✚=Add-on Code

▶(Do not report 93742 in conjunction with 93745)◀

●**93745**　Initial set-up and programming by a physician of wearable cardioverter-defibrillator includes initial programming of system, establishing baseline electronic ECG, transmission of data to data repository, patient instruction in wearing system and patient reporting of problems or events

▶(Do not report 93745 in conjunction with 93741, 93742)◀

 Rationale

Code 93745 was established to report the initial set-up and programming of a wearable cardioverter-defibrillator by a physician. Codes 93741 and 93742 were revised to include the wearable cardioverter-defibrillator system with the devices included in the electronic analysis described by these codes. Exclusionary cross-references have been added following codes 93741 and 93742 to indicate that these codes would not be appropriately reported in addition to code 93745. It would not be appropriate for an Evaluation and Management service to be reported by the same provider on the same day as code 93745 which is reported for the initial set-up and programming of the wearable cardioverter-defibrillator device.

The wearable cardioverter-defibrillator is a system that is worn outside the body rather than implanted in the chest by patients who are at risk for sudden cardiac arrest and are not candidates for an implantable cardiac defibrillator. The wearable device is capable of monitoring electrocardiographic (ECG) information; storing data; and delivering shock when indicated.

 Clinical Example (93741)

A 72-year-old female with ventricular tachycardia and chronic atrial fibrillation has previously undergone insertion of a combination implantable cardioverter-defibrillator (ICD)/rate-responsive, single-chamber pacemaker. Due to recurrent ventricular tachycardia, an antiarrhythmic drug is initiated. In follow-up analysis, the device is interrogated to determine the number of defibrillator shocks delivered, the associated shock impedance, and review of the electrograms documenting episodes of tachycardia treated with either antitachycardia pacing or an internal shock. The sensing, pacing, and impedance characteristics along with the rate responsive characteristics of the lead are evaluated. Capacitors are reformed and charge times assessed. The results of the interrogation are reviewed with the patient and family, documented in the patient's history, and a report is sent to the referring physician.

Description of Procedure (93741)

The procedure is performed under continuous electrocardiographic (ECG) recording. The device is interrogated to assess program parameters and stored data. The battery voltage and/or charge time is assessed to confirm adequate battery reserve. The pacing lead impedance, sensing, and pacing thresholds are determined. The patient is walked to assess the rate-responsive settings of the defibrillator/pacemaker. Stored electrogram data documenting treated episodes of ventricular tachycardia or ventricular fibrillation are reviewed to make certain that the device is functioning properly. The services are documented, a report is generated, and the results are communicated with the referring physician, patient, and the patient's family.

Clinical Example (93742)

A 72-year-old female with spontaneous and electrically inducible ventricular tachycardia and chronic atrial fibrillation has previously undergone insertion of a combination implantable cardioverter defibrillator (ICD)/rate-responsive, single-chamber pacemaker. Due to recurrent ventricular tachycardia, an antiarrhythmic drug is initiated. In follow-up analysis, the device is interrogated to determine the number of defibrillator shocks delivered, the associated shock impedance, and review of the electrograms documenting episodes of tachycardia treated with either antitachycardia pacing or an internal shock. The sensing, pacing, and impedance characteristics along with the rate responsive characteristics of the lead are evaluated. Capacitors are reformed and charge times assessed. Interrogation of the device documents that one shock was delivered for atrial fibrillation, and the maximum heart rate achieved with moderate exercise today is only 80 beats per minute. Therefore, stability criteria is programmed in to help discriminate between atrial fibrillation and ventricular tachycardia, and the rate response parameters are readjusted to allow a more rapid heart rate during exercise. The results of the interrogation are reviewed with the patient and family, documented in the patient's history, and a report is sent to the referring physician.

Description of Procedure (93742)

The procedure is performed under continuous electrocardiographic (ECG) recording. The device is interrogated to assess program parameters and stored data. The battery voltage and/or charge time is assessed to confirm adequate battery reserve. The pacing lead impedance, sensing, and pacing thresholds are determined. The patient is walked to assess the rate-responsive settings of the defibrillator/pacemaker. Stored electrogram data documenting treated episodes of ventricular tachycardia or ventricular fibrillation are reviewed to make certain that the device is functioning properly. The device is reprogrammed to optimize the antitachycardia treatment parameters, tachycardia detection criteria, atrial and ventricular lead sensing and pacing thresholds, and rate responsive characteristics. The patient is then observed during light exercise to assess heart rate response. The services are documented, a report is generated, and the results are communicated with the referring physician, patient, and the patient's family.

Clinical Example (93745)

A 55-year-old female on the heart transplant list, with a history of ventricular fibrillation and cardiomyopathy, is hospitalized due to an infected implantable cardioverter defibrillator (ICD) pocket. The ICD has been explanted and the patient is put on prolonged antibiotic therapy. The patient is weak, especially on the right side from a previous stroke, though very alert. Her physician has prescribed the LifeVest to monitor abnormal heart rhythms that could lead to death from sudden cardiac arrest. The patient receives the LifeVest as a hospital inpatient. After the physician has completed the necessary LifeVest setup procedures, the patient will be discharged to her home.

Description of Procedure (93745)

The physician brings a laptop computer to the patient's hospital room for use in programming the patient's wearable cardio-defibrillator system device. The physician measures the patient's chest to determine proper belt size and electrode placement. Proper fit is necessary for optimum ECG signal clarity. The physician assembles the electrode belt, demonstrating this assembly process to the patient. The patient then assembles and reassembles the electrode belt herself while the physician assesses proper assembly procedure. Once the patient is comfortable in assembling the electrode belt, the physician demonstrates the various alarms and the proper use of the alarm module. The physician must demonstrate use of the various device components to educate the patient (ie, buttons, lights, signals).

The physician also provides an explanation of various messages that may appear on the device display and advises the patient on necessary response. The physician discusses the risk of sudden death caused by abnormal heart rhythms and the need to wear the device at all times, except when bathing. The physician allows the patient to hear and distinguish the arrhythmia alarms from the poor ECG signal alarm with the device in training mode. Once the patient demonstrates proficiency in use of the wearable cardio-defibrillator system and her questions are answered, the physician initiates programming of the customized patient parameters. The physician chooses these parameters based on assessment of the patient's cardiac condition.

This programming is done using the hyper terminal program. The physician demonstrates how to connect the electrode belt to the device, fits the electrode belt on the patient's chest and familiarizes her with the startup messages. With the device in baseline mode, the physician then takes a baseline ECG recording and the patient may view the ECG recording on the device display. The physician stresses the importance of holding the response button for any arrhythmia alarms received while the patient is conscious.

The physician removes the wearable cardio-defibrillator system device and downloads the baseline ECG data for internet analysis. The device is again connected to the electrode belt. The physician answers additional questions and shows the patient how she would transfer her ECG data by herself, via modem, to the internet, how to charge and when to change the monitor batteries, and how to wear the monitor holster. The physician instructs the patient to download her wearable cardio-defibrillator system data to the internet on a weekly basis. After the physician answers the patient's final questions, patient set-up is complete, and the patient may be discharged from the hospital to the home.

Noninvasive Vascular Diagnostic Studies

Cerebrovascular Arterial Studies

▶A complete transcranial Doppler (TCD) study (93886) includes ultrasound evaluation of the right and left anterior circulation territories and the posterior circulation territory (to include vertebral arteries and basilar artery). In a limited TCD study (93888) there is ultrasound evaluation of two or fewer of these territories. For TCD, ultrasound evaluation is a reasonable and concerted attempt to identify arterial signals through an acoustic window.◀

93886	Transcranial Doppler study of the intracranial arteries; complete study
93888	limited study
●**93890**	vasoreactivity study
●**93892**	emboli detection without intravenous microbubble injection
●**93893**	emboli detection with intravenous microbubble injection

▶(Do not report 93890-93893 in conjunction with 93888)◀

✍🏻 Rationale

The transcranial Doppler (TCD) study section has been updated to include explanatory notes to define the terms "complete" and "limited" utilized in codes 93886 and 93888. Additionally, three new TCD codes have been added for cerebrovascular reactivity testing (93890) and embolus detection monitoring (93892, 93893). These three tests require additional equipment, laboratory time and expertise not included in the standard TCD examinations (93886, 93888).

Cerebrovascular reactivity (93890) is performed to evaluate carotid and vertebrobasilar stenosis/occlusion (eg, transient ischemic attack (TIA), stroke, cerebral hemodynamic insufficiency) by measuring the presence and magnitude of changes in intracranial blood flow velocity induced by alteration in the level of carbon dioxide in the blood (eg inhalation of gas mixture with a higher percentage of carbon dioxide, breath holding, hyperventilation), or as a response to injection of a drug that alters cerebral blood flow (eg acetazolamide). It is also performed preoperatively to assess cerebrovascular reserve prior to carotid endarterectomy, carotid interventional treatment, coronary artery bypass graft surgery, or other vascular or cardiac procedures that can involve or affect flow to the brain. The typical cerebrovascular reactivity involves measuring bilateral middle cerebral arteries (MCA) continuously during the resting phase, hypercapnic (after hyperventilation) and hypocapnic (after administration of CO_2 inhalation). A calculation program determines the cerebrovascular reserve by calculating the percentage change in blood flow velocity from baseline to after the physiological challenge. This provides a measure of whether there is adequate cerebrovascular reserve (adequate collateral flow channels and function) to preserve and maintain blood flow to the brain, and avoid ischemic injury or stroke, in the face of unexpected physiological challenges (eg drop in blood pressure, cardiac arrhythmia, occlusion of the carotid artery), or procedures that might interrupt or impair normal blood flow to the brain (eg carotid surgery, carotid intervention, cardiac bypass).

Embolus detection monitoring is performed to detect embolic activity in arterial insufficiencies (eg, internal carotid artery atherothromboembolic disease, vertebrobasilar atherothromboembolic disease) and cardiac conditions (eg, atrial fibrillation, dilated cardiomyopathy, left ventricular thrombus, infectious endocarditis). Specialized hardware and software are utilized to detect each embolic event. The physician/interpreter, knowledgeable in embolus detection, must utilize his skills in classifying each event to determine if it is a genuine embolic signal.

Ø=Modifier 51 Exempt　　⊙=Conscious Sedation　　✚=Add-on Code

Embolus detection monitoring with intravenous injection of agitated saline is performed to identify right to left cardiac, pulmonary, and other extracardiac shunts potentially inherent in the following conditions: transient ischemic attack, stroke, deep vein thrombosis, pulmonary embolism, suspected intracardiac shunts (eg, patent foramen ovale and other atrial and ventricular septal defects) and suspected extracardiac shunts (ie, pulmonary arteriovenous malformations). Again this procedure requires the physician interpreter to utilize his knowledge base and skill to classify each event as consistent with a genuine microembolic signal.

 Clinical Example (93890)

A 66-year-old male is referred to the transcranial Doppler (TCD) laboratory because a carotid, duplex, ultrasound examination identified 90% left internal carotid artery stenosis. The patient is scheduled to undergo coronary artery bypass surgery. TCD vasoreactivity testing is ordered to assess cerebrovascular reserve adequacy of collateral flow, to assist with decision making about performing a left carotid endarterectomy during the heart surgery.

Description of Procedure (93890)

The physician reviews acquired Doppler spectral waveforms, flow direction, mean, systolic, and diastolic flow velocities, depth of sampling, pulsatility index values, and capnometer values in the resting values for the arterial segments studied. He/she documents procedure results and then integrates findings with clinical presentation to formulate and document exam interpretation.

 Clinical Example (93892)

A 44-year-old female is referred to the TCD laboratory after presenting with a moderate right hemisphere infarct, producing hemineglect, hemiparesis, and dysphagia. A computed tomography (CT) angiogram of the neck is normal. A transthoracic echocardiogram is normal. Although a transesophageal echocardiogram is attempted, it cannot be performed due to the patient's dysphagia, preventing passage of the esophageal probe. TCD embolus detection is ordered to assess evidence of a proximal embolic source and assist with decisions about the need for anticoagulation, further testing, and treatment.

Description of Procedure (93892)

The physician reviews acquired Doppler spectral waveforms, flow direction, mean, systolic, and diastolic flow velocity, depth of sampling, and pulsatility index values, including waveforms throughout the monitoring epoch. He/she identifies and reviews each high intensity transient signal event recorded and classifies it as a genuine embolic signal or artifact. The physician then counts the total number of embolic signals occurring spontaneously, and documents the vessel segment(s) in which they occurred, as well as the length of the period of monitoring. He/she documents procedure results and integrates findings with clinical presentation to formulate and document exam interpretation.

Clinical Example (93893)

A 36-year-old male experienced a 20-minute episode of aphasia and right hemiparesis, which spontaneously cleared with no residual deficits. Magnetic resonance imaging (MRI) shows scattered T2 hyperintensities bilaterally, while carotid ultrasound, TCD, and routine transthoracic echocardiogram are unremarkable. A TCD with agitated, saline injection is ordered to assess for a patent foramen ovale, or other right to left intracardiac shunt.

Description of Procedure (93893)

The physician reviews acquired Doppler spectral waveforms, flow direction, mean, systolic, and diastolic flow velocity, depth of sampling, and pulsatility index values, including waveforms obtained before, during, and after the agitated saline injection(s). He/she identifies and reviews any high intensity transient signal events and classifies it as embolic or artifact. Then the total number of post-injection embolic signals are counted and any shower or curtain appearance of embolic signals is noted and the vessel segment(s) in which they were identified. The physician records the relationship to time after intravenous injection and to Valsalva maneuver. The physician then documents the procedure results and integrates findings with clinical presentations to formulate and document exam interpretation.

Pulmonary

▲**94060**   Bronchodilation responsiveness, spirometry as in 94010, pre- and post-bronchodilator administration

▶(Report bronchodilator supply separately with 99070 or appropriate supply code)◀

▲**94070**   Bronchospasm provocation evaluation, multiple spirometric determinations as in 94010, with administered agents (eg, antigen(s), cold air, methacholine)

▶(Report antigen(s) administration separately with 99070 or appropriate supply code)◀

✐ Rationale

Codes 94060 and 94070 have been revised to clarify that administration of the bronchodilator is not included in spirometry. The previous language was misleading, since the term "evaluation" included in the descriptor of 94060 and 94070 was often interpreted to exclude use of an E&M code, and thus bundling of services occurred. The supply of the bronchodilator and antigen(s) should be reported with 99070 or appropriate HCPCS supply codes(s).

94450   Breathing response to hypoxia (hypoxia response curve)

▶(For high altitude simulation test (HAST), see 94452, 94453)◀

●**94452**   High altitude simulation test (HAST), with physician interpretation and report;

▶(For obtaining arterial blood gases, use 36600)◀

▶(Do not report 94452 in conjunction with 94453, 94760, 94761)◀

●**94453**   with supplemental oxygen titration

▶(For obtaining arterial blood gases, use 36600)◀

▶(Do not report 94453 in conjunction with 94452, 94760, 94761)◀

○=Modifier 51 Exempt   ⊙=Conscious Sedation   ✚=Add-on Code

Rationale

Codes 94452 and 94453 were added to the Pulmonary subsection of the Medicine section to describe high altitude simulation testing (HAST). An instructional note was added following code 94450 directing users to codes 94452 and 94453 for the HAST test. Instructional notes were added below codes 94452 and 94453 directing users to code 36600 to report obtaining arterial blood gases. Exclusionary notes were also added following codes 94452 and 94453 instructing users not to report codes 94452 and 94453 together, and not to report them with codes 94760 or 94761. Code 94453 should be reported when the HAST test is performed with supplemental oxygen titration.

Clinical Example (94452)

A 65-year-old male with known chronic obstructive lung disease reports to his physician that he became short of breath during a commercial airflight. The physician orders a high altitude simulation test. The patient breathes a hypoxic gas mixture (ie, 15% oxygen and 85% N_2) at rest of 15 minutes. Oxygen saturation remains above 88% throughout the procedure so that supplemental oxygen is not felt to be necessary. Test results are analyzed and a report written by the performing physician and sent to the ordering physician (if appropriate).

Description of Procedure (94452)

Following the patient's breathing of the hypoxic gas mixture for 15 minutes, the physician determines if oxygen titration is necessary.

Clinical Example (94453)

A 66-year-old female with documented chronic obstructive lung disease and prior blood gases has revealed mild hypoxemia. She reports to her physician that she became short of breath during a commercial airflight. The physician orders a high altitude simulation test. The patient breathes a hypoxic gas mixture (ie, 15% oxygen and 85% N_2) at rest of 15 minutes. Oxygen saturation drops below 88%, necessitating supplemental oxygen. Oxygen is supplied by nasal cannula, and flow rate is titrated until saturation is approximately 90%. Test results are analyzed and a report is written by the performing physician and sent to the ordering physician (if appropriate). An air travel prescription is written and the appropriate documentation is sent both to the ordering physician (if appropriate) and the commercial airline.

Description of Procedure (94453)

Following the patient's breathing of the hypoxic gas mixture for 15 minutes, the physician determines if oxygen titration is necessary.

Neurology and Neuromuscular Procedures

Neurologic services are typically consultative, and ...

In addition, services and skills outlined under **Evaluation and Management** levels of service appropriate to neurologic illnesses should be reported similarly.

The EEG, autonomic function, evoked potential, ►reflex tests, EMG, NCV, and MEG◄ services (95812-95829 and ►95860-95967◄) include recording, interpretation by a physician, and report. For interpretation only, use modifier 26.

(For repetitive transcranial magnetic stimulation for treatment of clinical depression, use Category III code 0018T)

(Do not report codes 95860-95875 in addition to 96000-96004)

 Rationale

The Neurology and Neuromuscular Procedures guidelines have been revised to clarify, with an expanded list of neurology testing procedures, those codes which include recording and interpretation by a physician.

Intraoperative Neurophysiology

(Use 95920 in conjunction with the study performed, 92585, 95822, 95860, 95861, 95867, 95868, ►95870,◄ 95900, 95904, 95925►–95937◄)

(Code 95920 describes ongoing electrophysiologic testing and monitoring performed during surgical procedures. Code 95920 is reported per hour of service, and includes only the ongoing electrophysiologic monitoring time distinct from performance of specific type(s) of baseline electrophysiologic study(s) (95860, 95861, 95867, 95868, ►95870,◄ 95900, 95904, ►95928, 95929,◄ 95933–95937) or interpretation of specific type(s) of baseline electrophysiologic study(s) (92585, 95822, ►95870, 95925-95928, 95929, 95930◄). The time spent performing or interpreting the baseline electrophysiologic study(s) should not be counted as intraoperative monitoring, but represents separately reportable procedures. Code 95920 should be used once per hour even if multiple electrophysiologic studies are performed. The baseline electrophysiologic study(s) should be used once per operative session.)

(For intraoperative neurostimulator programming and analysis, see 95970-95975)

 Rationale

The parenthetical notes following code 95920 were revised to indicate that the new electrophysiologic codes (95928, 95929) should be reported in conjunction with code 95920, when performed. In addition, the needle electromyography code 95870 was added to the series of codes appropriate for separate reporting, as this was previously missed.

Evoked Potentials and Reflex Tests

●**95928**   Central motor evoked potential study (transcranial motor stimulation); upper limbs

●**95929**   lower limbs

 Rationale

Two new codes, 95928 and 95929, were established to describe central motor evoked potential studies for the upper and lower limbs. Code 95928 is reported for central motor evoked potential studies on the upper limbs, while 95929 should be reported for studies on the lower limbs. Also, the parenthetical notes following code 95920 were revised to include new codes 95928 and 95929 as part of the list of procedure codes that 95920 may be reported in conjunction with, when intraoperative testing is performed. In addition, code 95870 was also added to the parenthetical note for procedure codes in which code 95920 may be reported with, as this was previously missed.

Transcranial electrical motor stimulation is a method that allows for stimulation of the motor area of the cerebral cortex and recording from peripheral muscles of the upper and lower extremities. It allows for assessment of motor pathway function and integrity. During surgical procedures typically involving the spinal cord, there is a potential for compromise of the motor and the sensory tracts. Somatosensory evoked potential recording is typically done to monitor the sensory tracts during these surgeries. However, this method does not monitor the motor tracts, which may be impaired leading to paresis or paralysis. Intraoperatively, transcranial electrical motor stimulation is a method that allows for physician interpretation of motor responses in order to determine if a significant change in the responses has occurred.

Central motor evoked potential studies may be used intraoperatively to monitor procedures involving scoliosis instrumentation, intramedullary spinal cord tumors, brain tumor resection, laminectomies, or other surgical procedures to repair spondylosis and spinal stenosis.

In the outpatient setting, these studies are used as a diagnostic test which can assist in identifying upper motor neuron involvement in many disorders including motor neuron diseases such as amyotrophic lateral sclerosis (ALS) and multiple sclerosis (MS). A non-invasive technique called transcranial magnetic stimulation (TMS) is used in which a magnetic coil is placed over the vertex and used to stimulate the motor cortex as peripheral muscles record surface electromyographic signals.

 Clinical Example (95928)

This 47-year-old male presents with subacute arm and leg weakness without sensory disturbances. Imaging shows spondylotic cervical myelopathy. After examination, electromyography (EMG) and other testing, his diagnosis remains uncertain. The differential diagnosis includes cervical myelopathy, amyotrophic lateral sclerosis (ALS), and several, peripheral, neuromuscular disorders. He is referred for central motor evoked potential testing to assess whether his disorder includes central motor pathway impairment and to provide a baseline for measurement of progression.

Description of Procedure (95928)

The physician applies electrodes over the patient's biceps, triceps, abductor pollicis brevis and abductor digiti minimi muscles in belly-tendon, recording derivation. The gel is applied. The electrodes are secured. He/she checks impedances, and reapplies electrodes as needed. Prior to performing transcranial magnetic stimulation, routine motor nerve conduction studies of the ulnar and/or median nerves are performed to establish baseline compound muscle action potentials (CMAP). This should include stimulation at Erb's point and distal segments of the nerve. Next, the optimal scalp location is determined for head coil using stepwise stimulus location changes and adjustments of intensity. At the optimal location for the first muscle tested, usually abductor digiti minimi, the resting motor-evoked potential (MEP) threshold is determined using 5% increments of maximal stimulator output. After determining the threshold, MEPs are recorded during modest tonic isometric contraction using stimulation 25% of maximum output above threshold. The transcranial MEP amplitude and onset latency is measured and compared to the baseline nerve conduction studies. Then, the abductor digiti minimi CMAP obtained with supramaximal electrical stimulation of the ulnar nerve is measured. Next, the relative abductor digiti minimi MEP amplitude, as a percentage of the CMAP amplitude, is measured. The MEP to cervical stimulation is measured. The central motor conduction time (CMCT) is calculated by subtracting latencies for scalp and cervical stimulation tests. He/she measures the dissociation between MEP threshold and the cortical stimulation silent period (CSSP) by reducing the stimulator output in 5% increments until stimulation no longer alters the appearance of the average rectified abductor digiti minimi EMG. The physician measures the dissociation between excitatory and inhibitory effects of transcranial stimulation (MEP facilitation failure) as EMG inhibition without a preceding MEP at 2 or more stimulus intensities. The data are replicated. The signals are stored for later review and analysis. This procedure is repeated for 3 to 4 selected muscles on the same limb. Finally, this procedure is repeated on the other upper extremity.

 Clinical Example (95929)

This 63-year-old female presents with subacute leg weakness without sensory disturbances. Imaging shows lumbar stenosis with myelopathy. After examination, electromyography (EMG), and other testing, her diagnosis remains uncertain. The differential includes lumbar myelopathy, lumbar stenosis with secondary code compression, and several peripheral neuromuscular disorders. She is referred for central, motor-evoked potential, testing to assess whether her disorder includes central motor pathway impairment and to provide a baseline for measurement of progression.

Description of Procedure (95929)

The physician applies electrodes over appropriate muscles and checks impedances. Motor-nerve conduction studies are performed and the baseline compound muscle action potentials (CMAP) are established. He/she determines the optimal scalp location for the head coil. Next, he/she determines the resting motor-evoked potential (MEP) threshold and records the MEP during modest tonic isometric contraction. The physician also measures the transcranial MEP amplitude and onset latency and compares this to the baseline nerve conduction studies. The physician measures CMAP obtained with supramaximal electrical stimulation and calculates the relative MEP amplitude. He/she measures the MEP to lumbar stimulation and calculates the relative MEP amplitude. The dissociation between MEP threshold and the cortical stimulation silent period (CSSP) is measured as is the dissociation between excitatory and inhibitory effects of transcranial stimulation (MEP facilitation failure). Next, the data is replicated and the signals stored for later review and analysis. The procedure is repeated for selected muscles on the same limb. Finally, this procedure is repeated for the other lower extremity.

⊘=Modifier 51 Exempt   ⊙=Conscious Sedation   ✚=Add-on Code

Neurostimulators, Analysis-Programming

A simple neurostimulator pulse . . .

Code 95970 describes subsequent electronic analysis of a previously implanted simple or complex brain, spinal cord, or peripheral neurostimulator pulse generator system, without reprogramming. Code 95971 describes intraoperative or subsequent electronic analysis of an implanted simple spinal cord or peripheral (ie, peripheral nerve, autonomic nerve, neuromuscular) neurostimulator pulse generator system, with programming. Codes 95972 and 95973 describe intraoperative (at initial insertion/revision) or subsequent electronic analysis of an implanted complex spinal cord or peripheral (except cranial nerve) neurostimulator pulse generator system, with programming. Codes 95974 and 95975 describe intraoperative (at initial insertion/revision) or subsequent electronic analysis of an implanted complex cranial nerve neurostimulator pulse generator system, with programming. ▶Codes 95978 and 95979 describe initial or subsequent electronic analysis of an implanted brain neurostimulator pulse generator system, with programming.◀

(For insertion of neurostimulator pulse generator, see 61885, 63685, 63688, 64590)

(For revision or removal of neurostimulator pulse generator or receiver, see 61888, 63688, 64595)

(For implantation of neurostimulator electrodes, see 61850-61875, 63650-63655, 64553-64580. For revision or removal of neurostimulator electrodes, see 61880, 63660, 64585)

95970 Electronic analysis of implanted neurostimulator pulse generator system (eg, rate, pulse amplitude and duration, configuration of wave form, battery status, electrode selectability, output modulation, cycling, impedance and patient compliance measurements); simple or complex brain, spinal cord, or peripheral (ie, cranial nerve, peripheral nerve, autonomic nerve, neuromuscular) neurostimulator pulse generator/transmitter, without reprogramming

▲**95971**   simple spinal cord, or peripheral (ie, peripheral nerve, autonomic nerve, neuromuscular) neurostimulator pulse generator/transmitter, with intraoperative or subsequent programming

▲**95972**   complex spinal cord, or peripheral (except cranial nerve) neurostimulator pulse generator/transmitter, with intraoperative or subsequent programming, first hour

+▲**95973**   complex spinal cord, or peripheral (except cranial nerve) neurostimulator pulse generator/transmitter, with intraoperative or subsequent programming, each additional 30 minutes after first hour (List separately in addition to code for primary procedure)

(Use 95973 in conjunction with 95972)

●**95978** Electronic analysis of implanted neurostimulator pulse generator system (eg, rate, pulse amplitude and duration, battery status, electrode selectability and polarity, impedance and patient compliance measurements), complex deep brain neurostimulator pulse generator/transmitter, with initial or subsequent programming; first hour

+●**95979**   each additional 30 minutes after first hour (List separately in addition to code for primary procedure)

▶(Use 95979 in conjunction with 95978)◀

Rationale

The 95970 series of codes for electronic analysis and programming of implanted neurostimulator pulse generator/transmitter has been revised and expanded to differentiate stimulation of deep cerebral structures (ie, globus pallidus, subthalamic nucleus) apart from other target sites (ie, spinal cord, peripheral nerve, neuromuscular or cranial nerve (vagus). Deep brain stimulator systems are implanted predominantly in patients with chronic Parkinson's disease and Essential Tremor who are not adequately controlled with medications. Deep brain stimulation (DBS) involves more complex technology, with more side effects, risk, and clinical features to measure. Additionally, it requires an interactive adjustment of anti-Parkinsonian medications during programming to minimize side effects which may occur in managing both the medications and the neurostimulation. To capture this more complex technology, two new codes (95978, 95979) have been added for analysis and programming of DBS, and the existing codes 95971, 95972 and 95973 have been revised to exclude brain stimulation which will now be coded as 95978 and 95979.

Deep brain stimulation (DBS) therapy improves many of the symptoms of Parkinson's disease, essential tremor, or dystonia when implanted in patients experiencing symptoms that are not adequately controlled by medications. The therapy includes implanted components consisting of stimulating electrodes connected to pulse generator(s) located in the subclavicular area. The stimulating electrodes are placed in various deep brain structures depending on the symptoms and disease being treated. Once implanted, the pulse generators can be programmed by the physician to reduce symptoms. As symptoms evolve due to disease progression, the pulse generators can be reprogrammed to improve symptom control and reduce disability.

Clinical Example (95971)

A 53-year-old male requires intraoperative electronic analysis and programming of an implanted neurostimulator pulse generator/transmitter. His history includes intractable right leg pain (rated 8/10) in an L5 distribution despite a lumbar diskectomy and a laminectomy, oral narcotic and non-narcotic medication, physical therapy, back brace trial, and various injection blocks. At operation, electronic analysis and programming of an implanted permanent single array electrode system and subcutaneous generator/transmitter is performed. The programming system is checked to ensure proper functioning, the physician tests limited combinations of the implant parameters, while assessing the degree of symptom and side effect improvement or worsening after each programming change. After the patient's device is programmed to achieve maximal comfortable stimulation, the physician provides the patient and family members with detailed instructions regarding stimulator operation and precautions.

Description of Procedure (95971)

Electronic analysis and programming of an implanted permanent single array electrode system and subcutaneous generator/transmitter is performed. With this system, there is one lead and four contacts. The physician tests limited combination of the implant parameters, while assessing the degree of symptom and side effect improvement or worsening after each programming change.

⊘=Modifier 51 Exempt   ⊙=Conscious Sedation   ✦=Add-on Code

Clinical Example (95972)

A 45-year-old male requires intra-operative electronic analysis of an implanted neurostimulator pulse generator. His history includes intractable chronic low back pain and right leg pain despite a laminectomy and a lumbar spine fusion, oral narcotic and non-narcotic medications, physical therapy, back brace trial, and various injection blocks. At operation, electronic analysis and programming of an implanted permanent multiple array electrode system and subcutaneous generator/transmitter is performed. After the patient's device is programmed to achieve maximal comfortable stimulation, the physician provides the patient and family members with detailed instructions regarding stimulator operations and precautions.

The patient presents for follow-up programming of an implanted permanent spinal cord multiple array electrode system and subcutaneous generator/transmitter. At the visit, the programming system is checked to ensure proper functioning, the physician tests multiple combinations of the implant parameters, while assessing the degree of symptom and side effect improvement or worsening after each programming change. After the patient's device is programmed to achieve maximal comfortable stimulation, the physician provides the patient and family members with detailed instructions regarding stimulator operations and precautions.

Description of Procedure (95972)

The actual programming is a cognitive type of service. High levels of analytic and interpretation skills are used in addition to the physical work of making each programming change. Of the 60 million or more combinations of the different parameters for an individual patient, the physician tests 30-60 of these combinations in a typical session. Much of the complexity of the programming comes from deciding which 30-60 combinations to test. Extensive patient feedback is utilized by the physician for this programming. Assessing the degree of symptom improvement or worsening after a single programming change can be complex. The physician will interact with the patient to determine whether the most recent change has reduced the patient's pain rating (where 10 is the worst pain imaginable) to perhaps a 6. This would be only a modest reduction but suggestive that the parameter change is on the right track. In addition to pain, the physician also evaluates the stimulation pattern and stimulation side effects such as motor changes (spasm, weakness) with each change and works to program the patient's device to achieve adequate, comfortable stimulation. During this time, the physician adjusts the electrode combinations, amplitude, pulse width, rate, one or multiple stimulation channels, multiple programs, phase angle, and pattern of alternating polarities.

The physician will typically begin the programming session by making changes, one at a time, in four to five of the parameters. This is done to discover which one or two parameters are the key, at least for that patient at that time. This discovery process can typically take 30-40 minutes of programming and much complexity to begin to find the right parameters to pursue further for the best programming result. The physician assesses symptom (eg, degree of pain) modification, based on experience with the type of patient and all the different parameters (eg, phase angle). For example, based upon 12 very similar previous patients where multiple programs seemed to provide the most powerful improvements in symptom relief, the physician would pursue in more detail changes in phase angle in this specific patient. After each change in any parameter, it will typically take 30-60 seconds to see symptom (eg, pain) relief or worsening. Thus, it typically will take one to two minutes per change. There may be 50 or more changes per session when programming a complex neurostimulator. The process typically takes one to two minutes per change. The process typically requires one programming session for about 60-90 minutes. The physician also provides the patient and family members with detailed instructions regarding stimulator operations and limited modifications of stimulation parameters (pulse width and amplitude) at home. The patient's device is reprogrammed to achieve adequate, comfortable stimulation. During this time, the physician adjusts the electrode combinations, amplitude, pulse width, rate, one or multiple stimulation channels, multiple programs, phase angle, and pattern of alternating polarities. The physician will typically begin the programming session by making changes, one at a time, in four to five of the parameters. This is done to discover which one or two parameters are the key, at least for that patient at that time. This discovery process can typically take 30-40 minutes of programming and much complexity to begin to find the right parameters to pursue further for the best programming result. The physician assesses symptom (eg, degree of pain) modification, based on experience with the types of patient and all the different parameters (eg, phase angle). For example, based upon 12 very similar previous patients where multiple programs seemed to provide the most powerful improvements in symptom relief, the physician would pursue in more detail changes in phase angle in this specific patient. After each change in any parameter, it will typically take 30-60 seconds to see symptom (eg, pain) relief or worsening. Thus, it typically will take one to two minutes per change. There may be 50 or more changes per session when programming a complex neurostimulator. The process typically requires detailed instructions regarding stimulator operations and limited modifications of stimulation parameters (pulse width and amplitude) at home.

 ### Clinical Example (95973)

A 45-year-old male requires intraoperative electronic analysis of an implanted neurostimulator pulse generator. His history includes intractable chronic low back pain and right leg pain (rated 8/10) despite a laminectomy and a lumbar spine fusion, oral narcotic and non-narcotic medications, physical therapy, back brace trial, and various injection blocks. At operation, electronic analysis and programming of an implanted permanent multiple array electrode system and subcutaneous generator/transmitter is performed. After the patient's device is programmed to achieve maximal comfortable stimulation, the physician provides the patient and family members with detailed instructions regarding stimulator operations and precautions.

The patient presents for follow-up programming and monitoring of an implanted permanent spinal cord multiple-array electrode system and subcutaneous generator/transmitter. At the visit, the programming system is checked to ensure proper functioning, the physician tests multiple combinations of the implant parameters, while assessing the degree of symptom and side effect improvement or worsening after each programming change. After the patient's device is programmed to achieve maximal comfortable stimulation, the physician provides the patient and family members with detailed instructions regarding stimulator operations and precautions.

Description of Procedure (95973)

Please see description for primary code 95972.

 Clinical Example 1 (95978)

A 71-year-old female with a 15-year history of idiopathic Parkinson's disease with disability for many activities of daily living is inadequately controlled with multiple medications. She returns 4 weeks following bilateral implantation of a deep brain neurostimulator system in both subthalamic nuclei as well as subcutaneous implantation of two neurostimulator devices. The neurostimulators have not been activated since surgery and she presents for initiation of neurostimulation during a programming session while off anti-Parkinson medications.

 Clinical Example 2 (95978)

A 71-year-old female with a 15-year history of idiopathic Parkinson's disease with disability for many activities of daily living returns for follow-up programming of implanted, deep, brain, neurostimulator devices. She is taking her usual doses of medications.

Description of Procedure (95978)

The physician checks the programming system to ensure proper functioning. He/she performs device and lead diagnostic testing, as needed. Each side of the brain has a lead with four contacts. The integrity of all eight contacts (four on each side of the brain) is evaluated by testing impedance. Next, the physician interrogates the device and determines the percentage of time the device has been in use since the last programming session to evaluate patient compliance and determine if the device may have been unintentionally inactivated. He/she evaluates the patient's experience to date with the device. Then the action/interaction of individual anti-Parkinson medications and deep brain stimulation and their combined effect on individual Parkinsonian symptoms is reviewed. During a programming session, the physician considers each contact along both electrode leads, stimulation amplitude, pulse width, rate, cathode/anode effects on current, gradual stimulator parameters on a case by case basis, symptom benefit or worsening, and side effects. The physician then considers 200 of a possible one million combinations of the different parameters for an individual patient with a deep brain stimulator. The physician decides which of the 200 combinations to test for an optimal effect while minimizing adverse side effects.

Clinical Example (95979)

A 71-year-old female with a 15-year history of idiopathic Parkinson's disease with disability for many activities of daily living returns for follow-up programming of implanted deep brain neurostimulator devices. She is taking her usual doses of medications.

Description of Procedure (95979)

The physician continues to review the action/interaction of individual anti-Parkinson medications and deep brain stimulation and their combined effect on individual Parkinsonian symptoms. During a programming session, he/she considers each contact along both electrode leads, stimulation amplitude, pulse width, rate, cathode/anode effects on current, gradual stimulator parameters on a case by case basis, symptom benefit or worsening, and side effects. The physician then considers 200 of a possible one million combinations of the different parameters for an individual patient with a deep brain stimulator. The physician decides which of the 200 combinations to test for an optimal effect while minimizing adverse side effects.

Motion Analysis

Codes 96000-96004 describe services performed as part of a major therapeutic or diagnostic decision making process. Motion analysis is performed in a dedicated motion analysis laboratory (ie, a facility capable of performing videotaping from the front, back and both sides, computerized 3-D kinematics, 3-D kinetics, and dynamic electromyography). Code 96000 may include 3-D kinetics and stride characteristics. Codes 96002–96003 describe dynamic electromyography.

Code 96004 should only be reported ...

96000   Comprehensive computer-based motion analysis by video-taping and 3-D kinematics;

96001   with dynamic plantar pressure measurements during walking

96002   Dynamic surface electromyography, during walking or other functional activities, 1-12 muscles

96003   Dynamic fine wire electromyography, during walking or other functional activities, 1 muscle

(Do not report 96002, 96003 in conjunction with 95860-▶95864, 95869-95872◀)

 Rationale

The cross-reference following code 96003 has been revised to exclude 95875. Code 95875 was revised in 2002 with removal of the electromyography component and is no longer appropriately included in this cross-reference. The Motion Analysis guidelines were also revised to clarify that the electromyography codes (95860-95875) are not inherent in codes 96000, 96001, and 96004.

Ø=Modifier 51 Exempt   ☉=Conscious Sedation   ✚=Add-on Code

Central Nervous System Assessments/Tests (eg, Neuro-Cognitive, Mental Status, Speech)

96110   Developmental testing; limited (eg, Developmental Screening Test II, Early Language Milestone Screen), with interpretation and report

▲96111   extended (includes assessment of motor, language, social, adaptive and/or cognitive functioning by standardized developmental instruments) with interpretation and report

🖎 Rationale

Code 96111 was revised in the code descriptor, as this code may be used to report any extensive developmental testing. Code 96111 was further revised by having the "per hour" specification removed, as this type of testing takes an average of 85 minutes.

🩺 Clinical Example (96111)

A 45-year-old male who is 3 months status post cerebrovascular accident (CVA) in the distribution of the left middle cerebral artery. A careful language evaluation is required to determine the nature and extent of aphasia deficits and to make recommendations for rehabilitation. This code includes work in addition to and separate from the neurological evaluation.

Description of Procedure (96111)

Intra-service includes administration of assessment procedures and clinical observations of the patient's behavior during the actual testing process.

Chemotherapy Administration

96545   Provision of chemotherapy agent

      (For radioactive isotope therapy, ▶use 79005◀)

🖎 Rationale

In tandem with the revisions to the radiopharmaceutical therapy subsection of Radiology, the cross-reference following code 96545 has been revised to refer the user to the appropriate code for oral administration of radioactive isotope therapy.

Physical Medicine and Rehabilitation

▶Codes 97001-97755 should be used to report each distinct procedure performed. Do not append modifier 51 to 97001-97755.◀

(For muscle testing, range of joint motion, electromyography, see 95831 et seq)

(For transcutaneous nerve stimulation (TNS), use 64550)

97001   Physical therapy evaluation

 Rationale

New instructional language was added at the beginning of the Physical Medicine and Rehabilitation subsection of the Medicine section to clarify that modifier 51 Multiple Procedures should not be appended to codes 97001-97755.

Modalities

SUPERVISED

97010   Application of a modality to one or more areas; hot or cold packs

97012   traction, mechanical

97014   electrical stimulation (unattended)

(For acupuncture with electrical stimulation, ▶see 97813, 97814◀)

 Rationale

In tandem with the establishment of two new codes to report performance of acupuncture with electrical stimulation, the cross-reference following code 97014 for unattended electrical stimulation has been revised to include the new electrical stimulation acupuncture services codes.

Active Wound Care Management

Active wound care procedures are performed to ▶remove devitalized and/or necrotic tissue and◀ promote healing. ▶Provider is required to have direct (one-on-one) patient contact.◀

(Do not report ▶97597◀-97602 in conjunction with 11040-11044)

●**97597**   Removal of devitalized tissue from wound(s), selective debridement, without anesthesia (eg, high pressure waterjet with/without suction, sharp selective debridement with scissors, scalpel and forceps), with or without topical application(s), wound assessment, and instruction(s) for ongoing care, may include use of a whirlpool, per session; total wound(s) surface area less than or equal to 20 square centimeters

●**97598**   total wound(s) surface area greater than 20 square centimeters

▶(97601 has been deleted. To report, use 97597, 97598)◀

97602   Non-selective debridement, without anesthesia (eg, wet-to-moist dressings, enzymatic, abrasion), including topical application(s), wound assessment, and instruction(s) for ongoing care, per session

●**97605**   Negative pressure wound therapy (eg, vacuum assisted drainage collection), including topical application(s), wound assessment, and instruction(s) for ongoing care, per session; total wound(s) surface area less than or equal to 50 square centimeters

●**97606**   total wound(s) surface area greater than 50 square centimeters

---

⃠=Modifier 51 Exempt   ⊙=Conscious Sedation   ✛=Add-on Code

Rationale

The Active Wound Care Management subsection of Medicine has been updated to include revised introductory guidelines, revised codes to report selective debridement based on total surface area of wound(s) size and new procedures to describe negative pressure wound therapy techniques based on total surface area wound(s) size. In addition, the cross-reference below the guidelines was revised to include the new codes (97597, 97598) which should not be reported in conjunction with debridement codes 11040-11044.

Codes 97597 and 97598 have been established to report selective debridement based on total surface area of wound(s) size.

Codes 97605 and 97606 have been established to report negative pressure wound therapy based on total surface area of wound(s) size.

Code 97601 has been deleted and a related cross-reference added to direct the user to the new codes 97597 and 97598. Code 97602 has been revised as a standalone code.

New codes 97605 and 97607 represent negative pressure wound therapy services. Negative pressure wound therapy is a procedure that manages wound exudates and promotes wound closure. The vacuum cleanses the wound and stimulates the wound bed, reduces localized edema and improves local oxygen supply. It places mechanical stress on the tissue that increases the rate of cellular proliferation, granular tissue formation and new vessel growth. This procedure requires work and practice expense different than any of the procedures considered to be selective debridement in the 97000 series codes. Also, it is a procedure that has different clinical indications.

Clinical Example (97597)

The patient is a 68-year-old female who has developed a pressure ulcer on the sacrum and reports pain from the ulcerated area. Examination reveals that the wound is covered with black eschar and is surrounded by chronic inflammation with dark pigmentation. It is determined that the patient is not a candidate for surgery due to several comorbidities, however, would benefit from sharp debridement of the necrotic tissue.

Description of Procedure (97597)

The wound is lightly cleansed and then measured. The sacral wound measures 6.5 cm x 2.0 cm, with 100% black wound bed and no obvious drainage. The surrounding tissue is palpated with the wound margin observed as being inflamed and indurated. The wound is wiped with an anti-microbial solution, followed by sharp debridement using scissors, scalpel and forceps to remove the devitalized tissue and facilitate subsequent wound healing. An enzymatic agent, saline gauze and a composite dressing are placed directly on the wound bed.

The last component related to this intervention is instruction to the patient/caregiver regarding application of dressing, frequency of dressing change and signs of wound deterioration.

Clinical Example (97598)

The patient is a 72-year-old male who developed a pressure ulcer on the left hip and a venous ulcer of the left medial lower leg just proximal to the ankle. The wounds are lightly cleansed and then measured.

Examination of the left hip wound reveals a stage III ulcer measuring 5.0 cm x 4.4 cm x 3.2 cm. The wound bed is obscured with semi-adherent, yellow necrotic tissue. The wound margin is indurated with non-blanchable redness noted. Moderate amounts of serosanguineous drainage is noted.

The left lower leg wound measures 10.0 cm x 6.8 cm x 1.5 cm. This is a full thickness wound. Seventy-five percent is covered with adherent yellow necrotic tissue. Twenty-five percent is dull pink tissue. The wound margins are irregular and macerated. Copious serosanguineous drainage is evident. Circumferential measurements taken at the calf and ankle reveals 2 centimeters of measurable edema on the left compared to the right lower extremity.

Description of Procedure (97598)

A more thorough cleansing of the left hip wound is performed utilizing high pressure waterjet with suction in order to facilitate loosening of the tissue. The wound is then wiped with an antimicrobial solution followed by sharp debridement with scissors, scalpel and forceps to remove devitalized tissue. The wound is then dressed with saline moistened gauze, lightly packed and a composite dressing applied.

The ankle wound is wiped with an antimicrobial solution followed by sharp debridement utilizing scissors, scalpel and forceps to remove the devitalized tissue. A barrier cream is applied to protect the tissue around the wound and prevent further breakdown. The wound is dressed with an absorbent dressing that promotes further autolytic debridement and covered with a composite dressing.

The last component related to this intervention is instruction to the patient/caregiver regarding appropriate exercise and limb elevation.

Clinical Example (97605)

The patient is a 73-year-old male with a stage III pressure ulcer of the sacrum. The base of the wound is clean and red and presents with heavy amount of serous drainage. There is also significant induration of the entire wound periphery with 1.5 cm of undermining proximally. The wound measures 8.5 x 5.0 x 3.2 centimeters.

Description of Procedure (97605)

Prior to application of the negative pressure therapy, the wound is thoroughly cleansed. The wound is assessed to assure no sinus tracts and/or fistulas are present. The skin around the wound is cleansed thoroughly and prepared for the application of transparent film. The foam sponge is cut to fit the size and depth of the wound as well as the undermined areas.

The foam is secured in the wound using an adhesive transparent film. The film is applied with ample border to assure a tight seal. The suction feet and tubing are then inserted into the foam. Additional transparent film is placed around the suction feet to secure the seal. The tubing is then connected to the negative pressure therapy pump. The negative pressure parameters are set on intermittent application at 100mm/Hg. The pump is activated and the dressing is inspected for appropriate negative pressure suction and no evidence of leaks.

The patient/caregiver is instructed in the maintenance of the pump, technique for canister replacement, proper inspection of the dressing and signs or symptoms of wound deterioration. The patient continues to be monitored for tolerance, and the tubing and film monitored for leaks, clogs, and the need for canister replacement.

 Clinical Example (97606)

The patient is a 68-year-old female who underwent gastric surgery. Four days after surgery, the abdominal post-op site dehisced revealing a proximal wound measuring 4.0 cm x 6.2 cm x 2.5 cm and a distal wound measuring 8.4 cm x 4.6 cm x 3.5 cm. The proximal wound has a 100% red granulating wound bed with indurated wound margins and moderate amounts of serosanguineous drainage. The distal wound presents with a 25% yellow necrotic wound bed, indurated wound margins, localized redness and copious amounts of purulent drainage.

Description of Procedure (97606)

The wounds are cleansed. The wounds are then assessed to assure no sinus tracts and/or fistulas are present. The skin around the wound is cleansed thoroughly and prepared for the application of transparent film. The foam sponges are cut to fit the size and depth of each wound.

The foam is secured in the wounds using an adhesive, transparent film. The film must be applied with ample border to assure a tight seal. The suction feet and tubing are then inserted into the foam at each site. Additional transparent film is placed around the suction feet to secure the seal. The tubing of both wounds is joined to the negative pressure therapy pump by a "Y" connector. The pump parameters are set at continuous pressure of 125 mm/Hg. The pump is activated and the dressing is inspected for appropriate negative pressure suction and no evidence of leaks.

The patient continues to be monitored for tolerance, and the tubing and film monitored for leaks, clogs, and the need for canister replacement.

Other Procedures

(For extracorporeal shock wave musculoskeletal therapy, use Category III code 0019T)

▶(97780 has been deleted. To report, see 97810, 97811)◀

▶(97781 has been deleted. To report, see 97813, 97814)◀

97799   Unlisted physical medicine/rehabilitation service or procedure

►Acupuncture is reported based on 15 minute increments of personal (face-to-face) contact with the patient, not the duration of acupuncture needle(s) placement.◄

►If no electrical stimulation is used during a 15 minute increment, use 97810, 97811. If electrical stimulation of any needle is used during a 15 minute increment, use 97813, 97814.◄

●**97810**   Acupuncture, one or more needles, without electrical stimulation; initial 15 minutes of personal one-on-one contact with the patient

+●**97811**   each additional 15 minutes of personal one-on-one contact with the patient, with re-insertion of needle(s) (List separately in addition to code for primary procedure)

►(Use 97811 in conjunction with 97810)◄

►(Do not report 97810, 97811 in conjunction with 97813 or 97814)◄

►(Evaluation and Management services may be reported separately, using modifier 25, if the patient's condition requires a significant separately identifiable E/M service, above and beyond the usual preservice and postservice work associated with the acupuncture services. The time of the E/M service is not included in the time of the acupuncture service.)◄

●**97813**   Acupuncture, one or more needles, with electrical stimulation; initial 15 minutes of personal one-on-one contact with the patient

+●**97814**   each additional 15 minutes of personal one-on-one contact with the patient, with re-insertion of needle(s) (List separately in addition to code for primary procedure)

►(Use 97814 in conjunction with 97813)◄

► (Do not report 97813, 97814 in conjunction with 97810 or 97811)◄

►(Evaluation and Management services may be reported separately, using modifier 25, if the patient's condition requires a significant separately identifiable E/M service, above and beyond the usual preservice and postservice work associated with the acupuncture services. The time of the E/M service is not included in the time of the acupuncture service.)◄

Rationale

Codes 97780 and 97781 were deleted and codes 97810-97814 were established to more clearly describe acupuncture and electroacupuncture services and to more accurately capture the varying times required to perform these services. Codes 97810 and 97811 describe acupuncture services without electrical stimulation. Code 97810 is intended to report the primary service, and 97811 is intended to be reported for each additional 15 minutes of one-on-one contact with the patient.

Similarly, codes 97813 and 97814 describe acupuncture services with electrical stimulation. Code 97813 is intended to report the primary service, and 97814 is intended to be reported for each additional 15 minutes of one-on-one contact with the patient. A parenthetical note has been added following codes 97811 and

Note: The misplacement of the semicolons for new codes 97810 and 97813 as shown in the CPT 2005 book have been corrected here. This corrected version will appear in the CPT 2006 book.

97814 to instruct that the acupuncture services without electrical stimulation would not be additionally reported at the same session in addition to the acupuncture services with electrical stimulation. The descriptor language of the new codes clarifies that they describe personal one-on-one contact with the patient. Two cross-references were also added to each of the new sets of acupuncture modality codes to indicate that significant and separately identifiable Evaluation and Management (E/M) services performed during the same session as the acupuncture services may be separately reported using modifier 25, and that the time of the E/M service is not included in the time of the acupuncture service.

Clinical Example 1 (97810)

A 17-year-old male presents for repeat treatment of non-traumatic cervicalgia of three days' duration. The patient reports cervical pain and limited range of motion.

Description of Procedure (97810 Example 1)

The practitioner reviews the chart, greets the patient and obtains a brief account of the results of the previous treatment and any significant changes that have occurred since the last visit. Three points are selected for today's treatment (trigger points in the levator scapula, trapezius and splenius capitus muscles). The patient is placed in the prone position. The points are located by careful palpation, identifying the tightest, most tender nodules in the affected muscles. Once the points are located, they are marked by pressing the skin and then cleaned with alcohol swabs. The practitioner selects the appropriate needle lengths and gauges for this treatment. After hand-washing, the practitioner inserts and mildly stimulates the needles. The process of insertion requires care to actually obtain the dull, aching sensation of a correctly needled point, while at the same time avoiding puncture of vital structures, in this case, the lungs. The patient is instructed to rest for 20 minutes while the needles are retained.

After charting the procedure, the practitioner leaves the patient to rest while the needles are retained. The practitioner returns periodically to monitor the patient and to re-stimulate the needles and to inquire about patient comfort and treatment response. When the desired effect is achieved, the practitioner removes the needles and presses on the points with a cotton ball to prevent bruising or bleeding. The needles are disposed in accordance with Occupational Safety and Health Administration (OSHA) guidelines. The practitioner then assists the patient to an upright position, making sure that the patient does not feel faint. Any final charting that may be required is then performed.

Clinical Example 2 (97810)

A 26-year-old female with a diagnosis of migraine presents for a return office visit. The patient is currently symptomatic, presenting with a unilateral headache of one days' duration.

Description of Procedure (97810 Example 2)

After reviewing the chart, greeting the patient and obtaining a brief account of the results of the previous treatment and any significant changes that have occurred since the last visit, a series of points are selected to address the migraine. The points are located by palpation, then marked and cleaned with alcohol swabs, bilaterally. The patient is instructed to lie in the supine position, so that needles may be inserted in the temporal region, hands and feet bilaterally. The practitioner selects the appropriate needle lengths and gauges for this treatment. After hand-washing, the practitioner inserts the needles to the proper depth and obtains the desired dull, radiating sensation. Care is taken to prevent puncture to the temporal nerve or artery, or any other sensitive anatomical structures. The practitioner manually stimulates the needles by lifting, thrusting and twisting them. The patient is instructed to rest for 20 minutes while the needles are retained. The practitioner charts the point selection and leaves the room.

The practitioner returns periodically to monitor the patient and to re-stimulate the needles. When that portion of the treatment is complete, the practitioner removes the needles, pressing on each point to prevent bleeding, then instructs the patient to turn to the prone position. The needles are disposed in accordance with Occupational Safety and Health Administration (OSHA) guidelines and additional points are selected in the sub-occipital region to complete the treatment. After palpating to locate these points, they are marked and cleaned with alcohol swabs, bilaterally. New needles are selected, inserted and manipulated to obtain the desired effect. The patient is instructed to rest for 20 minutes while these needles are retained. Periodically, the practitioner returns to manipulate these needles. When the treatment is complete, the practitioner removes the needles and presses cotton on the points to prevent bleeding or bruising. The needles are disposed in accordance with OSHA guidelines. The patient is assisted to an upright position. Any final charting is completed and the patient is instructed to avoid known migraine triggers.

 ### Clinical Example 3 (97810)
A 65-year-old male presents for a return office visit with acute, severe renal colic, which was diagnosed four days previously. His pain comes in waves and is accompanied by nausea. He also has previously diagnosed, chronic osteoarthritis of the knee, which affects his gait.

Description of Procedure (97810 Example 3)
After reviewing the chart, greeting the patient and charting a brief account of the results of the previous treatment and any significant changes that have occurred since the last visit, the patient is instructed to lie in the prone position. The practitioner palpates to locate tender points in the lower back and related points in the lower extremity. Palpation involves feeling for areas of localized muscle spasm that elicit pain when pressed. As some points are only about a millimeter across, palpation requires skill and patience. The practitioner selects the appropriate needle lengths and gauges for this treatment. The points are marked and cleaned with alcohol swabs bilaterally. The practitioner performs handwashing. The needles are inserted and manipulated to produce a deep, aching sensation. The patient is instructed to rest while the needles are retained.

⊘=Modifier 51 Exempt   ⊙=Conscious Sedation   ✚=Add-on Code

The practitioner returns periodically to re-manipulate the needles and check on the progress of the patient. When the abdominal spasm and pain has subsided, the needles are removed and the points are closed with pressure from a cotton ball to prevent bruising. The needles are disposed in accordance with OSHA guidelines. The patient is assisted to a sitting position and asked to move in ways that test the effectiveness of treatment. The pain has reduced but is still significant, and the nausea persists. The practitioner selects additional points on the hands, lower legs and feet. The practitioner palpates to locate, then marks and cleans those points. The practitioner washes hands again, selects and inserts six additional needles in the hands, and six in the lower extremities. The practitioner remains in the room and continues to stimulate the needles during this phase of treatment, until the pain and nausea are improved to an acceptable level.

The patient is instructed to lie supine with the osteoarthritic knee flexed. The practitioner palpates and locates points to treat the knee, then marks and cleans those points with alcohol swabs. The practitioner selects the appropriate needle lengths and gauges for this treatment. After re-washing, the practitioner selects and inserts a fresh set of needles into and around the knee. The patient is instructed to rest in the supine position. The practitioner leaves the room while the needles are retained. The practitioner returns to monitor the patient and re-stimulate the needles. When the pain and swelling are reduced to an acceptable level, the needles are removed and the points closed using a cotton ball to prevent bleeding or bruising. The needles are disposed in accordance with Occupational Safety and Health Administration (OSHA) guidelines. The patient is assisted to his feet and checked to be sure that he is ambulatory. Final charting is performed. The patient is instructed in home care measures including avoidance of lumbar flexion, lifting and other activities that might exacerbate the condition.

Clinical Example (97811)

A 26-year-old female with a diagnosis of migraine presents for a return office visit. The patient is currently symptomatic, presenting with a unilateral headache of one day's duration.

Description of Procedure (97811)

Following the initial 15-minute session of acupuncture, the needles are removed and the practitioner instructs the patient to turn to the prone position. New points are selected to complete the treatment. After palpating to locate these points, they are marked and cleaned with alcohol swabs, bilaterally. Six needles are selected, inserted and manipulated to obtain the desired effect. The patient is instructed to rest for 20 minutes while these needles are retained. Periodically, the practitioner returns to manipulate these needles. When the treatment is complete, the practitioner removes the needles and presses cotton on the points to prevent bleeding or bruising. The needles are disposed in accordance with OSHA guidelines. The patient is assisted to an upright position. Follow-up instructions are given to the patient. Final documentation is recorded in the patient chart.

Clinical Example 1 (97813)

A 49-year-old female receiving chemotherapy for breast cancer was previously referred for acupuncture to relieve post-chemo nausea. This treatment is part of an ongoing series of treatments for this condition. The patient is weak but not faint, and has not vomited since chemotherapy was received earlier in the day.

Description of Procedure (97813 Example 1)

The practitioner reviews the chart, greets the patient and obtains a brief account of the results of the previous treatment and any significant changes that have occurred since the last visit. One point is selected for today's treatment (proximal to the palmar surface of the wrist, bilaterally). The patient is placed in the supine position. The points are located by palpation. As points may be no larger than a millimeter in diameter, the process of point location requires considerable skill. Once the points are located, they are marked by pressing the skin and then cleaned with alcohol swabs. The practitioner selects the appropriate needle lengths and gauges for this treatment. After hand-washing, the practitioner inserts and mildly stimulates the needles. The process of insertion requires care to actually obtain the dull, aching sensation of a correctly needled point, while at the same time avoiding puncture of vital structures. In this case, the point P6 is on the medial wrist, between the flexor carpi tendons and blood vessels and directly over the median nerve. Electrodes are then attached to the shafts of the needles and an appropriate frequency (Hz) and waveform are selected. The practitioner then slowly increases the amplitude of the signal until patient tolerance is reached. The patient is instructed to rest for 20 minutes while the needles are retained.

After charting the procedure, the practitioner leaves the patient to rest while the needles are retained. The practitioner returns periodically to monitor the patient, re-adjust the electrical stimulation and to inquire about patient comfort and treatment response. When the desired effect is achieved, the practitioner removes the electrodes and needles, and presses on the points with a cotton ball to prevent bruising or bleeding. The needles are disposed in accordance with Occupational Safety and Health Administration (OSHA) guidelines. The practitioner then assists the patient to an upright position, making sure that the patient does not feel faint. Any final charting that may be required is then performed. The patient is instructed to maintain hydration and be careful about the possibility of fainting.

Clinical Example 2 (97813)

A 65-year-old male returns for a repeat visit to treat lumbalgia.

Description of Procedure (97813 Example 2)

After reviewing the chart, greeting the patient and charting a brief account of the results of the previous treatment and any significant changes that have occurred since the last visit, the patient is instructed to lie in the prone position. The practitioner palpates to locate tender points in the lower back and related points in the lower extremity. Palpation involves feeling for areas of localized muscle spasm that elicit pain when pressed. As some points are only about a millimeter across, palpation requires skill and patience. The practitioner selects the appropriate needle lengths and gauges for this treatment. The points are marked and cleaned with alcohol swabs bilaterally. The practitioner performs hand-washing. The needles are inserted and manipulated to produce a deep, aching sensation. Electrodes are then attached to the shafts of the needles and an appropriate frequency (Hz) and waveform is selected. The practitioner then slowly increases the amplitude of the signal until patient tolerance is reached. The patient is instructed to rest while the needles are retained.

The practitioner returns periodically to re-adjust the frequency and amplitude of the electrical stimulation to the needles, and to check on the progress of the patient. When the lumbar spasm and tenderness has subsided, the electrodes are disconnected, the needles are removed, and the points are closed with pressure from a cotton ball to prevent bruising. The needles are disposed in accordance with Occupational Safety and Health Administration (OSHA) guidelines.

The patient is assisted to his feet and asked to walk around the room to test the effectiveness of treatment. The pain has reduced but is still significant, so the practitioner selects additional points on the hands, palpates to locate, then marks and cleans those points. The practitioner washes hands again, selects and inserts six additional needles in the hands. The needles are manipulated to produce a deep, aching sensation. Electrodes are then attached to the shafts of the needles and an appropriate frequency (Hz) and waveform are selected. The practitioner then slowly increases the amplitude of the signal until patient tolerance is reached. The patient is instructed to walk in place, bend and twist to test the degree of improvement and to facilitate the treatment. The practitioner remains in the room and continues to stimulate the needles during this phase of treatment by adjusting the electrical stimulation, until the pain and dysfunction are improved to an acceptable level.

 Clinical Example 3 (97813)
A 37-year-old female returns for ongoing treatment of cervical spondylosis, carpal tunnel syndrome and fibromyalgia.

Description of Procedure (97813 Example 3)
After reviewing the chart, greeting the patient and obtaining a brief account of the results of the previous treatment and any significant changes that have occurred since the last visit, a series of points are selected to address the cervical and wrist/hand pain. The points are located by palpation, then marked and cleaned with alcohol swabs. The patient is instructed to lie in the supine position, so that needles may be inserted in the palmar wrist, ulnar side of the hand, and cervical region. The practitioner selects the appropriate needle lengths and gauges for this treatment. After hand-washing, the practitioner inserts the needles to the proper depth and obtains the desired dull, radiating sensation. Care is taken to prevent puncture to the brachial plexus, brachial artery, median nerve or artery, or any other sensitive anatomical structures. Electrodes are then attached to the shafts of the needles and an appropriate frequency (Hz) and waveform are selected. The practitioner then slowly increases the amplitude of the signal until patient tolerance is reached. The patient is instructed to rest for 20 minutes while the needles are retained. The practitioner charts the point selection and leaves the room.

The practitioner returns periodically to monitor the patient and re-stimulate the needles by adjusting the frequency, waveform and amplitude of the electrical stimulation. When that portion of the treatment is complete, the practitioner disconnects the electrodes and removes the needles, pressing on each point to prevent bleeding. The needles are disposed in accordance with Occupational Safety and Health Administration (OSHA) guidelines.

The patient is instructed to lie supine with the osteoarthritic knee flexed. The practitioner palpates and locates points to treat the knee, then marks and cleans those points with alcohol swabs. The practitioner selects the appropriate needle lengths and gauges for this treatment. After re-washing, the practitioner selects and inserts a fresh set of needles into and around the knee. The patient is instructed to rest in the supine position. The practitioner leaves the room while the needles are retained. The practitioner returns to monitor the patient and re-stimulate the needles by adjusting the frequency, waveform and amplitude of the electrical stimulation. When the pain and swelling are reduced to an acceptable level, the electrodes are disconnected. The needles are then removed and the points closed using a cotton ball to prevent bleeding or bruising. The needles are disposed in accordance with OSHA guidelines. The patient is assisted to her feet and checked to be sure that she is ambulatory. Final charting is performed. The patient is instructed in home care measures including avoidance of lumbar flexion, lifting, squatting and other activities that might exacerbate the condition.

 Clinical Example (97814)
65-year-old male returns for a repeat visit to treat lumbalgia.

Description of Procedure (97814)
Following the initial 15-minute session of electroacupuncture (97813), the needles are removed and the practitioner assists the patient to his feet and asks him to walk around the room to test the effectiveness of treatment. The pain has reduced but is still significant, so the practitioner selects four additional points, palpates to locate, then marks and cleans those points. The practitioner inserts the four additional needles, and they are manipulated to produce a deep, aching sensation. Electrodes are then attached to the shafts of the needles and an appropriate frequency (Hz) and waveform is selected. The practitioner then slowly increases the amplitude of the signal until patient tolerance is reached. The patient is instructed to rest. The practitioner remains in the room and continues to stimulate the needles during this phase of treatment by adjusting the electrical stimulation, until the pain and dysfunction are improved to an acceptable level. At the conclusion of this service the electrodes and needles are removed. Follow-up instructions are given to the patient. The needles are disposed in accordance with OSHA guidelines. Final documentation is recorded in the patient chart.

⊘ =Modifier 51 Exempt   ⊙ =Conscious Sedation   ✚ =Add-on Code

Category II

For 2005, all of the 2004 Category II codes have been deleted and renumbered. Four new codes have been added to represent Maternity Care Management. Eight new categories of codes have been added to accommodate the addition and organization of the existing and future Category II codes.

Category II Codes

The following section of Current Procedural Terminology (CPT) contains a set of supplemental tracking codes that can be used for performance measurement. ▶It is anticipated that the use of Category II◀ codes for performance measurement will decrease the need for record abstraction and chart review, and thereby minimize administrative burden on physicians, ▶other health care professionals, hospitals, and entities seeking to measure the quality of patient care. These codes are intended to facilitate data collection about the quality of care rendered by coding certain services and test results that support nationally established performance measures and that have an evidence base as contributing to quality patient care.◀

▶These codes describe clinical components that may be typically included in evaluation and management services or other clinical services and, therefore, do not have a relative value associated with them. Category II codes may also describe results from laboratory tests and procedures, select processes intended to address patient safety practices, or services reflecting compliance with state or federal law.◀

▶Category II codes described in this section make use of an alphabetical character as the 5th character in the string (ie, 4 digits followed by the letter F). These digits are not intended to reflect the placement of the code in the regular (Category I) part of CPT. To promote understanding of these codes and their associated measures, users are referred to Appendix H, which contains information about the measures and their origins. CPT Category II codes are arranged according to the following categories derived from standard clinical documentation format:◀

▶Composite Measures — To begin with 0001F (no measures at this time)◀

▶Patient Management — 0500F-0503F◀

▶Patient History — 1000F-1002F◀

▶Physical Examination — 2000F◀

▶Diagnostic/Screening Processes or Results — 3000F (no codes at this time)◀

▶Therapeutic, Preventive or Other Interventions — 4000F-4011F◀

▶Follow-up or Other Outcomes — To begin with 5000F (no codes at this time)◀

▶Patient Safety — To begin with 6000F (no codes at this time)◀

▶Cross-references to the measures associated with each Category II code and their origins are included for reference in Appendix H. Users should review the complete measure(s) associated with each code prior to implementing its use.◀

▶Category II codes are reviewed by the Performance Measures Advisory Group (PMAG), an advisory body to the CPT Editorial Panel and the CPT/HCPAC Advisory Committee. The PMAG is comprised of performance measurement experts representing the Agency for Healthcare Research and Quality (AHRQ), the American Medical Association (AMA), the Centers for Medicare and Medicaid Services (CMS), the Joint Commission on Accreditation of Healthcare Organizations (JCAHO), the National Committee for Quality Assurance (NCQA), and the Physician Consortium for Performance Improvement. The PMAG may seek additional expertise and/or input from other national health care organizations, as necessary, for the development of Category II codes. These may include national medical specialty societies, other national health care professional associations, accrediting bodies, and federal regulatory agencies.◀

▶Category II codes are published biannually: January 1 and July 1. The most current listing, along with guidelines and forms for submitting code change proposals for Category II codes, may be accessed on the Internet at http://www.ama-assn.org/go/cpt.◀

▶(0001F has been deleted. To report, use 2000F)◀

▶(0002F has been deleted. To report, use 1000F)◀

▶(0003F has been deleted. To report, use 1001F)◀

▶(0004F has been deleted. To report, use 4000F)◀

▶(0005F has been deleted. To report, use 4001F)◀

▶(0006F has been deleted. To report, use 4002F)◀

▶(0007F has been deleted. To report, use 4006F)◀

▶(0008F has been deleted. To report, use 4009F)◀

▶(0009F has been deleted. To report, use 1002F)◀

▶(0010F has been deleted)◀

▶(0011F has been deleted. To report, use 4011F)◀

▶Composite Measures◀

▶Composite measures codes combine several measures grouped within a single code descriptor to facilitate reporting for a clinical condition when all components are met. If only some of the components are met, or if services are provided in addition to those included in the composite code, they may be reported individually using the corresponding CPT Category II codes for those services.◀

▶No measures at this time.◀

▶Patient Management◀

▶Patient management codes describe utilization measures or measures of patient care provided for specific clinical purposes (eg, prenatal care, pre- and post-surgical care).◀

●0500F   Initial prenatal care visit (report at first prenatal encounter with health care professional providing obstetrical care. Report also date of visit and, in a separate field, the date of the last menstrual period - LMP)[2]

●0501F   Prenatal flow sheet documented in medical record by first prenatal visit (documentation includes at minimum blood pressure, weight, urine protein, uterine size, fetal heart tones, and estimated date of delivery). Report also: date of visit and, in a separate field, the date of the last menstrual period - LMP (Note: If reporting 0501F Prenatal flow sheet, it is not necessary to report 0500F Initial prenatal care visit)[1]

Ø=Modifier 51 Exempt   ⊙=Conscious Sedation   ✚=Add-on Code

● 0502F   Subsequent prenatal care visit

▶[Excludes: patients who are seen for a condition unrelated to pregnancy or prenatal care (eg, an upper respiratory infection; patients seen for consultation only, not for continuing care)]◀

● 0503F   Postpartum care visit[2]

▶Patient History◀

▶Patient history codes describe measures for select aspects of patient history or review of systems.◀

● 1000F   Tobacco use, smoking, assessed[1]

● 1001F   Tobacco use, non-smoking, assessed[1]

● 1002F   Anginal symptoms and level of activity, assessed[1]

▶Physical Examination◀

▶Physical examination codes describe aspects of physical examination or clinical assessment.◀

● 2000F   Blood pressure, measured[1]

▶Diagnostic/Screening Processes or Results◀

▶Diagnostic/screening processes or results codes describe results of tests ordered (clinical laboratory tests, radiological or other procedural examinations).◀

▶No codes at this time.◀

▶Therapeutic, Preventive or Other Interventions◀

▶Therapeutic, preventive or other interventions codes describe pharmacologic, procedural, or behavioral therapies, including preventive services such as patient education and counseling.◀

● 4000F   Tobacco use cessation intervention, counseling[1]

● 4001F   Tobacco use cessation intervention, pharmacologic therapy[1]

● 4002F   Statin therapy, prescribed[1]

- 4006F   Beta-blocker therapy, prescribed[1]

- 4009F   Angiotensin converting enzyme (ACE) inhibitor therapy, prescribed[1]

- 4011F   Oral antiplatelet therapy, prescribed (eg, aspirin, clopidogrel/Plavix, or combination of aspirin and dipyridamole/Aggrenox)[1]

▶Follow-up or Other Outcomes◀

▶Follow-up or other outcomes codes describe review and communication of test results to patients, patient satisfaction or experience with care, patient functional status, and patient morbidity and mortality.◀

▶No codes at this time.◀

▶Patient Safety◀

▶Patient safety codes that describe patient safety practices.◀

▶No codes at this time.◀

▶Footnotes◀

▶[1] Physician Consortium for Perfomance Improvement, www.ama-assn.org/go/quality◀

▶[2] National Committee on Quality Assurance (NCQA), Health Employer Data Information Set (HEDIS), www.ncqa.org◀

Rationale

A number of changes have been implemented for the continued development of the Category II Codes in the CPT coding book. In addition to four new codes, the Category II Codes section has received a make-over, utilizing a taxonomy to organize the codes included in this section into specific groups. It also includes a section that will list codes representing "groups" of performance measurement services that are commonly performed together (similar to the Organ or Disease Oriented Panels included in the Pathology and Laboratory section of the CPT book). Finally, Appendix H has been added to provide additional information regarding the performance measure itself, including a brief description of the performance measure and source (title, numerator, denominator, inclusion/exclusion criteria), the code number, a brief listing of the code descriptors, and website information for the origin of the source of the performance measure (to allow access to the organization that developed the measure as well as to obtain more detailed information regarding the measure).

The sectioning, or taxonomy, provided for Category II codes has been included to allow easier location of the appropriate Category II code(s) for the procedure being "measured". To create this new "sectioning", the eleven codes included in the Category II section have been deleted to allow relocation of ten of these codes into more appropriate sections (one of the codes, 0010F Anginal symptoms and level of activity, assessed using a standardized instrument (eg, Canadian Cardiovascular Society Classification-CCSC-System, Seattle Angina Questionnaire-SAQ) has been eliminated from CPT - see explanation that follows). To facilitate this relocation, parenthetic notes have been included after each deleted Category II code to guide the user to the new section and specific code for the previous listing. Similar to other listings in the CPT coding book, this cross-reference includes reference to the deleted code as well as the new code listing. In addition, a brief guideline has been included prior to each section to provide a brief description of the common identifying characteristics for the codes included in this section, including the anticipated addition of future codes. As is true for other codes included in the CPT book, the codes included in this section are listed as a "nomenclature" rather than a strict classification system. As a result of this, there may be some procedures that appear in sections other than in those where they ordinarily might be "classified". From a historical perspective, the CPT code set has always placed procedures in general sections according to where physicians will most conveniently find them.

The relocated codes, in addition to the new codes added for CPT 2005, have been arranged into the various sections of the Category II code set according to the following categories:

Composite Measures

Composite measures codes combine several measures grouped within a single code descriptor to facilitate reporting for a clinical condition when all components are met. If only some of the components are met, or if services are provided in addition to those included in the composite code, they may be reported individually using the corresponding CPT Category II codes for those services.

Presently, there are no composite measures codes.

Patient Management: 0500F-0503F

Patient management codes describe utilization measures or measures of patient care provided for specific clinical purposes (eg, prenatal care, pre- and post-surgical care).

Patient History: 1000F-1002F

Patient history codes describe measures for select aspects of patient history or review of systems.

Physical Examination: 2000F

Physical examination codes describe aspects of physical examination or clinical assessment.

Diagnostic/Screening Processes or Results

Diagnostic/screening processes or results codes describe results of tests ordered (clinical laboratory tests, radiological or other procedural examinations).

Presently, there are no diagnostic/screening processes or results codes.

Therapeutic, Preventive or Other Interventions: 4000F – 4011F

Therapeutic, preventive or other interventions codes describe pharmacologic, procedural, or behavioral therapies, including preventive services such as patient education and counseling.

Follow-up or Other Outcomes

Follow-up or other outcomes codes describe review and communication of test results to patients, patient satisfaction or experience with care, patient functional status, and patient morbidity and mortality.

Presently, there are no follow-up or other outcomes codes

Patient Safety

Patient safety codes describe patient safety practices.

Presently, there are no patient safety codes.

Four prenatal care codes have been added and 10 of the previous eleven Category II codes have been renumbered. Code 0010F has been deleted, as code 0009F will now be used to identify assessment of anginal symptoms and level of activity with or without use of a standardized instrument.

An additional appendix (Appendix H) has been added to the CPT coding book. This appendix has been added to promote understanding of the Category II code set and their associated measures. This new appendix provides information about the measures and their origins.

All Category II information, including the listing of Appendix H are included on the American Medical Association website at www.ama-assn.org/go/cpt. In addition, information regarding the source of the original measure as well as the website location of the measure organization is also included in a footnote subsequent to both the listing of the Category II codes and the Appendix H section.

Ⓢ =Modifier 51 Exempt   ⊙ =Conscious Sedation   ✚ =Add-on Code

Category III

A series of codes has been added for reporting percutaneous transcatheter placement of extracranial vertebral or intrathoracic carotid artery stents; ultrasound ablation of uterine leiomyomata; acoustic heart sound recording and computer analysis; computed tomographic colonography; and percutaneous intradiscal annuloplasty. Guidelines have been added to the Category III codes specifically to instruct appropriate reporting for Category III code 0074T for online evaluation and management service. Many Category III codes have been converted to Category I codes for 2005. In addition, 27 codes have been added, and one code revised for *CPT 2005*.

Category III Codes

▶(0001T has been deleted. To report, use 34803)◀

(0002T has been deleted. To report, use 34805)

✍ Rationale

With the addition of Category I code 34803 to report endovascular abdominal aortic aneurysm repair, Category III code 0001T has been deleted.

▶(0005T-0007T have been deleted. To report, see 0075T, 0076T)◀

✍ Rationale

With the addition of Category I codes 37215, 37216 for reporting percutaneous stent placement in the cervical portion of the extracranial carotid artery, Category III codes 0005T, 0006T and 0007T have been deleted and renumbered to Category III codes 0075T and 0076T to report transcatheter placement of extracranial vertebral or intrathoracic carotid artery stents.

▶(0009T has been deleted. To report, use 58356)◀

✍ Rationale

With the addition of Category I code 58356 to report endometrial cryoablation with ultrasonic guidance, including endometrial curettage, Category III code 0009T has been deleted.

▶(0012T has been deleted. To report, use 29866)◀

✍ Rationale

With the addition of Category I code 29866 to report arthroscopic osteochondral autograft harvest and implantation of femoral peripheral cartilage in the knee, Category III code 0012T has been deleted.

▶(0013T has been deleted. To report, see 29867, 27415)◀

✍ Rationale

With the addition of Category I code 29867 for arthroscopic repair of lesions of the femoral condyle with placement of osteochondral allograft arthroscopically and 27415 for open implantation of an osteochondral allograft in the knee for the treatment of moderate to large chondral or osteochondral knee defects, Category III code 0013T has been deleted.

▶(0014T has been deleted. To report, use 29868)◀

✍ Rationale

With the addition of Category I code 29868 to report arthroscopic meniscal knee transplantation in the medial or lateral compartments, Category III code 0014T has been deleted.

+▲ 0055T   Computer-assisted musculoskeletal surgical navigational orthopedic procedure, with image-guidance based on CT/MRI images (List separately in addition to code for primary procedure)

▶(When CT and MRI are both performed, report 0055T only once)◀

 Rationale

Category III code 0055T was revised to replace the word "and" with "/" (which means or) to clarify that 0055T describes utilization of only one type of imaging modality for navigating purposes during any single surgical procedure. Hence, either computed tomography (CT) imaging would be used to facilitate navigation or magnetic resonance imaging (MRI) or another type of image modality. Currently there is not a mechanism available to physicians to use two different imaging modalities.

A parenthetical note has been added to indicate that this procedure should be reported one time only, regardless of the type of images used.

▶(0057T has been deleted. To report, use 43257)◀

 Rationale

With the addition of Category I code 43257 to report the delivery of endoscopically guided radiofrequency thermal energy via electrodes to electrosurgically coagulate the muscle of the distal portion of the lower esophageal sphincter and/or gastric cardia for the treatment of gastroesophageal reflux disease, Category III code 0057T has been deleted.

● 0062T   Percutaneous intradiscal annuloplasty, any method, unilateral or bilateral including fluoroscopic guidance; single level

+● 0063T   one or more additional levels (List separately in addition to 0062T for primary procedure)

▶(For CT or MRI guidance and localization for needle placement and annuloplasty in conjunction with 0062T, 0063T, see 76360, 76393)◀

 Rationale

Category III codes 0062T and 0063T were added to describe percutaneous intradiscal destruction/neurolysis with stabilization of the annulus at single and multiple levels. "Fluoroscopic guidance" is included in the descriptor, as this is an integral component of the procedure and would not be separately reported. Code 0062T is intended to be reported for performance of percutaneous intradiscal annuloplasty at a single level. Add-on code 0063T is reported for percutaneous annuloplasty performed at any additional levels. As the descriptors for codes 0062T and 0063T include "unilateral or bilateral," it would not be appropriate to append modifiers 50 (bilateral) or 52 (reduced service).

The annuloplasty procedure entails the placement of either an electrothermal or a radiofrequency-powered catheter into the disc material, with placement verified by fluoroscopy (not separately reportable). Once positioned, resting against the posterior annular wall, electrothermal or radiofrequency energy is applied to the immediate area, causing a coagulation of disc material and decompression of the nerve root as well as ablation of pain receptors in the annulus fibrosis. A cross-reference was added to instruct that codes 76360 and 76393 would be separately reported in addition to codes 0062T and 0063T for computed tomography (CT) and magnetic resonance imaging (MRI) guidance for confirmation of needle placement.

 Clinical Example (0062T)

A 32-year-old female with low back pain referred into her right buttock, 9 months after a lifting injury at home. Conservative treatment has been unsuccessful. Physical examination reveals restricted spinal motion without signs of neurologic deficit. X-rays are negative. A magnetic resonance image (MRI) demonstrates a contained single level (L4-5) central disc protrusion with preservation of disc height without spinal nerve compression. A discogram confirms concordant pain provocation from that disc and the presence of annular disruption with adjacent discs being painless and morphologically normal. At operation a percutaneous annuloplasty is performed. Post operative hospital care and office visits are conducted as necessary throughout the 90-day global period.

Description of Procedure (0062T)

The medical record is reviewed to ensure that the patient is stable for the planned surgical procedure. The radiographic studies are reviewed. Imaging studies are correlated with the clinical exam and the surgical plan is confirmed. The surgeon confers with the patient and family re-explaining the current condition and the need for surgical intervention. Questions are answered, consent obtained and a note written in the record. He confers with the anesthesiologist and the operating room staff to review positioning, the intra-operative plan and equipment needs. After monitoring lines are placed, the patient is positioned on the operative table. Fluoroscopy (reported separately) is utilized to localize the correct level. The surgical site is prepped and draped into a sterile field. Intravenous antibiotics are administered under physician supervision.

The physician marks the skin at the point of intended entry and local anesthetic is injected. A spinal needle is placed adjacent to the L4-5 disc, depth is measured and local anesthetic is injected. Then, an introducer needle is placed into the disc and advanced obliquely into the anterolateral quadrant of the disc space. This position is confirmed by fluoroscopy. The annuloplasty catheter is checked for any defects and to ensure that it is in proper working condition. The catheter is then advanced through the introducer needle and navigated into the area of disc pathology. Final position is confirmed by fluoroscopy. The catheter is connected to the generator and the disc is treated. The patient is monitored during the procedure by the physician for pain response that may require adjusting treatment intensity or increasing the level of sedation. The patient is also monitored for any radicular symptoms that would indicate impending nerve injury and that would necessitate re-positioning of the catheter. If complete treatment of the disc can not be accomplished from a unilateral approach, the procedure is repeated from the contralateral side. At the completion of the procedure, antibiotic solution may be injected into the disc. The catheter and needle are then removed.

Dressings are applied. The patient is rolled onto a recovery bed and the neurologic status is checked. The patient is then transported to the recovery room and observed for approximately one hour. Post operative orders are written and a note is dictated. The family is met in the waiting room and questions answered. The referring physician is contacted and informed about the results of surgery. Arrangements are made for outpatient physiotherapy visits after discharge. The patient is re-examined for neurologic function and the dressing is inspected and changed as needed. Discharge planning and coordination occurs with the patient and family. A lumbar sacral orthosis is fitted prior to discharge.

After discharge, the patient returns to the office for follow-up visits. Questions regarding physiotherapy and activity levels are answered. Phone calls are answered concerning pain levels and activity restrictions. Subsequent follow-up office visits are scheduled to recommend progression of activity and monitor functional and work status. Prescription medication refills are reviewed and written. An exercise program is recommended and printed material regarding therapy is provided to the patient. Adjustments to the orthosis are made during the follow-up visits as necessary.

 Clinical Example (0063T)

A 38-year-old male with low back pain after a lifting injury at work. Conservative treatment for 7 months has been unsuccessful. Physical examination reveals restricted spinal motion without signs of neurologic deficit. X-rays are negative. A magnetic resonance image (MRI) demonstrates annular fissures in two lumbar discs (L4-L5, and L5/S1) without spinal nerve compression. A discogram confirms the presence of annular tears at L4/L5 and L5/S1 and reproduces concordant pain. The L3/L4 disc is painless and morphologically normal. At operation, a percutaneous annuloplasty is performed at both levels. Post operative hospital care and office visits are conducted as necessary throughout the 90-day global period.

Description of Procedure (0063T)

While the first level of annuloplasty (L5/S1-reported separately) is being treated, the physician marks the skin at the point of intended entry for the L4/L5 level and local anesthetic is injected. A spinal needle is placed adjacent to the disc, depth is measured and local anesthetic is injected. Then an introducer needle is placed into the disc and advanced obliquely into the anterolateral quadrant of the disc space. This position is confirmed by fluoroscopy. The annuloplasty catheter is checked for any defects and to ensure that it is in proper working condition. The catheter is then advanced through the introducer needle and navigated into the area of disc pathology. Final position is confirmed by fluoroscopy (reported separately). When treatment of the L5/S1 level is complete the catheter at L4/L5 is connected to the generator and the disc is treated. The patient is monitored during the procedure by the physician for pain response that may require adjusting treatment intensity or increasing the level of sedation. The patient is also monitored for any radicular symptoms that would indicate impending nerve injury and that would necessitate re-positioning of the catheter. If complete treatment of the disc can not be accomplished from a unilateral approach, the procedure is

⊘ =Modifier 51 Exempt ⊙ =Conscious Sedation ✦ =Add-on Code repeated from the contralateral side. At the completion of the procedure, antibiotic solution may be injected into the disc. The catheter and needle are then removed.

●**0064T**   Spectroscopy, expired gas analysis (eg, nitric oxide/carbon dioxide test)

Rationale

Code 0064T has been added to identify expired gas analysis via spectroscopy, a new procedure for analyzing minute levels (ie, parts-per-billion) of compounds in exhaled breath using laser spectroscopy. This procedure provides real-time, non-invasive and objective information for quantification of lower airway inflammation. The procedure directly assesses airway inflammation, the underlying cause of asthma. In addition, the test can be used in determining the response to and compliance with prescribed anti-inflammatory therapies.

Code 0064T identifies those procedures that are now clinically available for diagnosing asthma in children under the age of 8. It functions by measuring the amount of nitrous oxide (NO), an inflammatory marker that is exhaled. Studies have shown that exhaled nitric oxide levels in healthy patients are approximately 5-20 ppb. Patients suffering from lower airway inflammation (eg, untreated asthmatic patients) are characterized by nitric oxide levels above 20 ppb. Carbon dioxide concentrations are measured simultaneously with nitric oxide during an exhalation to normalize results and account for exhalation variations that may exist due to the differences between patients. Carbon dioxide breath trends also serve as a convenient measure to determine correct breath donations.

Measure of this marker can also be useful in monitoring asthma response to corticosteroid treatments.

Clinical Example (0064T)

The patient is a 5-year-old child with complaints from parents of periodic waking at night with trouble breathing along with other periods of persistent wheezing. The attending physician has reviewed the clinical history, performed a physical examination, and has ruled out other chronic obstructive diseases, foreign body obstructions, upper airway obstructions, sinobronchitus, immune disorders, cardiac disease and other acute diseases. The physician orders spectroscopy, expired gas analysis of the lower airways to determine if the patient is suffering from chronic airway inflammation, a co-condition for hyper-reactive airway disease.

Description of Procedure (0064T)

The examination is performed with laser spectroscopy equipment that can perform real-time detection of nitric oxide and carbon dioxide concentrations in an exhaled breath sample. The equipment has the necessary sensitivity to enable the respiratory therapist (RT) to distinguish between upper airway and lower airway breath samples and corresponding nitric oxide concentrations.

The RT briefs the patient on the breath testing procedure that consists of a slow 15 second exhalation into the instrument. The RT evaluates the first exhalation in to the instrument and determines if the patient is capable of delivering the

---

breath sample based on the comparison of the patient's results from a normal carbon dioxide concentration curve. The respiratory therapist (RT) starts the spectroscopy instrument and coaches the patient to repeat the test three times to obtain consistent readings of lower airway nitric oxide concentrations. The RT evaluates the three samples, reviews the results for statistical consistency, and prints the results for attending physician evaluation.

Results will help the physician identify underlying airway inflammation and monitor effects of anti-inflammatory treatments.

● **0065T** Ocular photoscreening, with interpretation and report, bilateral

▶(Do not report 0065T in conjunction with 99172 or 99173)◀

✍ Rationale

Category III code 0065T was added to describe ocular photoscreening, a new technology which makes it possible to detect a defect in a child's eye without the need of a response from the child during screening. This is a useful exam on children during their preverbal years. An exclusionary note was added following code 0065T instructing users not to report code 0065T in conjunction with codes 99172 and 99173.

🩺 Clinical Example (0065T)

An 18-month-old child is visiting with the pediatrician for a well-baby examination. Mother mentions that there is a strong family history of strabismus and amblyopia. Clinical examination with typical office instrumentation revealed no abnormality. In keeping with clinical practice guidelines, the pediatrician recommends the child be screened with a photoscreening device.

Description of Procedure (0065T)
The service includes physician performance or supervision of patient preparation and equipment set-up. The infant is positioned for the photoscreening device and an image is obtained. The image is transmitted or conveyed to an appropriate screening laboratory for interpretation to produce a reliable assessment of ocular abnormality vs abnormality. Conditions detected include esotropia, exotropia, anisometropia, cataracts, ptosis, hyperopia and myopia. The result is returned to the pediatrician for action.

● **0066T** Computed tomographic (CT) colonography (ie, virtual colonoscopy); screening

● **0067T**   diagnostic

▶(Do not report 0066T or 0067T in conjunction with 72192-72194, 74150-74170, 76375)◀

✍ Rationale

Codes 0066T and 0067T are used to identify colonography (also known as virtual colonoscopy), identifying screening (0066T) and diagnostic (0067T) services. Use of these codes will help to distinguish the use of computed tomography (CT) colonography procedures from noncolonography CT procedures performed for the abdomen and pelvis, as separate codes are used for the imaging (72192-72194, 74150-74170) and reconstruction and analysis (76375) of these procedures.

Computed tomography (CT) colonography is one of several procedures employed for the purpose of detecting colonic polyps and colon cancer. This procedure can be specifically useful for a subset of patients for whom colonoscopy was attempted but failed (failed colonoscopy), or for whom contraindications for colonoscopy exist, such as sedation risk. This procedure can also be useful for determining the extraluminal extent of a colon tumor. This code is therefore useful in linking this exam with appropriate clinical indications.

Parenthetical notes are included subsequent to the code listing to exclude use of these codes with CT imaging and/or analysis procedures performed for the pelvis or abdomen. A similar cross-reference is included with the appropriate related codes in the radiology section (72192-72194, 74150-74170, and 76375).

Clinical Example (0066T)

A 65-year-old male presents with a family history of colon cancer in which conventional colonoscopy was unable to reach the right colon. CT colonography is ordered.

Clinical Example 2 (0066T)

A 75-year-old female presents with heme-positive stools. She could not undergo conventional colonoscopy due to risk of sedation. CT colonography is ordered.

Clinical Example 3 (0066T)

A 55-year-old male presents on Coumadin for valve replacement needs screening colonoscopy, but clinicians do not want to stop anticoagulation. CT colonography is ordered.

Description of Procedure (0066T)

The procedure is described to the patient and informed consent is obtained where applicable. A review of any prior applicable studies is also performed.

Rectal tube is inserted (or supervision provided during insertion) and the colon is insufflated with either air or carbon dioxide. Next, a scout topogram of abdomen and pelvis is obtained/interpreted to ensure adequate colonic distention. Additional air is added if necessary. The non-contrast CT images of the abdomen and pelvis performed in the supine position are obtained/reviewed. The patient is then turned to the prone position. The axial images of both the supine and prone data sets are interpreted.. Three-dimensional reconstructions of the colon including endoluminal fly-throughs are supervised and/or created. An adjustment of the projection of the three-dimensional reconstructions is provided to optimize visualization of anatomy or pathology. The 3D endoluminal views are interpreted and compared to axial images. These are also compared to all pertinent available prior studies.

The final report is dictated, audited, and signed. The relevant images from three dimensional (3D) colonic flythrough are printed. Alternatively, a small video clip can be created for the patient record or referring clinician.

Clinical Example (0067T)

An 82-year-old male presents with cancer detected in the sigmoid colon on conventional colonoscopy. Due to the size of the lesion, the endoscopist could not pass the scope and therefore could not visualize the colon proximal to the mass. Computed tomography (CT) colonography is ordered.

Clinical Example 2 (0067T)

A 64-year-old male presents with severe diverticular disease. The endoscopist was unable to maneuver the scope past the sigmoid stricture. CT colonography is ordered.

Description of Procedure (0067T)

The procedure is described to the patient and informed consent is obtained where applicable. A review of any prior applicable studies is also performed.

Rectal tube is inserted (or supervision provided during insertion) and the colon is insufflated with either air or carbon dioxide. Next, a scout topogram of abdomen and pelvis is obtained/interpreted to ensure adequate colonic distention. Additional air is added if necessary. The non-contrast CT images of the abdomen and pelvis performed in the supine position are obtained/reviewed. The patient is then turned to the prone position. The axial images of both the supine and prone data sets are interpreted.. Three-dimensional reconstructions of the colon including endoluminal fly-throughs are supervised and/or created. An adjustment of the projection of the three-dimensional reconstructions is provided to optimize visualization of anatomy or pathology. The 3D endoluminal views are interpreted and compared to axial images. These are also compared to all pertinent available prior studies.

The final report is dictated, audited, and signed. The relevant images from three dimensional (3D) colonic fly-through are printed. Alternatively, a small video clip can be created for the patient record or referring clinician.

+●0068T Acoustic heart sound recording and computer analysis; with interpretation and report (List separately in addition to codes for electrocardiography)

▶(Use 0068T in conjunction with 93000)◀

+●0069T acoustic heart sound recording and computer analysis only (List separately in addition to codes for electrocardiography)

▶(Use 0069T in conjunction with 93005)◀

+●0070T interpretation and report only (List separately in addition to codes for electrocardiography)

▶(Use 0070T in conjunction with 93010)◀

Rationale

Three Category III add-on codes (0065T, 0069T, 0070T) were established to report acoustic heart sound (phonocardiographic) recording and computer analysis when performed in addition to the electrocardiogram services reported with codes 93000-93010 and are used for substantiation of the diagnosis of symptomatic patients with left ventricular hypertrophy, acute myocardial infarction and detection of S3, S4 heart sounds in the identification of cardiac conditions associated with left ventricular dysfunction. Acoustic heart sound recording is achieved through acoustic sensors. Parenthetical notes were added to each add-on code to instruct the users to report the add-on code in conjunction with the listed primary procedure.

 Clinical Example (0068T)

A previously asymptomatic 56-year-old Caucasian female with the major cardiac risk factor of a 40 pack-year smoking history presents to the emergency department complaining of shortness of breath that began approximately an hour before arrival. The skin of the patient is prepped and the combined electrocardiogram (ECG) and phonocardiographic electrodes are properly placed on the patient's chest as are the electrocardiographic electrodes. Correlated audioelectric cardiographic signals are then obtained and computer analysis performed. The results are then reviewed by the physician, interpreted, and a report generated.

Description of Procedure (0068T)

Service includes prepping the skin, applying the electrodes in their customary ECG positions, determining the proper positioning of the dual sensors in the V3 and V4 positions, reviewing the raw recording to verify proper placement and appropriateness of signals, acquisition of the signals, reviewing the computer analysis (sound and ECG), and generating a report.

●**0071T**   Focused ultrasound ablation of uterine leiomyomata, including MR guidance; total leiomyomata volume less than 200 cc of tissue

●**0072T**   total leiomyomata volume greater or equal to 200 cc of tissue

▶(Do not report 0071T, 0072T in conjunction with 51702 or 76394)◀

 Rationale

Codes 0071T and 0072T were established to describe new technology for magnetic resonance-guided focused ultrasound (MRgFUS) ablation. MRgFUS is the first non-invasive thermal ablation device that produces coagulative necrosis of soft tissue at a precise focal point within a soft tissue target in the body. It is also the only ablation system that is fully integrated with a magnetic resonance (MR) imaging system that provides continuous guidance and monitoring. It provides accurate volumetric therapy planning through the utilization of system specific therapy planning software, which computes the time and number of sonifications required for therapeutic efficacy. It has the ability to provide on-line thermometric imaging that provides "real time" feedback and treatment verification. MR images taken during the sonification provide a diagnostic image of the target tissue and a quantitative "real time" temperature map overlay to confirm the therapeutic effect of the ablation treatment. MRgFUS is a safe and effective noninvasive alternative to hysterectomy, myomectomy, and uterine fibroid embolization in the treatment of uterine fibroids.

Code 0071T should be reported when the total leiomyomata volume is less than 200 cc of tissue and code 0072T should be reported if it's greater or equal to 200 cc of tissue.

Total leiomyomata should be documented in the medical record when this procedure is performed.

A parenthetical note with exclusionary codes has been added and a corresponding cross-reference in the Radiology subsection has been added following code 76394 directing users to the new codes.

Description of Procedure (0071T)

The patient is evaluated by the treating physician for the procedure, and specifically for administration of intra-venous conscious sedation (IVCS). A repeat focused history and physical exam is performed to rule out any interval pertinent changes since the last office visit and as IVCS is still deemed appropriate by the physician, additional informed consent for the sedation is obtained.

At that time then a nurse inspects the skin surface, if necessary further pre-operative preparation is performed, and an IV and a Foley catheter in the urinary bladder are placed.

On completion of all the preparatory steps, the patient enters the magnetic resonance imaging (MRI) suite, is placed on the treatment table, and a 3-plane localizer scan is completed to confirm that the patient is positioned correctly on the table to allow a complete treatment. If necessary, the patient is re-positioned and a second series is run. Multi-planar T2W images are then obtained of the entire pelvis, spine and skin anteriorly.

The treating physician and team review all MR images, (the original ones and the new current ones). The skin contact is evaluated and then the target fibroid (s) is identified and the selected volume is outlined by the operating physician in the treatment software program. Computer analysis of the MR images is performed by the treating physician to calculate the safety of the treatment routes and dose delivery mechanism through the tumor(s) to be treated.

3D renderings are created within the computer by the treating physician, and dose simulations are reviewed.

The treatment plan and all beam path simulations in three dimensional (3D) are then reviewed by the operating physician prior to proceeding with therapy. The beam path (before and after the target) is evaluated carefully to ensure safe passage of the thermal therapy. If necessary adjustments can be made to the position of the patient, or the transducer in the table. The transducer is tilted or rolled as necessary to ensure optimal angulation of the beam. The spine and posterior pelvis are carefully evaluated as the beam should avoid the sacral nerve plexus.

Conscious sedation is administered and vital signs monitored by a nurse under the direct supervision of the operating physician throughout the procedure. The nurse remains in the room with the patient at all times. Prior to the first sonication the patient is instructed to communicate all sensations to the treating physician during or after each sonication. The patient is given an emergency shut off button to hold and she can terminate the procedure at any time. The nurse and treating physician can also do this. The patient remains awake and in regular communication with the treating physician through out the entire procedure.

⊘=Modifier 51 Exempt ⊙=Conscious Sedation ✚=Add-on Code

During treatment, continuous magnetic resonance (MR) imaging is performed as described above to acquire anatomic and quantitative thermal information to control the therapy and to incrementally determine if any treatment parameters need to be altered. If more than one site is to be treated (ie a complex case), the new fibroid is retargeted, as necessary, and all of the preceding imaging and analysis steps are repeated, as necessary.

When the treatment is complete, a final set of MR images with T1-weighting with intravenous (IV) gadolinium contrast is completed to evaluate the volume of non-perfused tissue vs. the pre-treatment images. These images are reviewed by the radiologist at the end of the procedure to immediately assess the completeness of treatment, assess for any potential damage, and to decide if a second treatment at a later date is warranted.

The vignettes for the simple and complex services are exactly the same, except that the more complex targets (as defined previously) require more treatment planning time and more treatment time as well. The risks and the decision-making contribution are also greater in the more complex cases.

●0073T Compensator-based beam modulation treatment delivery of inverse planned treatment using three or more high resolution (milled or cast) compensator convergent beam modulated fields, per treatment session

▶(For treatment planning, use 77301)◀

▶(Do not report 0073T in conjunction with 77401-77416, 77418)◀

Rationale
Category III code 0073T was established to report compensator-based beam modulation treatment delivery. Compensator beam modulation technique is clinically different than existing techniques used in radiotherapy. For delivery of this mode of radiotherapy, another form of beam modulation is used instead of multileaf collimation as described in code 77418. For consistency purposes, the descriptor in code 77418 was revised to omit the "eg" parenthetical.

A parenthetical note with the list of exclusionary codes has been added and a cross-reference directing users to report 77310 for treatment planning.

Clinical Example (0073T)
A 71-year-old male with T2a, Gleason 7, prostate specific antigen (PSA) 12 ng/ml, prostate cancer. Elected to undergo external beam radiation to the prostate with dose escalation to 80 Gy. The clinical target volume included the prostate and seminal vesicles and the planning target volume with a 8mm margin around the prostate and seminal vesicles. The prescribed dose was to the planning target volume. Dose constraints for the rectum, bladder and femoral heads were defined. A fluence map was generated for a 5-field compensator-based beam modulation technique to treat this patient meeting the required constraints. Once this was approved, the final plan was generated using a single compensator for each beam of varying thickness throughout its area to generate the required fluence map. The compensator was milled according to specifications. The treatment was delivered

to a film phantom using these compensators and images overlaid well with the dose distributions. The treatments were delivered as prescribed 2 Gy daily 5 days a week for a total dose of 80 Gy to the PTV.

▶ONLINE MEDICAL EVALUATION◀

▶An online medical evaluation is a type of Evaluation and Management (E/M) service provided by a physician or qualified health care professional to a patient using internet resources in response to the patient's online inquiry. Reportable services involve the physician's personal timely response to the patient's inquiry and must involve permanent storage (electronic or hard copy) of the encounter. This service should not be reported for patient contacts (eg, telephone calls) considered to be pre-service or post-service work for other E/M or non E/M services. A reportable service would encompass the sum of communication (eg, related telephone calls, prescription provision, laboratory orders) pertaining to the online patient encounter or problem(s).◀

●0074T   Online evaluation and management service, per encounter, provided by a physician, using the Internet or similar electronic communications network, in response to a patient's request, established patient

Rationale

Code 0074T has been established to identify online evaluation and management service, with introductory language to clarify the intent of this service. The guidelines indicate that code 0074T is not intended to be reported for each online inquiry (eg email), but is rather intended to encompass the total interchange of online inquiries and other communications associated with a single patient encounter. In addition, the guidelines clarify that code 0074T is not intended to be reported for patient services which are considered to be part of the pre- and post-service for other services.

Clinical Example 1 (0074T)

A 2-year old child has a history of ear infections. The child's mother would like to speak the pediatrician to discuss the ongoing problems associated with ear infection and learn the long-term potential effects of chronic ear infections (i.e. hearing loss, etc.) The mother has had difficulty reaching the pediatrician by telephone and wishes to get substantial and detailed information related to ear infections and potential sequelae for her child. The mother would prefer not to wait weeks for the next available office appointment. The pediatrician has previously discussed the available option of online medical consultations with the patient.

Description of Procedure (0074T Example 1)

The mother and patient request an online medical consultation with the pediatrician over a secure, encrypted and Health Insurance Portability and Accountability Act (HIPAA)/eRisk-compliant communications network via a standard Web browser. The mother is presented with explicit service terms and charges that are understood and agreed to, as well as reminders that online medical consultation should not be used for emergent and/or urgent conditions presented with explicit service terms and charges that are understood and agreed to, and provides a credit card for billing, prior to initiation of the online medical consultation. During the consultation, the mother describes the patient's symptoms and the pediatrician uses this information plus prior information gathered, referencing the patient chart, to provide information and a proposed follow-up plan for the mother. As a result of this online medical consultation, the mother has new information about how to proactively manage her child's ear infections without having to take time out of her very busy day to for an office visit.

 ### Clinical Example 2 (0074T)

A 59-year-old post-menopausal female with a family history of breast cancer and personal history of mild osteopenia and borderline high cholesterol who is re-considering the safety and value of hormone replacement therapy (HRT) in light of recent publicity on the subject. Patient has been on HRT for past 8 years secondary to initial severe menopausal symptoms and ongoing management of long-term chronic symptoms. Patient has been tolerating the HRT and has no other medical complaints. Patient would like her physician's recommendation on the appropriate action to take given her family history and current medical status. Patient attempted to make an appointment with her physician but was informed that she would have to wait weeks before the next appointment was available at this busy office. She would like her doctor's opinion as well as patient information related to this therapy, but does not wish to take time off from work or wait weeks for an appointment at this very busy OB/GYN physician's office.

Description of Procedures/Services (0074T Example 2)

The patient request an online medical consultation with her physician over a secure, encrypted and HIPAA/eRisk-compliant communications network via a standard Web browser. The patient is presented with explicit service terms and charges that are understood and agreed to, as well as reminders that online medical consultation should not be used for emergent and/or urgent conditions. The patient is presented with explicit service terms and charges that are understood and agreed to, and provides a credit card for billing, prior to initiation of the online medical consultation. During the consultation, the patient poses a series of questions and concerns to her physician. The physician addresses these questions and issues referencing the patient chart, past medical problems, current meds, etc, to provide information and a proposed follow-up plan for the patient. The patient receives the information and recommendations online from her physicians including a list of hypertext links to articles produced by the American College of Obstetrics and Gynecology and the American Medical Association related to the subject of hormone replacement therapy. Physician provides an interpretation of recent publicity on HRT and opinion/recommendation on whether patient should continue HRT given family history and current medical issues. Physician reminds patient she is due for her annual mammogram screening and physical examination in 4 months. As a result of this online medical consultation, the patient has received more timely and complete care than would likely have occurred during a routine office visit including more complete access to valuable reference materials.

●**0075T** Transcatheter placement of extracranial vertebral or intrathoracic carotid artery stent(s), including radiologic supervision and interpretation, percutaneous; initial vessel

+●0076T   each additional vessel (List separately in addition to code for primary procedure)

▶(Use 0076T in conjunction with 0075T)◀

▶(When the ipsilateral extracranial vertebral or intrathoracic carotid arteriogram (including imaging and selective catheterization) confirms the need for stenting, then 0075T and 0076T include all ipsilateral extracranial vertebral or intrathoracic selective carotid catheterization, all diagnostic imaging for ipsilateral extracranial vertebral or intrathoracic carotid artery stenting, and all related radiologic supervision and interpretation. If stenting is not indicated, then the appropriate codes for selective catheterization and imaging should be reported in lieu of code 0075T or 0076T.)◀

Rationale

With the addition of Category I codes 37215, 37216 for reporting percutaneous stent placement in the cervical portion of the extracranial carotid artery, Category III codes 0005T, 0006T and 0007T have been deleted and renumbered to Category III codes 0075T and 0076T to report transcatheter placement of extracranial vertebral or intrathoracic carotid artery stents. An instructional parenthetical statement has been added to indicate that codes 0075T and 0076T include all diagnostic imaging for ipsilateral extracranial vertebral or intrathoracic carotid artery stenting, and all related radiological supervision and interpretation.

●0077T   Implanting and securing cerebral thermal perfusion probe, including twist drill or burr hole, to measure absolute cerebral tissue perfusion

▶(0078T-0081T should be reported in accordance with the Endovascular Abdominal Aneurysm Repair guidelines established for 34800-34826)◀

Rationale

Code 0077T was added to report surgical implantation of a cerebral thermal perfusion probe to measure cerebral tissue perfusion. It is used for patients with conditions including: subarachnoid hemorrhage (SAH); intracerebral hemorrhage; traumatic brain injury; malignant (hemispheric) stroke; and cerebral arteriovenous malformation (AVM). The procedure is performed for inpatients in the hospital setting.

The device used for the procedure consists of a monitor and a probe. The probe is surgically implanted and secured in the brain through either a twist drill hole or a burr hole. The monitor quantifies cerebral tissue perfusion in absolute units and in real-time at the patient's bedside. This procedure uses completely different equipment and resources than the laser Doppler scan, which is a different method of measuring cerebral perfusion.

In addition to the coding reference, a parenthetic note has been included subsequent to the listing of code 61107 to specify the use of this code when a twist drill or burr hole procedure is performed to place a thermal perfusion probe.

Clinical Example (0077T)

A 20-year-old female, who is cardiopulmonary stable, presents with a Glasgow Coma Score (GCS) of 8 or less following a nontraumatic subarachnoid hemorrhage. She is controlled to maintain an arterial oxygen concentration greater than 100mmHg and an arterial CO_2 of 35-40mmHg. Patients with meningitis, ventriculitis or other infection of the central nervous system are typically excluded from this type of monitoring.

Description of Procedure (0077T)

The scalp is shaved at the appropriate location. The area of insertion is disinfected and draped. Once the insertion site is determined, a small incision (0.5 cm) is made through the scalp to the cranium. A twist burr hole is made with a perpendicular trajectory through the skull and through the outer and inner tables of the skull until the dura is reached but not penetrated. Cotton tipped applicators are used to remove bone debris in the twist burr hole. The dura is perforated with a needle. The appropriate securing device is affixed and the thermal perfusion probe is inserted into the puncture hole in the dura, 20 to 25 mm below the level of the dura into the cerebral tissue. The probe is secured and the scalp incision is sutured.

The "start" button on the monitor is pressed and after four minutes the perfusion measurement begins. If the K value is greater than a defined threshold (indicating that the probe is close to a thermally significant vessel) the probe is moved back by about 1 mm and the "calibrate" button is pushed to recalibrate the probe. The probe is recalibrated until an acceptable K value is obtained.

●0078T   Endovascular repair of abdominal aortic aneurysm, pseudoaneurysm or dissection, abdominal aorta involving visceral vessels (superior mesenteric, celiac or renal), using fenestrated modular bifurcated prosthesis (two docking limbs)

     ▶(Do not report 0078T in conjunction with 34800-34805, 35081, 35102, 35452, 35454, 35472, 37205-37208)◀

     ▶(Report 0078T in conjunction with 35454, 37205-37208 when these procedures are performed outside the target zone of the endoprosthesis)◀

+●0079T   Placement of visceral extension prosthesis for endovascular repair of abdominal aortic aneurysm involving visceral vessels, each visceral branch (List separately in addition to code for primary procedure)

     ▶(Use 0079T in conjunction with 0078T)◀

     ▶(Do not report 0079T in conjunction with 34800-34805, 35081, 35102, 35452, 35454, 35472, 37205-37208)◀

     ▶(Report 0079T in conjunction with 35454, 37205-37208 when these procedures are performed outside the target zone of the endoprosthesis)◀

●0080T   Endovascular repair of abdominal aortic aneurysm, pseudoaneurysm or dissection, abdominal aorta involving visceral vessels (superior mesenteric, celiac or renal), using fenestrated modular bifurcated prosthesis (two docking limbs), radiological supervision and interpretation

     ▶(Do not report 0080T in conjunction with 34800-34805, 35081, 35102, 35452, 35454, 35472, 37205-37208)◀

     ▶(Report 0080T in conjunction with 35454, 37205-37208 when these procedures are performed outside the target zone of the endoprosthesis)◀

+●0081T Placement of visceral extension prosthesis for endovascular repair of abdominal aortic aneurysm involving visceral vessels, each visceral branch, radiological supervision and interpretation (List separately in addition to code for primary procedure)

▶(Use 0081T in conjunction with 0080T)◀

▶(Do not report 0081T in conjunction with 34800-34805, 35081, 35102, 35452, 35454, 35472, 37205-37208)◀

▶(Report 0081T in conjunction with 35454, 37205-37208 when these procedures are performed outside the target zone of the endoprosthesis)◀

✍ Rationale

Codes 0078T-0081T have been established with corresponding parenthetical notes for reporting placement of a fenestrated aortic endograft for treatment of abdominal aortic aneurysms (AAA) involving the visceral arteries. In addition, corresponding cross-references were added in the appropriate Category I sections referencing the new Category III codes.

Codes 0078T and 0079T are intended to report endovascular prosthesis insertion repair of aortic aneurysms with little or no normal infrarenal aortic neck and therefore unsuitable for infrarenal endovascular AAA repair due to compromised proximal aortic neck anatomy. Prior to this, endovascular infrarenal aortic aneurysm repair using the available devices required a 10-15 mm segment of relatively straight, minimally diseased, normal diameter aortic neck aorta below the renal artery origins. Fenestrated aortic endograft for treatment of abdominal aortic aneurysms (AAA) involving the visceral arteries is accomplished by deploying the proximal end of the stent-graft across the renal artery origins, and variably across the superior mesenteric and celiac origins. Pre-placed fenestrations in the aortic graft allow blood flow into these visceral arteries. Extension stent-grafts are then placed through the main body and into the visceral arteries as needed to achieve hemostatic seal. As is evident from this procedure description, the described components are a more complex module endograft system with fenestrations in the main endograft body to allow perfusion of the visceral arteries. In addition, extension endovascular prostheses are placed from inside the main endograft body into the visceral arteries. By analogy to open surgery, these procedures represent the endovascular version of open AAA repair involving visceral vessels (35091) compared to infrarenal repair (35081 or 35102).

Code 0078T is intended to be reported for deployment of the main fenestrated aortic device. Code 0079T is intended to be reported as a separate add-on code for deployment of each visceral extension prosthesis. Typically, the number of visceral extensions may vary from one to four, depending on the morphology of the aneurysm.

Codes 0080T and 0081T are intended to report radiological supervision and interpretation services for endovascular repair of abdominal aortic aneurysms involving visceral vessels. Code 0080T is reported for imaging services for placement of the main fenestrated aortic device. Code 0081T is reported one time for imaging services for each visceral branch extension.

Ⓢ=Modifier 51 Exempt   ⊙=Conscious Sedation   ✚=Add-on Code

A parenthetical instruction has been inserted at the beginning of these procedures to refer the user to the Endovascular Abdominal Aneurysm Repair guidelines to indicate that the Category I guidelines are applicable to the Category III set of procedure codes.

The exclusionary cross-references following codes 0078T and 0079T contain a listing of the procedure codes which would not be performed in the same patient during same encounter. Additional cross-references following codes 0078T and 0079T list endovascular abdominal aneurysm repair procedures which would be separately reportable if required and performed outside the target zone of the endoprosthesis. Examples of these procedures include treatment of dissections with external iliac stent deployments well below the endograft target zones, for 37205 and 37207; and for 37206, 37208 rarely performed bilateral external iliac stent deployment code.

The exclusionary cross-references following the imaging codes 0080T and 0081T indicate that these procedures are only reported in addition to the fenestrated aortic endograft procedures involving the visceral arteries.

Clinical Example (0078T)

A 67-year-old male who presents with coronary artery disease status post myocardial infarction (MI) and chronic obstructive pulmonary disease (COPD) was found to have a 6.8-cm diameter abdominal aortic aneurysm (AAA). Imaging studies (computed tomography [CT] scan, magnetic resonance imaging [MRI], and/or angiography) indicate that the aneurysm has a configuration unsuitable for infrarenal repair but amenable to a fenestrated aortic endograft with covered extension stents to both renals and the superior mesenteric artery. Distally the aneurysm extends to the very end of the aorta, indicating that a bifurcated prosthesis will be required.

Note: 0078T does not include open femoral or iliac artery exposure, arterial catheterization, placement of the fenestrated graft limbs to visceral vessels, or radiological supervision and interpretation. These services are reported separately. See CPT Instructions for Endovascular Repair of Abdominal Aortic Aneurysm (AAA).

Description of Procedure (0078T)

Work begins after the decision to operate is made, from the day before the operation until the skin incision. This activity includes obtaining and reviewing the previous work-up, with special attention to potential cardiovascular risks. In addition, an extensive and detailed review of the preoperative imaging studies (CT, CT angiogram, CT with three dimensional [3D] reconstructions, MRI, and/or contrast angiogram) is required to determine the exact measurements of the aneurysm. This is necessary because an accurate preoperative choice of component diameters and lengths is one of the primary determinants of whether the endovascular procedure will be successful.

Initial work for aneurysm repair involving the visceral arteries also includes determining the exact location of the visceral artery orifices so appropriate fenestrations can be placed in the main component of the endograft. There can be no error in loading the graft into the delivery system, because the graft fenestrations must align exactly with the visceral artery orifices when deployed.

Informed consent is obtained from the patient following a discussion of surgical risks and benefits with the patient and the family. Other pre-service work includes scrubbing, donning lead apparel, patient positioning, waiting for the anesthetic to become effective, prepping and draping the patient.

NOTE: Reporting the deployment of 0078T will follow the coding guidelines in the CPT introductory notes for Endovascular Repair of Abdominal Aortic Aneurysm. In addition, deployment of the visceral extension prostheses will be reported using 0079T. The intraservice work of 0078T includes performing road-mapping arteriogram with specific attention to renal artery origins, final examination of endovascular components for correct models, sizing, etc., exchange of soft J-wires for superstiff wires, and reconfirming that the appropriate device has been chosen. The main-body component is then unpackaged and the device is prepared for insertion. The patient is anticoagulated with intravenous (IV) heparin. The main-body component is then loaded onto the ipsilateral superstiff wire and advance to the femoral artery. The tip of main device is introduced into arteriotomy site, the proximal vascular clamp is opened and the from of the device is advanced into artery. Rubber constrictors are used to limit blood loss. Under fluoroscopic guidance, the main-body device is directed through external iliac and advanced into the common iliac artery and subsequently, into aorta. The device is pushed through the aneurysm carefully such that the tip lies above visceral artery origins and the circular orientation aligns fenestrations with visceral artery origins. Arteriography is repeated as needed to absolutely confirm orientation, and deployment is begun. Final precise adjustments are made to align top of device at desired visceral level with fenestrations lying exactly over visceral artery origins. The main body device is deployed with constant attention to exact positioning, making final position adjustments as needed, keeping the proximal anastomosis and fenestrations as required, and checking distally to determine that the position above the aortic bifurcation is correct. Next, the main body device is deployed to the point of opening the contralateral docking port. The contralateral docking port is cannulated using a selective catheter/guidewire combination, and the catheter advanced into the main body of the graft to the level of the proximal anastomosis. Inject contrast and image graft is provided to confirm placement of the catheter within the graft. A final angiogram is performed to confirm positioning of the proximal anastomosis, and any final adjustments to position of the proximal anastomosis are made at this time. The suprarenal fixation portion of the main body component is deployed. At this point in the procedure, 1-4 visceral artery extensions are deployed through the previously placed aortic graft fenestrations. This work is reported separately as 0079T for each vessel.

Sterile dressings are applied, and the physician ensures that the patient is stable and able to leave the suite. Help is provided to transfer the patient to a post procedure recovery unit.

Depending on the preexisting comorbidities and operative course, it is determined if the patient requires admission to the intensive care unit. The physician writes

⃠=Modifier 51 Exempt   ⊙=Conscious Sedation   ✚=Add-on Code orders, dictates the operative note, and communicates with the patient's family, referring, and consulting physicians. Assistance is provided for the anesthesiologist to ensure smooth emergence from anesthesia. After this, the physician discusses the procedure results with patient once he/she is fully awake and determines when the patient is adequately recovered for transfer to floor. Daily visits are provided during postoperative care, and orders and notes are written, etc.

Discharge day management includes communicating with all support services such as visiting nurse, meals on wheels, etc., communication with the referring physician, provision of activity advice, warnings to the patient and family, and arranging office follow ups for wound checks, suture/staple removal, etc. All related office visits for 90-days are included in the post-service work of 0078T

 Clinical Example (0079T)
Note: See Clinical Example for 0078T.

Description of Procedure (0079T)
Ensure all required guidewires and extension prostheses are available for use.

The appropriate combination of guidewire and guiding sheath are advanced through appropriate fenestration in aortic endograft, and into visceral artery. Angiogram is then performed through guiding sheath to ensure proper fenestration alignment. A visceral extension is then advanced through guiding sheath, through fenestration and into visceral artery. Exact positioning of extension is then checked to ensure proximal end in aortic graft and distal in visceral artery. The visceral extension is deployed, and angioplasty of all components is provided as needed for complete expansion and seating. Note: angioplasty within target zone is included in 0079T. An arteriogram is then performed to confirm patency and evaluate for endoleak. The stents are deployed, if needed, within body of extension prosthesis to seal endoleaks or treat kinks. Note: stent placement in body of graft is included in 0079T.

 Clinical Example (0080T)
Note: See Clinical Example for 0078T.

Description of Procedure (0080T)
A review of MR, CT, CT with 3D reconstructions, and arteriograms for final assurance of suitability for endovascular AAA repair using fenestrated visceral level device is performed. The physician then checks the suite to ensure proper function and configuration of the imaging equipment including compliance with all radiation safety issues. The physician also ensures that all technical personnel have been familiarized with the endovascular prosthesis and are fully familiar with all required wires, balloons, stents. In addition, the physician supervises selection of all equipment, including catheters, wires, balloons, stents, sheaths, contrast material, etc., and assures all needed equipment is available. Radiation protection is then applied (also ensures all others are adequately protected). The patient is then positioned (by provider or via supervision of staff)

Technical personnel are directed throughout procedure, and an interpretation of imaging of vessel being treated is provided. Accurate radiological views, exposures, shielding, image size, injection sequences, radiation protection and management are ensured for the patient and staff. Real-time analysis of all imaging during procedure is provided, including pre-treatment imaging, fluoroscopic and angiographic imaging throughout the procedure as required to perform the procedure, as well as post-procedure fluoroscopic and angiographic imaging. This includes all imaging to manipulate the wires, catheters, devices, into position, correct positioning and deployment of endoprosthesis, post-deployment ballooning, assessing post-op success and complications, complete study post-deployment, and removal of catheters. Continuous fluoroscopic imaging is also provided during all catheter/device/balloon/stent manipulations to assess proper position/performance/deployment of primary aortic endograft and iliac limbs

A review and interpretation of all image sequences for the main device positioning and deployment is provided. All radiologic images are post-processed and converted to an archived form for permanent record. A review and record of the patient fluoroscopic exposure time & contrast volume is documented. In addition, the procedure note is dictated, including interpretation of diagnostic and therapeutic imaging. The final report is then reviewed, revised, and sign final. A formal report is then sent to the primary care physician (PCP) and referring providers.

● **0082T**   Stereotactic body radiation therapy, treatment delivery, one or more treatment areas, per day

▶(Do not report 0082T in conjunction with 77401-77416, 77418)◀

● **0083T**   Stereotactic body radiation therapy, treatment management, per day

▶(Do not report 0083T in conjunction with 77427-77432)◀

 Rationale

Two new Category III codes were created to describe stereotactic body radiation therapy (SBRT) for the treatment of localized tumors or lesions anywhere in the body. Code 0082T is reported for SBRT treatment delivery and 0083T is reported for SBRT treatment management.

Two parenthetical notes were also added following these codes to indicate that they are not to be reported in conjunction with the standard radiation treatment and management codes found in the Radiation Oncology subsection of the CPT book. Code 0082T should not be reported in addition to treatment delivery codes 77401-77416, or 77418, and code 0083T should not be reported in conjunction with treatment management codes 77427-77432. Also, two parenthetical cross references were added in the Radiation Oncology subsection to direct users to the new Category III codes for reporting SBRT delivery and management.

Previously, the codes in the CPT book described stereotactic procedures for the brain only. SBRT expands the application to tumors throughout the body (beyond intracranial lesions) and necessitates completely different care processes. Also, the treatment management codes described services for patients undergoing conventional fractionated radiation delivery. SBRT treatment management requires additional and different work by the physician to evaluate and manage patients undergoing SBRT.

SBRT delivers potent target doses of radiation via numerous carefully directed fields, each with relatively low intensity in order to precisely identify targets and corresponding delivery of treatment to deep seated tumors. The radiation, which enters from a variety of angles, minimizes entrance exposure thereby avoiding harm to the healthy tissue around the target.

SBRT may be used as an alternative to conventional open surgery for treating various lesions and may be an alternative treatment to conventional radiation therapy for certain presentations of cancers, or other non-cancer targets.

 Clinical Example (0082T)

A 60-year-old female with long history of tobacco use is found to have a 3.5 cm peripheral nodule on chest x-ray. A computed tomography (CT)-guided biopsy shows non-small cell cancer. Staging including CT of mediastinum and upper abdomen and positron emission tomography shows only localized disease (stage T1b, N0, M0). Pre-operative evaluation indicated FEV1 < 40% predicted (medically inoperable). Treatment options include limited pulmonary resection with risk of being a pulmonary cripple, conventional fractionated radiation which will expose considerable lung volume to ionizing radiation, or stereotactic body radiation therapy. The choice of stereotactic body radiation therapy is made based on treatment to just the defined lesion while decreasing radiation exposure to normal lung.

Description of Procedure (0082T)

The patient will be treated with 2000 cGy per fraction for 6 fractions. Treatment is planned using either a frame based stereotactic system or imaging-based stereotactic unit to facilitate the precise identification of the target(s) (the tumor or area of interest) and may include comparison with or analysis of CT scans/magnetic resonance imaging/positron emission tomography scans (or other imaging and/or functional studies) with or without image fusion.

The final plan (using work currently described by CPT codes 77301 and 77295) will achieve stereotaxic treatment to the target (planned treatment volume (PTV)) and is usually associated with numerous beams that are arranged to deliver a high focal dose to the tumor target.

Under the direct supervision of the physician, the patient is set up on the treatment table and the positioning/immobilization devices are placed. All treatment parameters are verified by the physician. Appropriate accounting for patient movement, respiratory motion or other types of motion is verified. With the physician in attendance, this is followed by the delivery of the radiation dose for that fraction (which may last for an hour or more). The entire treatment process is repeated for each of the 6 fractions. Following each treatment, a patient assessment is performed by the physician.

 Clinical Example (0083T)

A 60-year-old female with long history of tobacco use is found to have a 3.5cm peripheral nodule on chest x-ray. CT-guided biopsy shows non-small cell cancer. Staging, including CT of mediastinum and upper abdomen and positron emission tomography, shows only localized disease (stage T1b, N0, M0). Pre-operative evaluation indicated FEV1 < 40% predicted (medically inoperable). Treatment options include limited pulmonary resection with risk of being a pulmonary cripple, conventional fractionated radiation which will expose considerable lung volume to ionizing radiation, or stereotactic body radiation therapy. The choice of stereotactic body radiation therapy is made based on treatment to just the defined lesion while decreasing radiation exposure to normal lung.

Description of Procedure (0083T)

The patient will be treated with 2000 cGy per fraction for 6 fractions. Treatment is planned using either a frame based stereotactic system or imaging-based stereotactic unit to facilitate the precise identification of the target(s) (the tumor or area of interest) and may include comparison with, or analysis of, computed tomography scans/magnetic resonance imaging/positron emission tomography scans (or other imaging and/or functional studies) with or without image fusion.

The final plan (using work currently described by CPT codes 77301 and 77295) will achieve stereotaxic treatment to the target planned treatment volume (PTV) and is usually associated with numerous beams that are arranged to deliver a high focal dose to the tumor target.

Under the direct supervision of the physician, the patient is set up on the treatment table and the positioning/immobilization devices are placed. All treatment parameters are verified by the physician. Appropriate accounting for patient movement, respiratory motion or other types of motion is verified. With the physician in attendance, this is followed by the delivery of the radiation dose for that fraction (which may last for an hour or more). The entire treatment process is repeated for each of the 6 fractions. Following each treatment, a patient assessment is performed by the physician.

●**0084T** Insertion of a temporary prostatic urethral stent

Rationale

Code 0084T is used to identify temporary prostatic urethral stent inserted in the prostatic urethra. This procedure is performed when permanent insertion of urethral stent is not clinically indicated, such as placement to manage voiding dysfunction during the healing phase of a condition being treated. Unlike a permanent endoprosthesis, which may be placed in more than one portion of the urethra, the temporary prostatic urethral stent is only inserted in the prostatic urethra.

Clinical Example (0084T)

Following transurethral microwave thermotherapy (TUMT) a 70-year-old male presents to his urologist for an evaluation of continuing lower urinary tract symptoms caused by benign prostatic hyperplasia (BPH). It is determined the patient is a candidates for a minimally invasive prostatic therapy. Following the minimally invasive therapy the patient presents with temporary worsening symptoms (e.g. decreased voided volume, increase in post void residual urine, urinary retention). A temporary prostatic urethral stent is placed to manage voiding dysfunction during the healing phase.

⊘=Modifier 51 Exempt   ⊙=Conscious Sedation   ✚=Add-on Code

Description of Procedure (0084T)

The patient is prepped and draped for a typical sterile urethral device insertion procedure.

To achieve the best results with the spanner, the appropriate length device must be selected to accommodate the patient's anatomical requirements. The length of the urethra from the bladder neck to the distal side of the external sphincter is measured using the surveyor urethral measurement device. Using the length measurement from the surveyor, the appropriate size spanner is selected.

The spanner and insertion tool are prepared for insertion, and inserted into the urethra until the distal tip and balloon are positioned in the bladder. The balloon is then inflated, the urethral stent is positioned in the prostatic urethra by applying gentle traction and then deployed. The insertion tool is slowly withdrawn from the urethra. The spanner's retrieval suture may be trimmed such that the distal end is just inside the urethra's meatus.

After inserting the spanner, the patient should be assessed to assure that the patient is able to void adequately prior to discharge from the clinic. This may be accomplished by uroflometry and a bladder ultrasound

●**0085T**   Breath test for heart transplant rejection

 Rationale

Code 0085T intended to identify non-invasive breath test for the detection of heart transplant rejection. The procedure is used as an aid in the diagnosis of grade 3 heart transplant rejection in first year heart transplant recipients. The Heartsbreath is intended to be used an adjunct to and not as a substitute for endomyocardial biopsy. The use of the device is limited to patients who are less than or equal to one year post-transplant.

This test most frequently is performed in the office or other outpatient, independent laboratory, hospital inpatient and outpatient and home settings. It involves the collection of volatile organic compounds in breath and air onto sorbent traps. These samples are then analyzed for breath markers of oxidative stress.

 Clinical Example (0085T)

A 44-year-old white male received a heart transplant two weeks ago, for the management of intractable congestive cardiac failure. The operation is successful, and he is followed intensively as an outpatient during the first postoperative year by a transplant cardiologist who performs serial endomyocardial biopsies. However, the transplant cardiologist is concerned about the limitations of endomyocardial biopsy—it is an expensive, invasive procedure, and its dependability is limited by subjectivity. There is poor interobserver reproducibility amongst the pathologists who read the slides and score the severity of rejection. The transplant cardiologist requests that the patient should have a breath test for heart transplant rejection performed every two weeks during the first postoperative year, as an objective marker of grade 3 rejection. During the course of the year, the transplant cardiologist employs the results of the breath test as an adjunct to endomyocardial biopsy, in order to determine whether or not the patient requires a change in immunosuppressant therapy.

Description of Procedure (0085T)

The patient breathes into a breath collection apparatus for 2.0 min, and the volatile organic compounds (VOCs) in 1.0 l alveolar breath are captured on to a sorbent trap. No expiratory effort is required beyond normal respiration. A second sample of 1.0 l ambient room air is similarly collected on to a second sorbent trap. There are no known risks to this procedure. The collection is supervised by a technician.

The sorbent traps are sent to the laboratory for analysis by automated thermal desorption with gas chromatography and mass spectroscopy (ATD/GC/MS).

Data are downloaded into a computerized data base. A subtraction chromatogram is constructed, comprising the abundance of VOCs in breath minus the abundance of VOCs in room air. The breath methylated alkane contour (BMAC) is constructed, a three-dimensional display of markers of oxidative stress. It comprises a three dimensional graph of the abundance of C4 to C20 alkanes and monomethylated alkanes in the subtraction chromatogram. The BMAC is interpreted by an algorithm derived from a clinical study, which generates the probability of grade 3 heart transplant rejection as a value between zero and one. Based on these findings, a report is sent to the requesting physician stating the probability of grade 3 heart transplant rejection, and the interpretation of the test (positive, negative, or intermediate for rejection). The positive or negative predictive value of the test is also provided, if the probability of grade 3 heart transplant rejection is greater than or less than 0.5 respectively.

●0086T   Left ventricular filling pressure indirect measurement by computerized calibration of the arterial waveform response to Valsalva maneuver

Rationale

Category III code 0086T has been established to describe measurement of left ventricular end-diastolic pressure (LVEDP) that can recognize the normal filling pressure range and deviations of filling pressure which exceed the normal range and therefore support the diagnosis of volume overload which could be associated with heart failure and can be useful in estimating the severity of such conditions. The LVEDP measurements are obtained by the analysis of the changes in the contour of the arterial waveform response to the Valsalva maneuver. In monitoring situations, as with the monitoring of patients with heart failure, significant declines in LVEDP may suggest excessive diuresis especially in the presence of a fall in blood pressure and other clinical manifestations. In addition, regular monitoring to maintain the LVEDP of the heart failure (HF) patient within a certain range can reduce hospitalizations.

Clinical Example (0086T)

A patient arrives in the emergency department with shortness of breath (SOB). The patient is known to have chronic lung disease and heart disease. The question is whether the SOB is secondary to lung disease, heart failure or a combination of the two. Within 15 minutes and with no risk to the patient, VeriCor can provide an accurate measurement of LVEDP which, if normal, virtually excludes heart failure as a cause. If this is significantly elevated, it would contribute to the diagnosis of heart failure. Furthermore, the severity of heart failure can be assessed and this can help to determine whether or not hospitalization is necessary.

Description of Procedure (0086T)

A digital expiratory manometer, a continuous arterial pressure monitor, and a medical grade computer, are integrated and controlled by state-of-the-art software and provide a series of prompts on a video screen. A tonometric sensor is attached to the patient's wrist with a blood pressure cuff attached to the arm. After an 8-minute tonometric calibration period is completed, the system is ready for use. For the test, the patient is prompted to perform a Valsalva maneuver by blowing into the mouthpiece of the digital manometer to produce an expiratory pressure of 20 to 30 mmHg for a minimum of eight seconds. The expiratory pressure and the arterial blood pressure measurements are recorded, stored and analyzed.

The patient is asked to perform a series of three Valsalva maneuvers over a period of 15 minutes. Total testing time is approximately 25 minutes. The LVEDP measurements are obtained via the analysis of the changes in the contour of the arterial waveform response to the Valsalva maneuver that have been calibrated by simultaneous left ventricular catheterization.

●0087T   Sperm evaluation, Hyaluronan binding assay

 Rationale

Category III code 0087T is intended to report a hyaluronan binding assay (HBA), which is a qualitative assay for the evaluation of sperm maturity. In addition, a cross reference has been added following code 89325 directing users to Category III code 0087T for sperm evaluation.

 Clinical Example (0087T)

A 34-year-old male and his partner were referred to the in vitro fertilization (IVF) laboratory after two years of unprotected sexual activity and no pregnancies. Fresh semen would be collected and the hyaluronic binding assay (HBA) would be run in addition to standard sperm count, motility, morphology and other measures to diagnose male infertility. The results from this assay in combination with those obtained from other diagnostic tests would assist the physician in determining the best course of treatment for the couple.

Description of Procedure (0087T)

The assay requires fresh liquefied semen less than three hours old. Semen should be obtained by masturbation, preferably following 203 days of abstinence. It should be collected in a sterile collection container and kept at room temperature (18-28° C) for 30 minutes to allow it to liquefy.

Gently mix the sample and pipette a drop, 7-10µL in volume, near to the center of chamber A or B. Place the Cell-Vu gridded cover slip over the sample.

Incubate the slide for at least 10 and not more than 20 minutes at room temperature. Count the total number of motile sperm, both bound and unbound. In the same number of grid squares count the number of bound motile sperm.

Calculate the percent hyaluronan-binding sperm using the equation below:

$$\%bound = 100x \frac{Boundmotile}{Boundmotile+unboundmotile}$$

A score of >80% indicates normal binding capacity: A score <80% and >60% indicates possible problems with binding capacity and a score <60% indicates poor binding capacity.

It is suggested that patients with poor binding capacity bypass intrauterine insemination and tradition IVF procedures and proceed directly to ICSI.

●**0088T**   Submucosal radiofrequency tissue volume reduction of tongue base, one or more sites, per session (ie, for treatment of obstructive sleep apnea syndrome)

Rationale

Category III code 0088T was added to describe submucosal radio-frequency tissue volume reduction of the tongue base. Radio-frequency tissue volume reduction is commonly performed for the treatment of obstructive sleep apnea syndrome by widening the oropharyngeal airway. Radio-frequency may be applied to multiple sites of the tongue during the same session; however, code 0088T should be reported only one time for the same session, regardless of the number of sites treated.

Clinical Example (0088T)

A 57-year-old, hypertensive male with a BMI of 35 kg/m^2 is diagnosed with severe obstructive sleep apnea by polysomnography. He exhibits an apnea-hypopnea index (AHI) of 52/hour and concomitant severe oxygen desaturation. He has failed both continuous positive airway pressure (CPAP) and bi-level positive airway pressure (BiPAP) due to non-compliance. Prior nasal surgery and uvulopalatopharyngoplasty also failed to produce subjective or objective improvement of his sleep apnea. Examination shows macroglossia and fiberoptic laryngoscopy demonstrates retrolingual airway narrowing and collapse.

Description of Procedure (0088T)

After topical oral and pharyngeal anesthesia, the surgeon has the patient rinse his mouth with antibacterial rinse. The mouth is secured open with bite blocks, the tongue is protruded and held in position and immobilized. The tongue midline and circumvallate papillae are marked with a skin marker to maintain orientation. Planned probe insertion sites are similarly marked. Planned treatment sites are injected with anesthetics. For each treatment site, the physician injects saline, inserts the probe, verifies proper position away from the neurovascular bundle, and radio frequency (RF) energy is delivered to the submucosal tissues. The surgeon actively monitors the treatment sites as energy is delivered to assure complete

⊘=Modifier 51 Exempt   ⊙=Conscious Sedation   ✚=Add-on Code

submucosal application and no mucosal overlap of applied energy. This procedure is performed on each subsequent target site until all planned sites have been treated for this session. The patient is observed for signs of bleeding or swelling that might lead to airway obstruction. The patient, once stable, is discharged on oral antibiotics, pain medication, and instructions for care. The patient is seen in about a week in the office and the surgical site inspected.

Appendixes F, G, H, and I

The most significant revisions to *CPT 2005* are in the Appendix section. Four new appendixes have been added to the CPT code set. The new appendixes list the codes exempt from use of the modifier 63; codes exempt from separately reporting the conscious sedation codes; full descriptions of the measures applicable to the Category II codes; and the new genetic testing modifiers for reporting with the molecular genetics testing and cytogenetic studies codes.

Appendix F

The listing is a summary of CPT codes that are exempt from the use of modifier 63. The codes listed below are additionally identified in the CPT code set with the parenthetical instruction "(Do not report modifier 63 in conjunction with …)"

30545	33694	36420	46715	49606
31520	33730	36450	46716	49610
33401	33732	36460	46730	49611
33403	33735	36510	46735	53025
33450	33736	36660	46740	54000
33472	33750	39503	46742	54150
33502	33755	43313	46744	54160
33503	33762	43314	47700	63700
33505	33778	43520	47701	63702
33506	33786	43831	49215	63704
33610	33918	44055	49491	63706
33611	33919	44126	49492	65820
33619	33922	44127	49495	
33647	33960	44128	49496	
33670	33961	46070	49600	
33690	36415	46705	49605	

Appendix G

The following list of procedures for *CPT 2005* includes conscious sedation as an inherent part of providing the procedure. The codes listed below are identified in CPT 2005 with a symbol. Conscious sedation is defined as moderate sedation/analgesia and is a drug-induced depression of consciousness during which patients respond knowingly and intentionally to verbal commands, either alone or accompanied by light tactile stimulation. No interventions are required to maintain a patent airway, spontaneous ventilation is adequate, and cardiovascular function is usually maintained. Conscious or moderate sedation is not the less intense minimal sedation ("anxiolysis") or the more intense deep sedation/analgesia.

Since these services include conscious sedation, it is not appropriate for the same physician to report both the service and one of the conscious sedation codes (99141 or 99142). It is expected that if conscious sedation is provided to the patient as part of one of these services, it is provided by the same physician who is providing the service. The provision of conscious sedation by the operating physician includes the oversight of personnel who are monitoring the patient.

The inclusion of a procedure on this list does not prevent separate reporting of an associated anesthesia procedure/service (CPT codes 00100-01999) when performed by a physician other than the operating physician or a qualified professional under the responsible supervision of a physician other than the operating physician. In such cases the person providing anesthesia services shall be present for the purpose of continuously monitoring the patient and shall not act as a surgical assistant. When clinical conditions of the patient require such anesthesia services, or in the circumstances when the patient does not require sedation, the operating physician is not required to report the procedure as a reduced service using modifier 52.

19298	33222	36583	43245	44369
20982	33223	36585	43246	44370
31615	33233	36590	43247	44372
31622	33234	36870	43248	44373
31623	33235	37203	43249	44376
31624	33240	37215	43250	44377
31625	33241	37216	43251	44378
31628	33244	43200	43255	44379
31629	33249	43201	43256	44380
31635	35470	43202	43258	44382
31645	35471	43204	43259	44383
31646	35472	43205	43260	44385
31656	35473	43215	43261	44386
31725	35474	43216	43262	44388
32019	35475	43217	43263	44389
32020	35476	43219	43264	44390
32201	36555	43220	43265	44391
33010	36557	43226	43267	44392
33011	36558	43227	43268	44393
33206	36560	43228	43269	44394
33207	36561	43231	43271	44397
33208	36563	43232	43272	44500
33210	36565	43234	43453	44901
33211	36566	43235	43456	45303
33212	36568	43236	43458	45305
33213	36570	43239	44360	45307
33214	36571	43240	44361	45308
33216	36576	43241	44363	45309
33217	36578	43242	44364	45315
33218	36581	43243	44365	45317
33220	36582	43244	44366	45320

45327	45386	92974	93505	93561
45332	45387	92975	93508	93562
45333	45391	92978	93510	93571
45334	45392	92979	93511	93572
45337	47011	92980	93514	93609
45338	48511	92981	93524	93613
45339	49021	92982	93526	93615
45340	49041	92984	93527	93616
45341	49061	92986	93528	93618
45342	50021	92987	93529	93619
45345	58823	92995	93530	93620
45355	66720	92996	93539	93621
45378	77600	93312	93540	93622
45379	77605	93313	93541	93624
45380	77610	93314	93542	93640
45381	77615	93315	93543	93641
45382	92953	93316	93544	93642
45383	92960	93317	93545	93650
45384	92961	93318	93555	93651
45385	92973	93501	93556	93652

Appendix H

Note: Prior to coding, the user must review the complete description of the code in the Category II section of the CPT coding book and the complete description of its associated measure by accessing the measure developer's Web site provided in the footnoted reference.

Brief Description of Performance Measure & Source: Title, Numerator, Denominator, Inclusion/Exclusion Criteria	CPT Code(s)	Brief Code Descriptor
Coronary Artery Disease (CAD)		
Blood Pressure Measurement[1] – Percentage of patients who had a blood pressure measurement during the last office visit **Numerator:** Patients who had a blood pressure measurement during the last office visit **Denominator:** All patients with CAD **Inclusion/Exclusion:** None	2000F	Blood pressure measured
Smoking Cessation Evaluation[1] –Percentage of patients evaluated for smoking or other tobacco use **Numerator:** Patients evaluated for smoking or other tobacco use **Denominator:** All patients with CAD **Inclusion/Exclusion:** None	1000F 1001F	Tobacco use, smoking, assessed Tobacco use, non-smoking, assessed
Smoking Cessation Intervention[1] – Percentage of patients identified as cigarette smokers who received smoking cessation intervention **Numerator:** Patients identified as smokers or other tobacco users who were offered an intervention for tobacco use cessation, either counseling or pharmacologic therapy during one or more office visits **Denominator:** All patients identified as smokers or other tobacco users **Inclusion/Exclusion:** None	4000F 4001F	Tobacco use cessation counseling Tobacco use cessation intervention, pharmacologic therapy

Brief Description of Performance Measure & Source: Title, Numerator, Denominator, Inclusion/Exclusion Criteria	CPT Code(s)	Brief Code Descriptor
Drug Therapy for Lowering Cholesterol[1] – Percentage of patients who were prescribed a statin (based on current ACC/AHA guidelines) **Numerator:** Patients who were prescribed a statin **Denominator:** All patients with CAD **Inclusion:** None **Exclusion:** Documentation that a statin was not indicated; documentation of medical or patient reason(s) for not prescribing a statin	4002F	Statin therapy prescribed
Beta-blocker Therapy- Prior Myocardial Infarction (MI)[1] – Percentage of CAD patients who also have prior MI who were prescribed beta-blocker therapy **Numerator:** Patients with CAD who had a prior MI who were prescribed beta-blocker therapy **Denominator:** All patients with CAD **Inclusion:** Only patients with prior MI <if ok by consortium, otherwise consider this as the denominator and use "none"> **Exclusion:** Documentation that a beta-blocker was not indicated; documentation of medical or patient reason(s) for not prescribing a beta-blocker	4006F	Beta-blocker therapy prescribed
Angiotensin Converting Enzyme (ACE) Inhibitor Therapy[1] – Percentage of CAD patients who also have diabetes and/or left ventricular systolic dysfunction (LVSD) who were prescribed ACE inhibitor therapy **Numerator:** Patients who were prescribed ACE inhibitor therapy **Denominator:** All patients with CAD who also have diabetes and/or LVSD **Inclusion:** Patients with CAD who also have diabetes and/or LVSD, left ventricular ejection fracture (LVEF) < 40% or moderately or severely depressed left ventricular systolic function) **Exclusion:** Documentation that ACE inhibitor was not indicated (eg, patients on angiotensin receptor blockers; documentation of medical or patient reason(s) for not prescribing ACE inhibitor	4009F	Angiotensin Converting Enzyme (ACE) Inhibitor therapy, prescribed

Brief Description of Performance Measure & Source: Title, Numerator, Denominator, Inclusion/Exclusion Criteria	CPT Code(s)	Brief Code Descriptor
Symptom & Activity Assessment[1] – Percentage of CAD patients who were evaluated for both level of activity and anginal symptoms during one or more office visits **Numerator:** Patients who were evaluated for both level of activity and anginal symptoms during one or more office visits **Denominator:** All patients with CAD **Inclusion/Exclusion:** None	1002F	Anginal symptoms and level of activity assessed
Antiplatelet Therapy[1] – Percentage of patients who were prescribed antiplatelet therapy **Numerator:** Patients who were prescribed antiplatelet therapy **Denominator:** All patients with CAD **Inclusion:** None **Exclusion:** Documentation that antiplatelet therapy was not indicated; documentation of medical or patient reason(s) for not prescribing a beta-blocker	4011F	Oral antiplatelet therapy prescribed

Prenatal-Postpartum Care

Timeliness of Prenatal Care[2] **Numerator:** Number of women in the denominator who received a prenatal care visit as a member of the managed care organization (MCO) in the first trimester or within 42 days of enrollment in the MCO **Denominator:** Women who had live births between November 6th of the year prior to the measurement year and November 5th of the measurement year, who were continuously enrolled at least 43 days prior to delivery through 56 days after delivery **Inclusion/Exclusion Criteria:** None	0500F	Initial prenatal care visit (report at first prenatal encounter with health care professional providing obstetrical care. Report also: date of visit and, in a separate field, the date of the last menstrual period – LMP. Note: MCO will determine membership and enrollment criteria. Consider all women receiving prenatal care to be eligible.)

Brief Description of Performance Measure & Source: Title, Numerator, Denominator, Inclusion/Exclusion Criteria	CPT Code(s)	Brief Code Descriptor
Prenatal Flow Sheet[1] **Numerator:** Number of patients in the denominator with a flow sheet in use by the date of the first physician visit, which contains at a minimum: blood pressure, weight, urine protein, uterine size, fetal heart tones, and estimated date of delivery **Denominator:** Pregnant women seen for prenatal care **Inclusion Criteria: None** **Exclusion Criteria:** Patients seen for consultation only, not for continuing care	0501F	Prenatal flow sheet documented (report also: date of visit and, in a separate field, the date of the last menstrual period – LMP. (Note: If reporting 0501F Prenatal flow sheet, it is not necessary to report 0500F Initial prenatal care visit) [*Excludes:* patients who are seen for a condition unrelated to pregnancy or prenatal care – eg an upper respiratory infection; patients seen for consultation only, not for continuing care]
Frequency of Ongoing Prenatal Care[2] **Numerator:** Number of women in the denominator who had an unduplicated count of less than 21%, 21%-40%, 41%-60%, 61%-80%, or greater than or equal to 81% of the expected number of prenatal care visits, adjusted for the month of pregnancy at the time of enrollment and gestational age **Denominator:** Women who had live births during the measurement year **Inclusion/Exclusion Criteria:** MCOs must exclude members for whom a prenatal visit is not indicated	0502F	Subsequent prenatal care visit Note: MCO will determine eligibility. Consider all women receiving prenatal care to be eligible.
Postpartum Care[2] - Percentage of women who received a postpartum care visit on or between 21 and 56 days after delivery. **Numerator:** Number of women in the denominator who had a postpartum visit on or between 21 days and 56 days after delivery **Denominator:** Women who had live births between November 6th of the year prior to the measurement year and November 5th of the measurement year, who were continuously enrolled at least 43 days prior to delivery through 56 days after delivery **Inclusion/Exclusion: None**	0503F	Postpartum care visit Note: MCO will determine eligibility. Consider all women receiving postpartum care to be eligible.

[1] Physician Consortium for Performance Improvement, www.ama-assn.org/go/quality

[2] National Committee on Quality Assurance (NCQA), Health Employer Data Information Set (HEDIS®), www.ncqa.org

Appendix I

Genetic Testing Code Modifiers

This listing of modifiers is intended for reporting with molecular laboratory procedures related to genetic testing. Genetic test modifiers should be used in conjunction with CPT and HCPCS codes to provide diagnostic granularity of service to enable providers to submit complete and precise genetic testing information without altering test descriptors. These modifiers are categorized by mutation. The first (numeric) digit indicates the disease category and the second (alpha) digit denotes gene type. Introductory guidelines in the molecular diagnostic and molecular cytogenetic code sections of CPT provide further guidance in interpretation and application of genetic test modifiers.

Neoplasia (solid tumor)

0A	BRCA1 (Hereditary Breast/Ovarian Cancer)
0B	BRCA2 (Hereditary Breast Cancer)
0C	Neurofibromin (Neurofibromatosis, type 1)
0D	Merlin (Neurofibromatosis, type 2)
0E	c-RET (Multiple endocrine neoplasia, types 2A/B, Familial medullary thyroid carcinoma)
0F	VHL (Von Hippel Lindau Disease)
0G	SDHD (Hereditary paraganglioma)
0H	SDHB (Hereditary paraganglioma)
0I	Her-2/neu
0J	MLH1 (HNPCC)
0K	MSH2 (HNPCC)
0L	APC (Hereditary polyposis coli)
0M	Rb (Retinoblastoma)
1Z	Solid Tumor, not otherwise specified

Neoplasia (lymphoid/hematopoetic)

2A	AML1 - also ETO (Acute myeloid leukemia)
2B	BCR - also ABL (Chronic myeloid, acute lymphoid leukemia)
2C	CGF 1
2D	CBFbeta (Leukemia)

2E	MML (leukemia)
2F	PML/RARalpha (Promyelocytic Leukemia)
2G	TEL (leukemia)
2H	bcl-2 (lymphoma)
2I	bcl-1 (lymphoma)
2J	c-myc (lymphoma)
2K	IgH (lymphoma/leukemia)
2Z	Lymphoid/hematopoetic neoplasia, not otherwise specified

Non-neoplastic hematology/coagulation

3A	Factor V (Leiden, Others) (Hypercoagulable state)
3B	FACC (Fanconi Anemia)
3C	FACD (Fanconi Anemia)
3D	Beta globin (Thalassemia)
3E	Alpha globin (Thalassemia)
3F	MTHFR (Elevated homocysteine)
3G	Prothrombin (factor II, 20210A) (Hypercoagulable state)
3H	Factor VIII (Hemophilia A/VWF)
3I	Factor IX (Hemophilia B)
3J	Beta globin
3Z	Non-neoplastic hematology/coagulation, not otherwise specified

Histocompatability/blood typing

4A	HLA-A
4B	HLA-B
4C	HLA-C
4D	HLA-D
4E	HLA-DR
4F	HLA-DQ
4G	HLA-DP
4H	Kell
4Z	Histocompatability/blood typing, not otherwise specified

Neurologic, non-neoplastic

5A	Aspartoacylase A (Canavan disease)
5B	FMR-1 (Fragile X, FRAXA, syndrome)
5C	Frataxin (Freidreich's ataxia)
5D	Huntingtin (Huntington's Disease)
5E	GABRA (Prader Willi-Angelman syndrome)
5F	Connexin-26 (GJB2) (Hereditary Deafness)
5G	Connexin-32 (X-linked Charcot-Marie-Tooth Disease)
5H	SNRPN (Prader Willi-Angelman syndrome)
5I	Ataxin-1 (Spinocerebellar Ataxia type 1)
5J	Ataxin-2 (Spinocerebellar Ataxia type 2)
5K	Ataxin-3 (Spinocerebellar Ataxia type 3, Machado-Joseph Disease)
5L	CACNA1A (Spinocerebellar Ataxia type 6)
5M	Ataxin-7 (Spinocerebellar Ataxia type 7)
5N	PMP-22 (Charcot-Marie-Tooth Disease, type 1A)
5O	MECP2 (Rett syndrome)
5Z	Neurologic, non-neoplastic, not otherwise specified

Muscular, non-neoplastic

6A	Dystrophin (Duchenne/Becker Muscular dystrophy)
6B	DMPK (Myotonic Dystrophy, type 1)
6C	ZNF-9 (Myotonic Dystrophy, type 2)
6D	SMN (Autosomal recessive spinal muscular atrophy)
6Z	Muscular, not otherwise specified

Metabolic, other

7A	Apolipoprotein E (Cardiovascular disease, Alzheimer's disease)
7B	Sphingomyelin phosphodiesterase (Nieman-Pick Disease)
7C	Acid Beta Glucosidase (Gaucher Disease)
7D	HFE (Hemochromatosis)
7E	Hexosaminidase A (Tay-Sachs Disease)
7Z	Metabolic, other, not otherwise specified

Metabolic, transport

8A	CFTR (Cystic fibrosis)
8Z	Metabolic, transport, not otherwise specified

Metabolic-pharmacogenetics

9A	TPMT (thiopurine methyltransferase) (patients on antimetabolite therapy)
9L	Metabolic-pharmacogenetics, not otherwise specified

Dysmorphology

9M	FGFR1 (Pfeiffer and Kallman syndromes)
9N	FGFR2 (Crouzon, Jackson-Weiss, Apert, Saethre-Chotzen syndromes)
9O	FGFR3 (Achondroplasia, Hypochondroplasia, Thanatophoric dysplasia, types I and II, Crouzon syndrome with acanthosis nigricans, Muencke syndromes)
9P	TWIST (Saethre-Chotzen syndrome)
9Q	CATCH-22 (22q11 deletion syndromes)
9Z	Dysmorphology, not otherwise specified

The Tabular Review
of the Changes

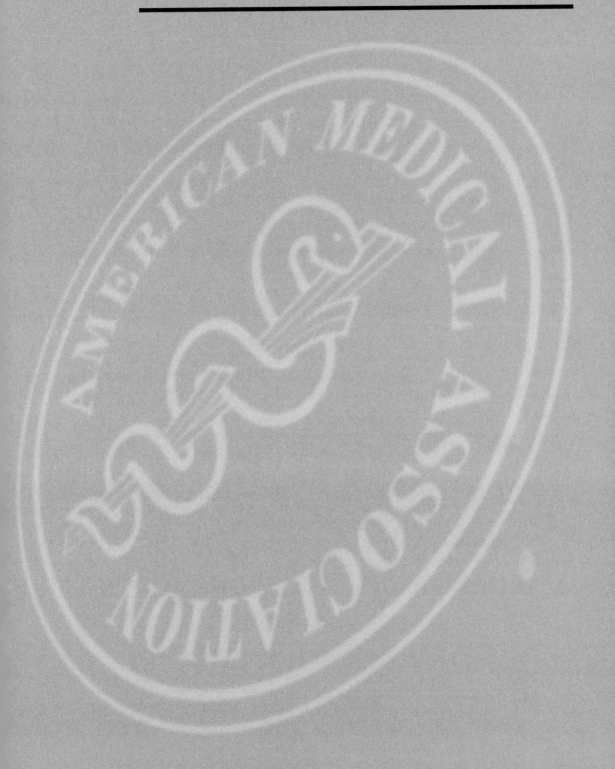

The Tabular Review of the Changes

KEY: **Adds** = Added
Del = Deleted
Rev = Revised
Gr = Grammar revision
Cross = Cross-reference

Section/Code	Adds	Del	Rev	Gr	Cross

Anesthesia

Intrathoracic

Section/Code	Adds	Del	Rev	Gr	Cross
00561	X				X

Surgery

Integumentary System

Skin, Subcutaneous and Accessory Structures

Excision-Debridement

Section/Code	Adds	Del	Rev	Gr	Cross
11000					X
11004	X				
11005	X				
11006	X				
11008	X				X
11044					X

Breast

Excision

Section/Code	Adds	Del	Rev	Gr	Cross
19160			X		
19162					X

Introduction

Section/Code	Adds	Del	Rev	Gr	Cross
19296	X				
19297	X				X
19298	X				

Section/Code	Adds	Del	Rev	Gr	Cross

Musculoskeletal System

Femur (Thigh Region) and Knee Joint

Repair, Revision, and/or Reconstruction

27412	X				X
27415	X				X

Endoscopy/Arthroscopy

29866	X				X
29867	X				X
29868	X				X
29870					X
29871					X
29883					X

Respiratory System

Larynx

Endoscopy

31545	X				
31546	X				X

Trachea and Bronchi

Endoscopy

31620	X				X
31630			X		
31631			X		X
31636	X				
31637	X				X
31638	X				

Lungs and Pleura

Incision

32019	X				X

Section/Code	Adds	Del	Rev	Gr	Cross
Lung Transplantation					
32850			X		
32855	X				
32856	X				X

Cardiovascular System

Heart and Pericardium

Section/Code	Adds	Del	Rev	Gr	Cross
Heart/Lung Transplantation					
33930			X		
33933	X				
33940			X		
33944	X				X

Arteries and Veins

Section/Code	Adds	Del	Rev	Gr	Cross
Endovascular Repair of Abdominal Aortic Aneurysm					
34803	X				X
34808					X
Direct Repair of Aneurysm or Excision (Partial or Total) and Graft Insertion for Aneurysm, Pseudoaneurysm, Ruptured Aneurysm, and Associated Occlusive Disease					
35161		X			
35162		X			X
Bypass Graft					
Vein					
35572					X
In-Situ Vein					
35582		X			X
35583					X
Venous					
36475	X				
36476	X				X
36478	X				
36479	X				X

Section/Code	Adds	Del	Rev	Gr	Cross

Hemodialysis Access, Intervascular Cannulation for Extracorporeal Circulation, or Shunt Insertion

Section/Code	Adds	Del	Rev	Gr	Cross
36818	X				X
36819					X

Transcatheter Procedures

Section/Code	Adds	Del	Rev	Gr	Cross
37205			X		X
37206					X
37215	X				
37216	X				X

Hemic and Lymphatic Systems

General

Bone Marrow or Stem Cell Services/Procedures

Section/Code	Adds	Del	Rev	Gr	Cross
38215					X

Digestive System

Esophagus

Endoscopy

Section/Code	Adds	Del	Rev	Gr	Cross
43257	X				

Stomach

Laparoscopy

Section/Code	Adds	Del	Rev	Gr	Cross
43644	X				X
43645	X				X

Other Procedures

Section/Code	Adds	Del	Rev	Gr	Cross
43845	X				X
43846			X		X

Intestines (Except Rectum)

Excision

Section/Code	Adds	Del	Rev	Gr	Cross
44132			X		
44133					X
44137	X				
44138					X

Section/Code	Adds	Del	Rev	Gr	Cross
Other Procedures					
44715	X				
44720	X				
44721	X				
Rectum					
Endoscopy					
45391	X				X
45392	X				X
Anus					
Excision					
46262					X
Introduction					
46500					X
Destruction					
46936					X
Suture					
46947	X				X
Liver					
Liver Transplantation					
47133			X		
47140			X		
47143	X				
47144	X				
47145	X				
47146	X				
47147	X				X
Pancreas					
Pancreas Transplantation					
48550			X		
48551	X				

Section/Code	Adds	Del	Rev	Gr	Cross
48552	X				X

Urinary System

Kidney

Renal Transplantation

Section/Code	Adds	Del	Rev	Gr	Cross
50300			X		
50320			X		
50323	X				X
50325	X				
50327	X				
50328	X				
50329	X				
50360			X		
50380					X

Introduction

50391	X				

Laparoscopy

50547			X		X

Endoscopy

50559		X			X
50578		X			X

Ureter

Endoscopy

50959		X			X
50978		X			X

Bladder

Transurethral Surgery

Urethra and Bladder

52234			X		

Ureter and Pelvis

52347		X			X

Section/Code	Adds	Del	Rev	Gr	Cross
Vesical Neck and Prostate					
52402	X				
Male Genital System					
Penis					
Incision					
54000					X
Testis					
Excision					
54500					X
Prostate					
Excision					
55859					X
Female Genital System					
Vagina					
Repair					
57267	X				X
57282			X		
57283	X				
Corpus Uteri					
Excision					
58263					X
Introduction					
58356	X				X
Laparoscopy/Hysteroscopy					
58565	X				X
Ovary					
Excision					
58956	X				X

Section/Code	Adds	Del	Rev	Gr	Cross

Endocrine System

Parathyroid, Thymus, Adrenal Glands, Pancreas, and Carotid Body

Excision

Section/Code	Adds	Del	Rev	Gr	Cross
60545					X

Nervous System

Skull, Meninges, and Brain

Twist Drill, Burr Hole(s), or Trephine

Section/Code	Adds	Del	Rev	Gr	Cross
61107					X

Neurostimulators (Intracranial)

Section/Code	Adds	Del	Rev	Gr	Cross
61885			X		
61888					X

Spine and Spinal Cord

Posterior Extradural Laminotomy or Laminectomy for Exploration/ Decompression of Neural Elements or Excision of Herniated Intervertebral Disks

Section/Code	Adds	Del	Rev	Gr	Cross
63050	X				
63051	X				X

Excision by Laminectomy of Lesion Other Than Herniated Disk

Section/Code	Adds	Del	Rev	Gr	Cross
63295	X				X

Neurostimulators (Spinal)

Section/Code	Adds	Del	Rev	Gr	Cross
63685			X		X

Extracranial Nerves, Peripheral Nerves, and Autonomic Nervous System

Neurostimulators (Peripheral Nerve)

Section/Code	Adds	Del	Rev	Gr	Cross
64590			X		X

Eye and Ocular Adnexa

Anterior Segment

Iris, Ciliary Body

Destruction

Section/Code	Adds	Del	Rev	Gr	Cross
66710			X		
66711	X				X

Section/Code	Adds	Del	Rev	Gr	Cross

Radiology

Diagnostic Radiology (Diagnostic Imaging)

Spine and Pelvis

Section/Code	Adds	Del	Rev	Gr	Cross
72194					X

Abdomen

74170					X

Vascular Procedures

Transcatheter Procedures

75952					X
75960			X		X

Other Procedures

76075			X		
76077	X				X
76375					X
76394					X

Diagnostic Ultrasound

76506					X

Head and Neck

76510	X				
76511			X		
76512			X		

Pelvis

Obstetrical

76820	X				
76821	X				
76827			X		

Radiation Oncology

Radiation Treatment Delivery

77401					X
77418			X		X

Section/Code	Adds	Del	Rev	Gr	Cross
Radiation Treatment Management					
77432					X
Clinical Brachytherapy					
77750			X		X

Nuclear Medicine

Diagnostic

Gastrointestinal System

78267			X		

Cardiovascular System

78464			X		
78465			X		

Other Procedures

78810		X			X
78811	X				
78812	X				
78813	X				
78814	X				
78815	X				
78816	X				X
78990		X			X

Therapeutic

79000		X			
79001		X			X
79005	X				
79020		X			
79030		X			
79035		X			X
79100		X			X
79101	X				X
79200			X		

Section/Code	Adds	Del	Rev	Gr	Cross
79300			X		
79400		X			X
79403					X
79420		X			X
79440			X		
79445	X				X
79900		X			X
79999			X		

Pathology and Laboratory

Chemistry

Section/Code	Adds	Del	Rev	Gr	Cross
82045	X				
82656	X				
83009	X				X
83013			X		
83014			X		X
83630	X				
84163	X				
84165			X		
84166	X				

Hematology and Coagulation

Section/Code	Adds	Del	Rev	Gr	Cross
85046			X		

Immunology

Section/Code	Adds	Del	Rev	Gr	Cross
86064	X				X
86334			X		
86335	X				
86353					X
86379	X				X
86587	X				X

Microbiology

Section/Code	Adds	Del	Rev	Gr	Cross
87046			X		

Section/Code	Adds	Del	Rev	Gr	Cross
87335					X
87807	X				

Cytopathology

Section/Code	Adds	Del	Rev	Gr	Cross
88180		X			X
88184	X				
88185	X				X
88187	X				
88188	X				
88189	X				

Surgical Pathology

Section/Code	Adds	Del	Rev	Gr	Cross
88342					X
88360	X				
88361			X		X
88365			X		X
88367	X				
88368	X				

Reproductive Medicine Procedures

Section/Code	Adds	Del	Rev	Gr	Cross
89321					X
89346			X		

Medicine

Immunization Administration for Vaccines/Toxoids

Section/Code	Adds	Del	Rev	Gr	Cross
90465	X				X
90466	X				X
90467	X				X
90468	X				X
90471			X		
90472					X
90474					X

Vaccines, Toxoids

Section/Code	Adds	Del	Rev	Gr	Cross
90656	X				

Section/Code	Adds	Del	Rev	Gr	Cross
90700			X		

Therapeutic, Prophylactic or Diagnostic Injections

Section/Code	Adds	Del	Rev	Gr	Cross
90782					X

Biofeedback

Section/Code	Adds	Del	Rev	Gr	Cross
90911					X
Dialysis					
90918				X	

Gastroenterology

Section/Code	Adds	Del	Rev	Gr	Cross
91032		X			
91033		X			X
91034	X				
91035	X				
91037	X				
91038	X				
91040	X				X
91065			X		X
91120	X				X

Special Otorhinolaryngologic Services

Audiologic Function Tests With Medical Diagnostic Evaluation

Section/Code	Adds	Del	Rev	Gr	Cross
92589		X			X

Evaluative and Therapeutic Services

Section/Code	Adds	Del	Rev	Gr	Cross
92620	X				
92621	X				X
92625	X				X
Cardiovascular					
Therapeutic Services					
92981					X
Other Vascular Studies					
93741			X		X
93742			X		X

Section/Code	Adds	Del	Rev	Gr	Cross
93745	X				X

Non-Invasive Vascular Diagnostic Studies

Cerebrovascular Arterial Studies

Section/Code	Adds	Del	Rev	Gr	Cross
93890	X				
93892	X				
93893	X				X

Pulmonary

Section/Code	Adds	Del	Rev	Gr	Cross
94060			X		X
94070			X		X
94450					X
94452	X				X
94453	X				X

Neurology and Neuromuscular Procedures

Intraoperative Neurophysiology

Section/Code	Adds	Del	Rev	Gr	Cross
95920					X

Evoked Potentials and Reflex Tests

Section/Code	Adds	Del	Rev	Gr	Cross
95928	X				
95929	X				

Neurostimulators, Analysis-Programming

Section/Code	Adds	Del	Rev	Gr	Cross
95971			X		
95972			X		
95973			X		
95978	X				
95979	X				X

Motion Analysis

Section/Code	Adds	Del	Rev	Gr	Cross
96003					X

Central Nervous System Assessments/Tests (eg, Neuro-Cognitive, Mental Status, Speech Testing)

Section/Code	Adds	Del	Rev	Gr	Cross
96111			X		

Chemotherapy Administration

Section/Code	Adds	Del	Rev	Gr	Cross
96545					X

Section/Code	Adds	Del	Rev	Gr	Cross
Physical Medicine and Rehabilitation					
Modalities					
Supervised					
97014					X
Active Wound Care Management					
97597	X				X
97598	X				
97601		X			X
97605	X				
97606	X				
Other Procedures					
97780		X			X
97781		X			X
Acupuncture					
97810	X				
97811	X				X
97813	X				
97814	X				X
Evaluation and Management					
Inpatient Pediatric Critical Care					
99293			X		
99294			X		
Inpatient Neonatal Critical Care					
99295			X		
99296			X		
Category II Codes					
0001F		X			X
0002F		X			X
0003F		X			X

Section/Code	Adds	Del	Rev	Gr	Cross
0004F		X			X
0005F		X			X
0006F		X			X
0007F		X			X
0008F		X			X
0009F		X			X
0010F		X			X
0011F		X			X

Patient Management

Section/Code	Adds	Del	Rev	Gr	Cross
0500F	X				
0501F	X				
0502F	X				
0503F	X				

Patient History

Section/Code	Adds	Del	Rev	Gr	Cross
1000F	X				
1001F	X				
1002F	X				

Physical Examination

Section/Code	Adds	Del	Rev	Gr	Cross
2000F	X				

Therapeutic, Preventive or Other Interventions

Section/Code	Adds	Del	Rev	Gr	Cross
4000F	X				
4001F	X				
4002F	X				
4006F	X				
4009F	X				
4011F	X				

Category III Codes

Section/Code	Adds	Del	Rev	Gr	Cross
0001T		X			X
0005T		X			
0006T		X			

Section/Code	Adds	Del	Rev	Gr	Cross
0007T		X			X
0009T		X			X
0012T		X			X
0013T		X			X
0014T		X			X
0055T			X		X
0057T		X			X
0062T	X				
0063T	X				X
0064T	X				
0065T	X				X
0066T	X				
0067T	X				X
0068T	X				X
0069T	X				X
0070T	X				X
0071T	X				
0072T	X				X
0073T	X				X

Online Medical Evaluation

Section/Code	Adds	Del	Rev	Gr	Cross
0074T	X				
0075T	X				
0076T	X				X
0077T	X				X
0078T	X				X
0079T	X				X
0080T	X				X
0081T	X				X
0082T	X				X
0083T	X				X

Section/Code	Adds	Del	Rev	Gr	Cross
0084T	x				
0085T	x				
0086T	x				
0087T	x				
0088T	x				